The Osteoporosis Primer

Osteoporosis is one of the leading causes of morbidity and mortality amongst the elderly. The rationale for *The Osteoporosis Primer* is to provide an introductory text that relates the clinical presentation of osteoporosis to its molecular biochemical basis. The text has been organized into four sections that deal with the molecular/cellular components of bone, the development of peak bone mass, the pathophysiology of aging bone and, finally, how all of these relate to the prevention, diagnosis and treatment of osteoporosis. The international team of authors includes many leading clinicians and scientists. They have provided the reader with a concise, yet comprehensive synopsis of bone development and skeletal homeostasis.

This will be an essential introduction for individuals working on osteoporosis, including students and doctors considering a career related to metabolic bone disease, physicians in general practice, geriatricians, rheumatologists, and endocrinologists.

Janet E. Henderson is Assistant Professor of Medicine at McGill University and a Project Director at the Lady Davis Institute for Medical Research, which is affiliated to the Sir Mortimer B. Davis–Jewish General Hospital in Montreal.

David Goltzman is Professor and Chair of the Department of Medicine of McGill University and Physician-in-Chief at the McGill University Health Centre (MUHC).

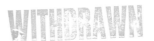

The Osteoporosis Primer

Edited by

Janet E. Henderson

McGill University and Lady David Institute for Medical Research
Montreal, Quebec, Canada

and

David Goltzman

McGill University and Royal Victoria Hospital
Montreal, Quebec, Canada

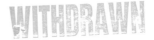
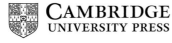
CAMBRIDGE
UNIVERSITY PRESS

PUBLISHED BY THE PRESS SYNDICATE OF THE UNIVERSITY OF CAMBRIDGE
The Pitt Building, Trumpington Street, Cambridge, United Kingdom

CAMBRIDGE UNIVERSITY PRESS
The Edinburgh Building, Cambridge CB2 2RU, UK   http://www.cup.cam.ac.uk
40 West 20th Street, New York, NY 10011–4211, USA   http://www.cup.org
10 Stamford Road, Oakleigh, Melbourne 3166, Australia
Ruiz de Alarcón 13, 28014 Madrid, Spain

First published 2000

Printed in the United Kingdom at the University Press, Cambridge

Typeface Minion (Adobe) 10.5/14pt.   *System* QuarkXPress® [SE]

A catalogue record for this book is available from the British Library

ISBN 0 521 64446 1 paperback

Every effort has been made in preparing this book to provide accurate and up-to-date information which is in accord with accepted standards and practice at the time of publication. Nevertheless, the authors, editors and publisher can make no warranties that the information contained herein is totally free from error, not least because clinical standards are constantly changing through research and regulation. The authors, editors and publisher therefore disclaim all liability for direct or consequential damages resulting from the use of material contained in this book. Readers are strongly advised to pay careful attention to information provided by the manufacturer of any drugs or equipment that they plan to use

Contents

Part 1   **Molecular and cellular environment of bone**

Contributors

Jonathan D. Adachi
Department of Medicine,
St Joseph's Hospital
501–25 Charlton Avenue East
Hamilton, Ontario L8N 1Y2, Canada

Jane E. Aubin
Department of Anatomy and Cell Biology,
University of Toronto, Faculty of Medicine,
6th Floor, Medical Sciences Building
1 King's College Circle, Toronto,
Ontario M5S 1A8, Canada

Debbie Chachra
Samuel Lunenfeld Research Institute of Mount
Sinai Hospital, University of Toronto,
600 University Avenue, Room 984B,
Toronto, Ontario M5G 1X5, Canada

David E. C. Cole
Department of Medicine and Genetics,
University of Toronto, Room 402, Banting Institute,
100 College Street, Toronto, Ontario M5G 1L5,
Canada

Felicia Cosman
Regional Bone Center, Helen Hayes Hospital,
Route 9 West, West Haverstraw, NY 10993, USA

Pierre D'Amour
Department of Medicine, Université de Montréal,
Centre de Recherche Clinique, Hôpital St Luc,
264 Rene-Levesque Boulevard East, Montréal,
Québec H2X 1P1, Canada

Patrick M. Doran
c/o Endocrine Research Unit, Division of
Endocrinology and Metabolism,
Mayo Clinic and Mayo Foundation
200 First Street, SW, Rochester, MN 55905, USA

Lawrence J. Fraher
Division of Medicine and Biochemistry,
Research Institute, Room 4–514,
St Joseph's Health Centre, 268 Grosvenor Street,
London, Ontario N6A 4V2, Canada

Marielle Gascon-Barré
Department of Pharmacology, Université de
Montréal
Centre de Recherche Clinique, Hôpital St Luc,
264 Rene-Levesque Boulevard East, Montréal,
Québec H2X 1P1, Canada

Francis H. Glorieux
Department of Medicine, McGill University,
Genetics Unit, Shriner's Hospital for Children,
1529 Cedar Avenue, Montréal, Québec H3G 1A6,
Canada

David Goltzman
Department of Medicine, McGill University,
Calcium Research Laboratory, Royal Victoria
Hospital,
687 Pine Avenue West, Room H4.67
Montréal, Québec H3A 1A1, Canada

Marc D. Grynpas
Samuel Lunenfeld Research Institute,
Mount Sinai Hospital,
600 University Avenue, Room 984B,
Toronto, Ontario M5G 1X5, Canada

David A. Hanley
Division of Endocrinology and Metabolism
Department of Medicine, University of Calgary,
Health Sciences Centre,
3330 Hospital Drive NW,
Calgary, Alberta T2N 4N1, Canada

Johan N. M. Heersche
Faculty of Dentistry Research Institute,
Department of Dentistry, University of Toronto,
124 Edward Street, Toronto, Ontario M5G 1G6,
Canada

Janet E. Henderson
Department of Medicine,
Lady Davis Institute for Medical Research,
3999 Cote Ste Catherine Road, Room 602,
Montréal, Québec H3T 1E2, Canada

Geoffrey N. Hendy
Department of Medicine, McGill University,
Calcium Research Laboratory, Royal Victoria
Hospital,
687 Pine Ave West, Room H4.67
Montréal, Québec H3A 1A1, Canada

Jacqueline C. Hodge
Department of Diagnostic Radiology,
Royal Victoria Hospital,
687 Pine Avenue West,
Montréal, Québec H3A 1A1, Canada

Anthony B. Hodsman
Osteoporosis Program, Department of Medicine,
St Joseph's Health Centre, 268 Grosvenor Street,
London, Ontario N6A 4V2, Canada

Karim M. Khan
School of Human Kinetics,
University of British Columbia,
210 War Memorial Gym,
6081 University Boulevard, Vancouver BC V6T
1Z1, Canada

Sundeep Khosla
Endocrine Research Unit, Division of
Endocrinology and Metabolism,
Mayo Clinic and Mayo Foundation,
200 First Street SW, Rochester, MN 55905, USA

Richard Kremer
Department of Medicine, McGill University,
Division of Biochemistry, Royal Victoria Hospital,
687 Pine Avenue West, Room H4.67
Montréal, Québec H3A 1A1, Canada

John D. Landoll
Bone and Mineral Metabolism Laboratory
Davis Medical Research Center,
The Ohio State University,
480 West 9th Avenue, Columbus,
OH 43210–1290, USA

Sheila Laverty
Faculty of Veterinary Medicine, University of
Montreal,
3200 rue Sicotte, Ste Hyacinthe, Québec J2S 7C6,
Canada

Hardy Limeback
Division of Preventive Dentistry, Faculty of
Dentistry,
University of Toronto, 124 Edward Street,
Toronto, Ontario M5G 1G6, Canada

Robert Lindsay
Columbia University College of Physicians and
Surgeons
Chief Internal Medicine, Helen Hayes Hospital,
Route 9 West,
West Haverstraw, NY 10993, USA

Heather A. McKay
School of Human Kinetics, Auditorium Annex
155,
1924 West Mall, University of British Columbia,
Vancouver, BC V6T 1Z2, Canada

Marc D. McKee
Faculty of Dentistry,
McGill University
Strathcona Building, Room M43,
3640 University Street
Montréal, Québec, H3A 2B2, Canada

Morris F. Manolson
Faculty of Dentistry Research Institute,
Department of Dentistry, University of Toronto,
124 Edward Street, Toronto, Ontario M5G 1G6,
Canada

Velimir Matkovic
Bone and Mineral Metabolism Laboratory,
Davis Medical Research Center,
Ohio State University, 480 West 9th Avenue,
Columbus, OH 43210–1290, USA

Paul D. Miller
Colorado Center for Bone Research,
3190 South Wadsworth Boulevard, Suite 250
Lakewood, CO 80227, USA

Payam Minoofar
Department of Endocrinology/Bone Disease
Program,
John Wayne Cancer Institute,
2200 Santa Monica Boulevard, Santa Monica, CA
90404, USA

Fackson Mwale
c/o Joint Diseases Laboratory,
Shriner's Hospital for Children,
1529 Cedar Avenue, Montreal, Québec H3G 1A6,
Canada

Alexandra Papaioannou
Hamilton Health Sciences Corporation, Chedoke
Site,
Box 2000, Hamilton, Ontario L8N 3Z5, Canada

Millan S. Patel
c/o Department of Medicine and Genetics,
University of Toronto, Banting Institute,
100 College Street, Toronto, Ontario M5G 1L5,
Canada

A. Robin Poole
Joint Diseases Laboratory, Shriner's Hospital for
Children
1529 Cedar Avenue, Montréal, Québec H3G 1A6,
Canada

Karen M. Prestwood
University of Connecticut Center on Aging
MC-5215,
University of Connecticut Health Center,
Farmington, CT 06030–5215, USA

Lawrence G. Raisz
University of Connecticut Center on Aging
MC-5215,
University of Connecticut Health Center,
Farmington, CT 06030–5215, USA

Frank Rauch
c/o Genetics Unit, Shriner's Hospital for Children,
1529 Cedar Avenue, Montréal, Québec H3G 1A6,
Canada

Laurence A. Rubin
Faculty of Medicine, University of Toronto and
Division of Rheumatology and Multidisciplinary
Osteoporosis Program,
Sunnybrook and Women's College Health Science
Center
60 Grosvenor Street, Suite 416,
Toronto, Ontario M5S 1B6, Canada

Frederick R. Singer
Department of Endocrinology/Bone Disease
Program,
John Wayne Cancer Institute,
2200 Santa Monica Boulevard, Santa Monica, CA
90404, USA

Jaro Sodek
MRC Group, Peridontal Physiology
University of Toronto, Fitzgerald Building Room
239,
150 College Street, Toronto, Ontario M5S 3E2,
Canada

Harriet S. Tenenhouse
MRC Genetics Group, Montreal Children's
Hospital,
2300 Tupper Street, Montréal, Québec H3H 1P3,
Canada

Patricia H. Watson
Department of Medicine, University of Western
Ontario,
Rm G444 Lawson Research Institute,
St Joseph's Health Center,
268 Grosvenor Street, London, Ontario N6A 4V2,
Canada

Carol Zapalowski
Colorado Center for Bone Research
3190 South Wadsworth Boulevard, Suite 250,
Lakewood, CO 80227, USA

Preface

Osteoporosis is one of the leading causes of morbidity and mortality amongst the elderly. With the prediction that the number of people who are 60 years or more will increase from ~300 million to greater than 700 million in the next 25 years, it can be appreciated that osteoporosis will rapidly reach epidemic proportions. This will not only represent a huge health care cost but also compromise the physical well-being and quality of life of a substantial segment of the world's population.

Osteoporosis has been defined as '. . . a systemic skeletal disease characterized by low bone mass and microarchitectural deterioration of bone tissue, with a consequent increase in bone fragility and susceptibility to fracture.' By World Health Organization standards, the term osteoporosis is used to designate bone mass values of 2.5 standard deviations below the young adult mean. Using this criterion, based on bone mass alone, 18 million North Americans have established osteoporosis and 10 million have osteopenia, which is a major risk factor for osteoporosis.

As a consequence of these alarming predictions there has been a steady increase in the attention focused on the physiology and pathophysiology of bone. Many excellent texts are now available, which deal in depth with topics related to the clinical presentation and management of osteoporosis. Likewise, specialized volumes on bone cell biology and the molecular biochemical mechanisms that regulate bone development and skeletal homeostasis are now available. While acting as comprehensive reference texts for physicians and scientists actively working in bone development and metabolism, they are less attractive to those who require a more general approach to the subject. The rationale for the *Osteoporosis Primer* is to provide an introductory text that relates the clinical presentation of osteoporosis to its molecular biochemical basis. It is aimed primarily at individuals who require an introduction to the domain of metabolic bone disease. This would include students considering a career related to metabolic bone disease, physicians in general practice, geriatricians, rheumatologists, and others.

The text of this volume has been organized into four sections that deal with the molecular/cellular components of bone, the development of peak bone mass, the pathophysiology of aging bone and, finally, how all of these relate to the prevention, diagnosis and treatment of osteoporosis. The authors who have contributed to this volume enjoy an international reputation for excellence in their area of expertise. They represent clinicians and scientists who are dedicated to the pursuit of improving our understanding of the etiology and pathogenesis of disorders of bone and mineral metabolism. As such, they have provided the reader with a concise, yet comprehensive, synopsis of bone development and skeletal homeostasis.

The reader is first introduced to endochondral bone formation, which is the process by which the vast majority of bones in the mammalian skeleton are formed. The recruitment and activity of cells that perform anabolic and catabolic functions in bone are described in relationship to the systemic hormones and locally derived factors which regulate these activities. The genetic and non-genetic determinants of peak bone mass are then outlined before describing age-related changes in the cellular and hormonal environment of bone that lead to a decline in bone mass. The final section deals with the epidemiology, laboratory diagnosis and treatment of osteoporosis. It includes discussion of the potential of antiresorptive agents, such as estrogen and bisphosphonates, anabolic agents, such as fluoride and PTH and nutritional therapy with calcium and vitamin D for the treatment and prevention of osteoporosis. These topics are related throughout the text to current research initiatives, using in vitro and in vivo models, which are aimed at improving the diagnosis and treatment of osteopenic disorders. It is hoped that the blend of clinical and basic science brings the reader to a more complete understanding of the complexity of the problem and an appreciation of the research efforts still required before prevention of osteoporosis is a reality.

Janet E. Henderson PhD
David Goltzman MD

Part I

Molecular and cellular environment of bone

Endochondral bone formation and development in the axial and appendicular skeleton

A. Robin Poole, Sheila Laverty and Fackson Mwale

Introduction

With the exception of the craniofacial skeleton and the clavicle, bone formation during development occurs through a process called endochondral ossification, whereby cartilage is formed as a skeletal tissue, calcified and replaced by bone. Much of the craniofacial skeleton consists of 'membrane' bones that form as a result of intramembranous ossification and without a cartilaginous intermediate. The clavicle is the only 'membrane' bone in mammals outside the craniofacial skeleton. The axial and appendicular skeletons and portions of the cranial skeleton (calvaria, otic capsule) arise from mesoderm.

In the embryo, bone formation occurs following an orderly and carefully orchestrated differentiation of mesenchymal cells into chondroblasts, perichondrium, periosteum and osteoblasts (Hall, 1987) (Fig. 1.1). Then growth plates are established, first to lengthen bones and then, in the case of long bones, to shape the forming epiphyses.

As part of this process, there is a complex series of events that involves the formation of chondroblasts and then their maturation into chondrocytes. Only mature hypertrophic chondrocytes establish a calcified extracellular matrix, which is then partly resorbed through a process involving angiogenesis. This first occurs early in development within the diaphysis and then later in the growth plates (Fig. 1.1). The calcified cartilage then acts as a template on which osteoblasts form woven bone, which is eventually resorbed and replaced with a mature trabecular bone within the epiphyses and the diaphysis. At the same time, these events are initially preceded by, but later always accompanied by, cortical bone formation.

The purpose of this chapter is to outline some aspects of these endochondral developmental processes and then review some of the key events and regulatory mechanisms which result in the formation of the majority of the skeleton. In line with the guidelines for these chapters, only selected references will be provided.

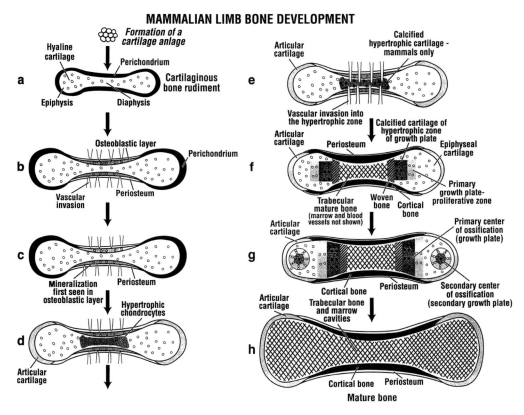

Fig. 1.1   The development of mammalian long bones from the cartilage anlage to the mature bone to show principal steps in cell and tissue differentiation, angiogenesis, growth plate formations and calcification.

The formation of the cartilage anlage in the embryo

Mesenchymal cells first form condensations, whereby cells in close proximity to each other and lacking vascularity, differentiate into chondroblasts (Fig. 1.2). Suppression of the proto-oncogene c-*myc* (which is upregulated in dividing cells) favors chondrogenesis. Around these sites where cartilage forms, blood vessels are present. Here mesenchymal cells differentiate into myogenic elements that form muscle. Distinctive alterations in fibroblast growth factor receptor (FGFR) gene expression in these mesenchymal cells and chondroblasts can be recognized prior to and during differentiation (Fig. 1.2; Szebenyi et al., 1995). These condensing cells transiently express the Osf2/Cbfa1 runt family transcription factor which is otherwise only subsequently expressed in osteoblasts (Ducy et al., 1997). The synthesis of type II procollagen, which defines the chondroblast/chondrocyte phenotype more than any other molecule, initially involves expression of type IIA procollagen in these condensing mesenchymal cells. As they differentiate, so the expression switches to the mature type IIB procollagen, characteristic of the chondroblast/chondrocyte phenotype.

When cells synthesize type IIB collagen, exon II is not expressed and the aminopropeptide is consequently shorter. The functional significance of this remains to be determined.

Abbreviations: GDF, growth differentiation factor; CDMP, cartilage-derived morphogenetic factor; SHH, Sonic hedgehog; IHH, Indian hedgehog; Ptc, patched; FGFR, fibroblast growth factor receptor; PTH, PTHrP, parathyroid hormone and parathyroid hormone-related peptide; GH, growth hormone; IGF-I, insulin-like growth factor-I; TGF, transforming growth factor; BMP, bone morphogenetic protein; T4, thyroxine; T3, triiodothyronine.

First bone formation

A recognizable perichondrium is formed (Fig. 1.1(*a*)) which serves as the principal site of chondroblast generation and differentiation. This process is called appositional growth. The perichondrium initially surrounds each forming epiphysis and newly formed cartilaginous diaphysis. These chondroblasts mature to chondrocytes and synthesize not only type IIB procollagen but also the large proteoglycan aggrecan link protein and many other specialized matrix molecules, which constitute the extensive extracellular matrix of mature hyaline cartilage.

With continuing development the most peripheral perichondrial tissue enveloping the diaphysis (the shaft of the forming bone) differentiates into the periosteum from which osteoblasts develop and form cortical bone (Fig. 1.1(*b*)). In mammals, capillaries must first invade the perichondrium before it transforms into the periosteum. These osteoblastic cells mature, establish and calcify an osteoid matrix which contains type I collagen and bone specific molecules, such as bone sialoprotein. Alkaline phosphatase, that is always present in increased amounts in mineralizing tissue, and is required for this process, is first found in the periosteal collar where mineralization, following angiogenesis, is first initiated (Fig. 1.1(*c*)). The absence of a functional alkaline phosphatase results in hypophosphatasia (see below). There are clear demarcations between the periosteal cellular layer and its underlying osteoid (which together constitute the periosteum) and between the osteoid and the cartilaginous diaphysis.

With maturation, the chondrocytes in the central diaphysis mature and enlarge in size to become 'hypertrophic' (Fig. 1.1(*d*)): they start to synthesize type X collagen and then calcify their matrix. This maturational change is dependent upon molecule(s) released from the more peripheral osteoblasts. Deletion of the osteoblast transcription factor Osf2/Cbfa1 (a runt family member) by homologous recombination results in impaired maturation of chondrocytes as well as of osteoblasts. This results in a lack of periosteal ossification and a very restricted and patchy cartilage calcification following chondrocyte hypertrophy (Fig. 1.1(*e*); Komori et al., 1997; Otto et al., 1997). Moreover, the calcified cartilaginous diaphysis is not vascularized (a feature characteristic of complete hypertrophic maturation) and fails to develop bone marrow cavities.

In birds, the cartilaginous diaphysis becomes hypertrophic but does not mineralize, but in mammals the cartilage starts to calcify following hypertrophy. The hypertrophy is ordinarily associated with the development of angiogenesis; blood vessels invade the hypertrophic cartilage from the periosteal collar, which has already been penetrated by capillaries. This vascular invasion is seen both at this stage in development and also in the primary and secondary centers of ossification within the growth plates. Hypertrophic chondrocytes produce angiogenic molecules (Alini et al., 1996b; Carlavaro et al., 1997) which probably also includes vascular–endothelial cell growth factor. These therefore serve to induce vascular invasion into this tissue.

With increasing osteoblastic activity, a collar of periosteal bone is formed which expands along the length of the diaphysis, fusing in the mid-diaphysis with the calcified core of the diaphysis. The primary growth plates are then established (at the ends of the long and vertebral bones (Fig. 1.1(*f*)) to provide accelerated growth in length. It is within these cartilaginous primary growth centers that this enhanced growth continues, both in the embryo and postnatally.

The growth plates

The proliferative zone

When the primary growth plates are first established, they abut the uncalcified epiphyseal cartilage and the calcified diaphysis. In these growth centers there is continuous formation of chondroblasts from a growth center abutting what is usually called the 'resting zone' of the epiphyseal cartilage. Cells become organized in an axial manner, giving rise to columns of proliferating cells, expressing c-*myc*. These cells actively establish an extensive extracellular cartilage matrix (Fig. 1.2). Both *c-jun* and c-*fos* proto-oncogene expression are then elevated later in the proliferative phase. These proliferating cells have receptors for growth hormone that generates insulin-like growth factor-I (IGF-I) synthesis that potently drives matrix synthesis as well as cell division (Poole, 1997). Thyroxine (T4), and more potently, triiodothyronine (T3), ensure the rapid maturation of these immature chondrocytes to the hypertrophic phenotype as well as regulating cell division. Vitamin D, both 1,25-dihydroxycholecalciferol and/or 24,25-dihydroxycholecalciferol, are required to ensure complete chondrocyte maturation, matrix calcification and vascular

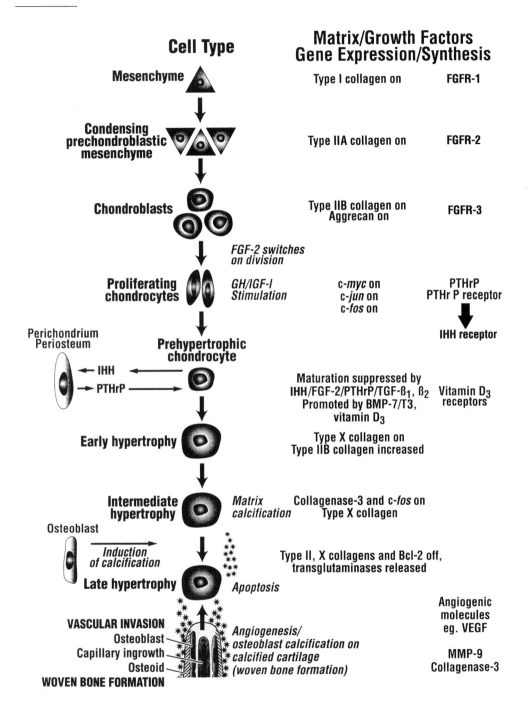

Fig. 1.2   A brief summary of the differentiation and maturation of mammalian chondrocytes, the synthesis of extracellular matrix, its remodeling and calcification and the regulation of these processes. The stages from chondroblasts to hypertrophic chondrocytes and vascular invasion of cartilage are represented in early development of the mammalian diaphysis as well as in the growth plates.

invasion. In the absence of vitamin D, maturation and mineralization is incomplete, the hypertrophic zone is extended and angiogenesis is impaired. The condition resembles hypophosphatasia. Each of these vitamin D metabolites can stimulate production of an angiogenic molecule from the maturing chondrocytes (Alini et al., 1996b) explaining the lack of angiogenesis in vitamin D deficiency.

The hypertrophic zone: early changes

In the proliferative zone, chondrocytes continue to synthesize the extracellular matrix. But then they suddenly upregulate synthesis of type IIB procollagen and start to synthesize type X collagen. The latter characterizes them as hypertrophic chondrocytes (Fig. 1.2). Type X collagen is found in both pericellular sites and in close association with type II collagen fibrils. Although its function is unclear, mutations that alter the structure of this molecule, such as those that give rise to Schmid-type metaphyseal dysplasia, reduce the rate of growth when patients are ambulatory, as compared with those undergoing bed rest. Thus type X collagen may play a structural role in maintaining collagen fibril organization and the mechanical properties of the matrix at a time when there is considerable resorption and remodeling of these type II collagen fibres and a reduction in fibril diameter (see below). Mutations in type II collagen also create a very marked disorganization of the growth plate with a loss of column formation, an irregular hypertrophic zone and disorganized mineralization. These chondrodysplasias are characterized by Kniest dysplasia and spondyloepiphyseal dysplasia (Poole, 1997). Mutations in cartilage oligomeric protein, that produce pseudoachondroplasia, also result in similar abnormalities in growth plates.

When these chondrocytes synthesize type X collagen, they exhibit a number of other fundamental changes. They lose functional receptors for basic fibroblast growth factor-2, which can suppress hypertrophy. Mutations in these receptors, leading to constitutive activity, produce growth abnormalities characterized by the most common skeletal dysplasia called achondroplasia. Ordinarily these hypertrophic chondrocytes also lose receptors for parathyroid hormone-related peptide (PTHrP), which is synthesized by the less mature chondrocytes of the proliferative zone. The loss of this gene, in knockout mice, or the gene for the PTH or PTH/PTHrP receptor, creates premature hypertrophy and disorganization in the growth plate (Amizuka et al., 1994). Thus PTHrP also serves to suppress the onset of hypertrophy.

At the time of early hypertrophy and type X collagen synthesis collagenase-3, a metalloproteinase (MMP-13) that potently degrades these type II collagen molecules, is also upregulated (Gack et al., 1995). The activity of this proteinase leads to a rapid and selective degradation of much of the extracellular type II collagen, resulting in an extensive resorption and remodeling of the extracellular matrix. This permits cellular enlargement or hypertrophy. Collagenase upregulation occurs in very close association with enhanced c-*fos* expression (Gack et al., 1994). C-*fos* is a component of the AP-1 transcription factor complex that regulates collagenase expression. This is a heterodimeric complex that also contains C-*jun*. Overexpression of the c-*fos* transgene causes formation of osteosarcomas and chondrosarcomas but suppresses hypertrophy. However, during natural development c-*fos* and c-*jun* expression are required. Increased expression of the latter is seen in prehypertrophic chondrocytes, and expression is enhanced by PTH which inhibits expression of the hypertrophic phenotype. Consistent with this, in c-*fos*$^{-/-}$ mice, there is premature hypertrophy (Wang et al., 1992). Thus both c-*jun* and c-*fos* are involved in the regulation of maturation. An imbalance in the activities of these oncogenes clearly impacts negatively on normal chondrocyte maturation.

Transforming growth factor β_1 can also upregulate collagenase-3 (but not collagenase-1) expression in fibroblasts and chondrocytes (Uría et al., 1998) and may also be involved in upregulation of collagenase-3 in the growth plate during hypertrophy when increased amounts of this growth factor are generated. In contrast, osteoblast collagenase-3 is upregulated by PTH (Selvamuragan et al., 1998) which suppresses hypertrophy in chondrocytes (Amizuka et al., 1994). Moreover, overexpression of c-*fos* and c-*jun* genes is observed in response to PTH activation of these genes in osteoblasts. It is likely that tissue specificity of collagenase regulation is achieved via the presence of a runt binding domain as well as an AP-1 site in bone cells.

Calcification of the hypertrophic zone

Following resorption and remodeling, the residual matrix, which is by now of minimal volume, then starts to calcify (Fig. 1.2). It is enriched in content in the proteoglycan aggrecan (Poole, 1997). Calcification occurs in focal sites in the longitudinal septa where these proteoglycan molecules are concentrated. The C-propeptide of type II collagen, a calcium-binding protein, accumulates in these mineralizing sites. Prior to calcification, matrix vesicles are produced by chondrocytes, starting in the proliferative zone. These apparently serve to generate local elevated concentrations of calcium and phosphate and ensure nucleation of mineral formation, that really increases later following hypertrophy. Mice, in which the gene for matrix Gla protein has been eliminated by homologous recombination, exhibit premature calcification in the proliferative zone, suggesting that this molecule restricts mineralization to the hypertrophic zone where expression of this gene is normally minimal (Luo et al., 1997).

Apoptosis as the end stage of hypertrophic phenotype

The mature hypertrophic cells represent terminally differentiated chondrocytes. Apoptosis occurs in advanced hypertrophy, when mineralization is maximal. This leads to the death of these cells in association with reduced expression of Bcl-2 a protein which negatively regulates programmed cell death (Amling et al., 1997). Apoptosis leads to the extracellular release of two transglutaminases, a tissue type and a plasma (avian factor XIIIA) form (Nurminskaya et al., 1998). The latter is markedly upregulated in hypertrophic chondrocytes, appears to cross-link matrix molecules and may contribute, like type X collagen, to matrix stabilization. It could alternatively enhance degradation since such cross-linked molecules (e.g., fibronectin) are more susceptible to proteolysis.

Vascular and chondroclastic erosion of hypertrophic zone

A striking feature of the hypertrophic zone, as in earlier development, is its vascular invasion. At this stage it is from the primary spongiosa and occurs in close association with apoptosis of hypertrophic chondrocytes. Following and accompanying the activity of the eroding multinucleate chondroclasts, capillary sprouts penetrate the largely uncalcified transverse septa (Fig. 1.2), accompanied by mononuclear cells rich in cathepsin B called septoclasts. This erosive angiogenic process leads to the progressive destruction of not only the transverse septa but also of many of the calcified septa. It involves the activity of extracellular proteases at the capillary invasion front where there is cleavage of type II collagen by collagenase cleavage of the proteoglycan aggrecan. Gelatinase B (MMP-9), a metalloproteinase present in these sites (Sakiyama et al., 1994; Vu et al., 1998) and produced by chondroclasts and osteoclasts, is involved in this process, since its removal by homologous recombination results in elongation of the hypertrophic zone. This is a consequence of impairment of apoptosis and of angiogenesis which is presumably dependent upon matrix degradation produced by this proteinase (Vu et al., 1998).

The formation of woven bone and its replacement with trabecular bone

As a consequence of this resorptive process in the lower hypertrophic zone, calcified cartilaginous trabeculae remain which extend into the diaphysis. Osteoblasts settle on these trabeculae, synthesize an extracellular matrix (osteoid) and then calcify it (Fig. 1.2). Initially bone sialoprotein is produced which acts as a nucleator for mineral formation. Eventually osteoclasts resorb this woven bone, and it is replaced by mature trabecular bone. Meanwhile, the periosteal bone collar gives rise to the mature cortical bone with its characteristic lamellae and Haversian canals. As osteoblasts mature, osteocalcin is also generated. This molecule somehow regulates bone formation since deletion of this gene results in an increase in bone formation without affecting bone resorption (Ducy et al., 1996). The calcified trabeculae on which woven bone forms are eventually replaced by a process of active osteoclastic resorption. This requires the presence of the osteoprotegerin ligand, without which osteoclasts fail to develop and the woven bone and trabeculae are not resorbed, causing osteopetrosis (Kong et al., 1999). The absence of the osteoclast proteinase cathepsin K also leads to osteopetrosis, revealing its essential role in osteoclast mediated bone resorption (Saftig et al., 1998).

The secondary center of ossification

The development of the epiphyses involves changes in shape and size. This is made possible by the formation of a secondary growth centre (Fig. 1.1(g)). The events that lead to its formation and function are essentially the same as those described for the primary centers of ossification or growth plates. At the outer edge there are germinal cells that give rise to proliferative cells which mature and form hypertrophic chondrocytes which calcify their extracellular matrix forming calcified trabeculae on which woven bone is formed. Subsequent events lead to trabecular bone formation. This secondary center appears following the development of hypertrophic chondrocytes in the uncalcified epiphyses: blood vessels invade towards these cells from the periosteum as in early development.

The regulation of chondrocyte development and chondrocyte interactions with the perichondrium and periosteum

Vitamin D

Vitamin D deficient (rachitic) animals exhibit abnormal development. The most pronounced changes are characterized by a lengthened hypertrophic zone and impaired angiogenesis. Nuclear receptors for 1,25-dihydroxycholecalciferol (1,25-dihydroxyvitamin D_3) have been detected in both hypertrophic and proliferative chondrocytes. Chondrocyte hypertrophy occurs in vitamin D deficiency but calcification of the extracellular matrix is restricted. Treatment of chondrocytes with either 1,25-dihydroxyvitamin D_3, or the metabolite 24, 25 dihydroxy vitamin D_3 causes increased production of an angiogenic molecule produced by the chondrocytes (Alini et al., 1996b). Both metabolites stimulate extracellular matrix synthesis (type II procollagen) and calcification.

Thyroid hormones

Thyroid hormones also play a key role in development. Untreated hypoparathyroidism in children results in marked retardation of growth because of incomplete skeletal maturation. Growth can be rapidly restored by thyroid hormone administration. Both T4 and T3 accelerate chondrocyte maturation and hypertrophy in vitro: T3 is much more potent than T4 and is considered to be the active metabolite (Alini et al., 1996) acting on the prehypertrophic chondrocytes that express receptors for thyroid hormones. Thyroid hormones also act directly on bone cells although this has received relatively little attention. Both osteoblast and osteoclast activity are stimulated by T3 and receptors have been reported to be present on both cell types, although this requires confirmation.

Estrogen

Estrogen also plays a key role in postnatal growth and during the growth spurt at puberty. It is required for epiphyseal growth plate fusion. This became obvious from a study of two male patients, one homozygous for a mutation in the estrogen receptor (Smith et al., 1994) and a second with aromatase deficiency (Morishima et al., 1995). Bone growth is also impaired by the lack of the estrogen receptor on osteocytes and osteoblasts, leading to net excessive resorption of bone.

Growth hormone (GH) and insulin-like growth factor-I (IGF-I)

These can each act directly to stimulate proliferation of prehypertrophic chondrocytes and expression of IGF-I receptor in immature proliferative cell development (Poole, 1997). GH probably acts to induce IGF-I synthesis and secretion which then acts in an autocrine and paracrine fashion in the proliferative zone.

Fibroblast growth factor (FGF)

Unlike IGF-I, FGF stimulates resting chondrocytes to proliferate during development (Wroblewski & Edwall-Arvidsson, 1995). FGF-2 is also a strong suppressor of terminal differentiation of the hypertrophic phenotype although it stimulates chondrocyte proliferation. Mature, hypertrophic chondrocytes fail to respond to FGF-2 (Iwamoto et al., 1991). This relates to a loss of receptor function. Disruption of the FGF receptor-3 (FGFR-3) gene (Deng et al., 1996) produces a severe and progressive bone dysplasia in mice with enhanced and prolonged endochondral growth, increased proliferation and expansion of the hypertrophic zone. These effects are observed postnatally and are restricted to bones that arise by endochondral ossification. Human mutations involving the FGFR-3 gene cause dominant heritable skeletal dysplasias such as achondroplasia, atotrophic dysplasia and hypochondroplasia (Deng et al., 1996; Poole, 1997). Dysplasias that result from a gain of function of this receptor include achondroplasia.

FGFR-1, 2 and 3 are all expressed during early development although postnatally FGFR-1 and 2 are not detectable in the growth plate in older mice. In the chick embryo FGFR-1 is expressed predominantly in undifferentiated proliferating mesenchyme, FGFR-2 in precartilage mesenchymal cell condensations and FGFR-3 in differentiating cartilage nodules (Szebenyi et al., 1995). FGF-4 can substitute for the presence of the apical ectodermal ridge in limb morphogenesis, leading to limb bud formation and limb development. FGF-4 induces a hedgehog gene (see below) as well as the homeobox gene Hoxd-13 (Reddi, 1994).

Bone morphogenetic proteins (BMPs)

These belong to a large family, members of which, such as the transforming growth factors, play key roles in skeletal development and maintenance. They work both individually and synergistically (Hogan, 1996; Reddi, 1994). Whereas platelet-derived growth factors are inhibitory, BMP-2, BMP-3 and BMP-4 can each induce differentiation of mesenchymal cells into chondrocytes. These BMPs, including BMP-7, can each promote chondrocyte maturation. In contrast, TGF-β_1 and TGF-β_2 can each arrest hypertrophy (Böhme et al., 1995). Maturing chondrocytes also express both BMP-4 and BMP-7. A mutation in the BMP-5 gene causes a condition observed in the *short ear* mouse (Kingsley et al., 1992). These mice have skeletal abnormalities that involve the long bones and xiphoid process of the sternum. BMP-5 is also expressed in early condensations of the pinnae and xiphoid processes and in the perichondria of limb bones.

Another family member, the growth differentiation factor 5 (GDF-5) gene, which is also known as cartilage-derived morphogenetic protein –CDMP-1, is involved in joint development. A mutation in this gene causes brachypodism in mice (Storm et al., 1994). The long bones are short and there are abnormalities in phalangeal development with lack of the development of some joints and joint abnormalities. GDF-5 (CDMP-1) is expressed in those sites where cartilage condensations occur prior to joint formation. The activity of this protein, and/or the product of its activity, is regulated (antagonized) by Noggin, another BMP. Mice lacking Noggin suffer a lack of joint development, although cartilage condensations form normally and skeletal cartilage maturation proceeds (Brunet et al., 1998).

Evidence for synergism in BMP activity has come from studies of double mutants of BMP-5 and GDF-5 (CDMP-1), where more severe skeletal defects are observed compared with those mice with single mutations (Storm & Kingsley, 1996).

The activities of BMPs are mediated by receptors at the cell surface (Hogan, 1996; Reddi, 1994). These are heterodimers or heterotetramers of the type I and type II receptors, which each contain intracellular serine/threonine kinase domains for signaling. Type IA, IB and II receptors are expressed by chondrocytes of the hypertrophic lineage. The type IB receptor is required for chondrogenesis and in combination with the type II receptor, is required for limb development. The type II receptor is necessary for expression of the chondrocyte phenotype (Iwamoto et al., 1991).

Hedgehogs, parathyroid hormone (PTH) and PTH related peptide (PTHrP)

The hedgehog gene family

This is involved in patterning and control of cell differentiation. The family includes Sonic hedgehog (SHH) and Indian hedgehog (IHH). Both proteins are synthesized as inactive precursors and require proteolysis for activation. In the case of Shh this is by an autoproteolytic mechanism producing amino-terminal and carboxy-terminal products. The receptor for hedgehog is called patched (Ptc). The amino-terminal portion of Sonic hedgehog can upregulate Ptc gene expression

and stimulate maturation of mesenchymal cells to express an osteoblastic phenotype.

Ihh is expressed in prehypertrophic chondrocytes, where it is involved in the regulation of hypertrophic differentiation by PTH/PTHrP (Fig. 1.2). It has been proposed that the direct target of IHH signaling is the perichondrium where the Ptc
receptor for Ihh flanks the cells in cartilage expressing IHH (Lanske et al., 1996).
PTHrP can be induced by the use of Sonic hedgehogs (as a substitute for IHH) in
both prehypertrophic chondrocytes and in the periarticular perichondrium. PTHrP
then signals to a receptor (PTHrPR) in prehypertrophic chondrocytes regulating
hypertrophic differentiation (Lanske et al., 1996). Shh as well as PTHrP, can suppress expression of the hypertrophic phenotype in wild-type mice but only PTHrP
can suppress in mice lacking the PTHrP gene. This suggests that SHH (IHH) operates upstream of PTHrP via induction of PTHrP leading to the suppression of
hypertrophy. In the growth plate, the PTHrP receptor is expressed proximal to IHH
in prehypertrophic cells although IHH expression overlaps with type X collagen
expression in hypertrophic cells. Mice that lack PTHrP ($^{-/-}$) or the PTHrP receptor
($^{-/-}$) exhibit accelerated differentiation of chondrocytes to the hypertrophic phenotype and are unresponsive to SHH and PTHrP indicating again that PTHrP acts at
the chondrocyte level to suppress hypertrophy via its receptor (Lanske et al., 1996).

In support of evidence for an interaction of the periosteum/perichondrium with
chondrocytes in the growth cartilage is the observation that removal of these
peripheral tissues leads to increased hypertrophy reflecting the suppressive regulatory effects of these tissues on chondrocyte hypertrophy (Long & Linsenmayer,
1998).

Consistent with its proposed function, overexpression of PTHrP causes prenatal suppression of bone formation and suppression of chondrocyte hypertrophy. At
birth, the skeleton is cartilaginous. However, by 7 weeks the delay in chondrocyte
differentiation and bone collar formation is largely corrected (Weir et al., 1996)
revealing once again that these regulatory mechanisms change with postnatal
development (as has been observed in other 'knockouts'). PTHrP overexpression
in transgenic mice is also associated not only with a major arrest in the onset of
hypertrophy but also of apoptosis. Bcl-2, the family of proteins that controls programmed cell death, shows reduced expression in PTHrP mice (Lee et al., 1996).
Moreover, Bcl-2 gene deletion causes accelerated maturation of chondrocytes and
shortening of long bones since the suppression of apoptosis by Bcl-2 is removed
(Amling et al., 1997). Interestingly, this gene ablation has been shown to result in
greater numbers of osteoblasts and altered morphology, coupled with disorganization of collagen deposition by the osteoblast.

Some of these changes, cellular interactions and regulatory molecules are summarized in Fig. 1.2.

Acknowledgements

Robin Poole's research is funded by Shriner's Hospital for Children, Medical Research Council of Canada, Canadian Arthritis Network and the National Institutes of Health. Fackson Mwale is a recipient of a Shriner's Hospital research fellowship. We thank Jane Wishart for her artwork.

REFERENCES

Alini, M., Kofsky, Y., Wu, W., Pidoux, I., & Poole, A. R. (1996a). In serum-free culture thyroid hormones can induce full expression of chondrocyte hypertrophy leading to matrix calcification. *J. Bone Miner. Res.*, **11**, 105–13.

Alini, M., Marriott, A., Chen, T., Abe, S., & Poole, A. R. (1996b). A novel angiogenic molecule produced at the time of chondrocyte hypertrophy during endochondral bone formation. *Dev. Biol.*, **176**, 124–32.

Amizuka, N., Warshawsky, H., Henderson, J. E., Goltzman, D., & Karaplis, A. C. (1994). Parathyroid hormone-related peptide-depleted mice show abnormal epiphyseal cartilage development and altered endochondral bone formation. *J. Cell Biol.*, **126**, 1611–23.

Amling, M., Neff, L., Tanaka, S., Inone, D., Kuida, K., Weir, E., Philbrick, W. M., Broadus, A. E., & Baron, R. (1997). Bcl-2 lies downstream of the parathyroid hormone-related peptide in a signalling pathway that regulates chondrocyte maturation during skeletal development. *J. Cell Biol.*, **136**, 205–13.

Böhme, K., Winterhalter, K.K., & Brückner, P. (1995). Terminal differentiation of chondrocytes in culture is a spontaneous process and is arrested by transforming growth factor-β2 and basic fibroblast growth factor. *Exp. Cell Res.*, **216**, 191–8.

Brunet, L.J., McMahon, J.A., McMahon, A.P., & Harland, R.M. (1998). Noggin, cartilage morphogenesis, and joint formation in the mammalian skeleton. *Science*, **280**, 1455–7.

Carlavaro, M.F., Albini, A., Ribatti, D., Gentilei, C., Benelli, R., Cermelli, S., Cancedda, R., & Descalzi Cancedda, F. (1997). Transferrin promotes endothelial cell migration and invasion: implication in cartilage neovascularization. *J. Cell Biol.*, **136**, 1375–84.

Deng, C., Wynshaw-Boris, A., Zhou, F., Kuo, A., & Leder, P. (1996). Fibroblast growth factor receptor 3 is a negative regulator of bone growth. *Cell*, **84**, 911–21.

Ducy, P., Desbois, C., Boyce, B., Pinero, G., Story, B., Dunstan, C., Smith, E., Bonadio, J., Goldstein, S., Gindberg, C., Bradley, A., & Karsenty, G. (1996). Increased bone formation in osteocalcin-deficient mice. *Nature*, **382**, 448–52.

Ducy, P., Zhang, R., Geoffroy, V., Ridall, A.L., & Karsenty, G. (1997). Osf2/Cbfal: a transcriptional activator of osteoblast differentiation. *Cell*, **89**, 747–54.

Gack, S., Vallon, R., Schaper, J., Rüther, U., & Angel, P. (1994). Phenotypic alterations in Fos-transgenic mice correlate with changes in Fos/Jun-dependent collagenase type I expression. Regulation of mouse metalloproteinases by carcinogens, tumor promoters, cAMP and Fos oncoprotein. *J. Biol. Chem.*, **269**, 10363–9.

Gack, S., Vallon, R., Schmidt, J., Grigoriadis, A., Tuckermann, J., Schenkel, J., Weiher, H., Wagner, E.F., & Angel, P. (1995). Expression of interstitial collagenase during skeletal development of the mouse is restricted to osteoblast-like cells and hypertrophic chondrocytes. *Cell Growth Differ.*, 6, 759–67.

Hall, B. K. (1987). Earliest evidence of cartilage and bone development in embryonic life. *Clin. Orthop. Rel. Res.*, 225, 255–72.

Hogan, B. L. M. (1996). Bone morphogenetic proteins: multifunctional regulators of vertebrate development. *Genes and Development*, 10, 1580–94.

Iwamoto, M., Shimazu, A., Nakashima, K., Suzuki, F., & Kato, Y. (1991). Reduction in basic fibroblast growth factor receptor is coupled with terminal differentiation of chondrocytes. *J. Bone Miner. Res.*, 10, 735–42.

Kingsley, D. M., Bland, A. E., Grubber, J. M., Marker, P. C., Russell, L. B., Copeland, N. G., & Jenkins, N. A. (1992). The mouse short ear skeletal morphogenesis locus is associated with defects in a bone morphogenetic member of the TGFbeta-superfamily. *Cell*, 71, 399–410.

Komori, T., Yagi, H., Nomura, S., Yamaguchi, A., Sasaki, K., Deguchi, K., Shimizu, Y., Bronson, R.T., Gao, Y-H., Inada, M., Sato, M., Okamoto, R., Kitimura, Y., Yoshik, S., & Kishimoto, T. (1997). Targeted disruption of Cbfa1 results in a complete lack of bone formation owing to maturational arrest of osteoblasts. *Cell*, 89, 755–64.

Kong, Y-Y., Yoshida, H., Sarosi, I., Tan, H.L., Timms, E., Capparelli, C., Morony, S., Oliveira-dos-Santos, A. J., Van, G., Itie, A., Khoo, W., Wakeham, A., Dunstan, C. R., Lacey, D. L., Mak, T. W., Boyle, W.J., & Penninger, J. M. (1999). OPGL is a key regulator of osteoclastogenesis, lymphocyte development and lymph-node organogenesis. *Nature*, 397, 315–23.

Lanske, B., Karaplis, A. C., Lee, K., Luz, A., Vortkamp, A., Pirro, A., Karperien, M., Defize, L. H. K., Ho, C., Mulligan, R. C., Abou-Samra, A-B., Jüppner, H., Segre, G. V., & Kronenberg, H. M. (1996). PTH/PTHrP receptor in early development and indian hedgehog-regulated bone growth. *Science*, 273, 663–6.

Lee, K., Lanske, B., Karapalis, A. C., Deeds, J. D., Kohno, H., Nissenson, R. A., Kronenberg, H. M., & Segre, G.V. (1996). Parathyroid hormone-related peptide delays terminal differentiation of chondrocytes during endochondral bone development. *Endocrinology*, 137, 5109–18.

Long, F. & Linsenmayer, T. F. (1998). Regulation of growth region cartilage proliferation and differentiation by perichondrium. *Development*, 125, 1067–73.

Luo, G., Ducy, P., McKee, M. D., Pinero, G.J., Loyer, E., Behringer, R. R., & Karsenty, G. (1997). Spontaneous calcification of arteries and cartilage in mice lacking matrix GLA protein. *Nature*, 386, 78–81.

Morishima, A., Grumbach, M. M., Simpson, E.R., Fisher, C., & Qin, K. (1995). Aromatase deficiency in male and female siblings caused by a novel mutation and the physiological role of estrogens. *J. Clin. Endocrinol. Meth.*, 80, 3689–98.

Nurminskaya, M., Magee, C., Nurminsky, D., & Linsenmayer, T. F. (1998). Plasma transglutaminase in hypertrophic chondrocytes: expression and cell-specific intracellular activation produce cell death and externalization. *J. Cell Biol.*, 142, 1135–44.

Otto, F., Thornell, A., Crompton, T., Denzel, A., Gilmour, K. C., Rosewell, I.R., Stamp, G. W. H., Beddington, R. S. P., Mundlos, S., Olsen, B. J., Selby, P. B., & Owen, M. J. (1997). Cbfal, a candidate gene for cleidocranial dysplasia syndrome, is essential for osteoblast differentiation and bone development. *Cell*, **89**, 765–71.

Poole, A. R. (1997). Cartilage in health and disease. In *Arthritis and Allied Conditions. A Textbook of Rheumatology*, ed. W. J. Koopman, pp. 255–308. Baltimore: Williams and Wilkins.

Reddi, H. (1994). Cartilage morphogenesis: role of bone and cartilage morphogenetic proteins, homeobox genes and extracellular matrix. *Mat. Biol.*, **14**, 599–606.

Saftig, P., Hunziker, E., Wehmeyer, O., Jones, S., Boyde, A., Rommerskirch, W., Moritz J. D., Schu, P., & von Figura, K. (1998). Impaired osteoclastic bone resorption leads to osteopetrosis in cathepsin-K-deficient mice. *Proc. Natl Acad. Sci., USA*, **95**, 13453–8.

Sakiyama, H., Inaba, N., Toyoguchi, T., Okada, Y., Matsumoto, M., Moriya, H., & Ohtsu, H. (1994). Immunolocalization of complement CIs and matrix metalloproteinase 9 (92KDa gelatinase/type IV collagenase) in the primary ossification center of the human femur. *Cell Tissue Res.*, **277**, 239–45.

Selvamuragan, N., Chou, W-Y., Pearman, A. T., Pulumati, M. R., & Partridge, N. C. (1998). Parathyroid hormone regulates the rat collagenase-3 promoter in osteoblastic cells through the cooperative interaction of the activator protein-1 site and the runt domain binding sequence. *J. Biol. Chem.*, **273**, 10647–57.

Smith, E. P., Boyd, J., Frank, G. R., Takahashi, H., Cohen, R. M., Specker, B., Williams, T. C., Labahn, D. B., & Korach, K.S. (1994). Estrogen resistance caused by a mutation in the estrogen-receptor gene in man. *New Engl. J. Med.*, **331**, 1056–61.

Storm, E. E. & Kingsley, D.M. (1996). Joint patterning defects caused by single and double mutations in members of the bone morphogenetic protein (BMP) family. *Development*, **122**, 3969–79.

Storm, E. E., Huynh, T. V., Copeland, N. G., Jenkins, N. A., Kingsley, D. M., & Lee, S. J. (1994). Limb alterations in brachypodism mice due to mutations in a new member of the TGF beta-superfamily. *Nature*, **368**, 639–43.

Szebenyi, G., Savage, M. P., Olwin, B. B., & Fallon, J. F. (1995). Changes in the expression of fibroblast growth factor receptors mark distinct stages of chondrogenesis in vitro and during chick limb skeletal patterning. *Dev. Dyn.*, **204**, 446–56.

Uría, J. A., Jiménez, M. G., Balbín, M., Freije, J. M. P., and López-Otin, C. (1998). Differential effects of transforming growth factor-β on the expression of collagenase-1 and collagenase-3 in human fibroblasts. *J. Biol. Chem.*, **273**, 9769–77.

Vu, T. H., Shipley, J. M., Berger, G., Berger, J. E., Helms, J. A., Hanahan, D., Shapiro, S. D., Senior, R. M., & Werb, Z. (1998). MMP-9/gelatinase B is a key regulator of growth plate angiogenesis and apoptosis of hypertrophic chondrocytes. *Cell*, **93**, 411–22.

Wang, Z. Q., Ovitt, C., Agamemnon, E., Grigoriadis, A. E., Möhle-Steinlein, U., Rüther, U., & Wagner, E.F. (1992). Bone and haematopoietic defects in mice lacking c-fos. *Nature*, **360**, 741–5.

Weir, E. C., Philbrick, W. M., Amling, M., Neff, L. A., Baron, R., & Broadus, A. E. (1996). Targeted overexpression of parathyroid hormone-related peptide in chondrocytes causes chondrodysplasia and delayed endochondral bone formation. *Proc. Natl Acad. Sci., USA*, **93**, 10240–5.

Wroblewski, J. & Edwall-Arvidsson, C. (1995). Inhibitory effects of basic fibroblast growth factor on chondrocyte differentiation. *J. Bone Miner. Res.*, **10**, 735–42.

2

The role of osteoblasts

Jane E. Aubin

Introduction

Bone formation takes place in the organism during embryonic development, growth, remodeling, fracture repair and when induced experimentally, e.g., by the implantation of decalcified bone matrix or purified or recombinant members of the bone morphogenetic protein family. This suggests there is a large reservoir of cells in the body capable of osteogenesis throughout life. The issues addressed in this chapter are the nature of these cells in younger vs. older animals, the identification of transitional steps from stem cell to committed osteoprogenitor to osteoblast, heterogeneity of the mature osteoblast phenotype, and how differentiation may be regulated in this lineage.

Osteoblast ontogeny

Mesenchymal stem cells and multipotential and restricted progenitors

Osteoprogenitor cells reside in bone marrow stroma and in the periosteal layers of bone. They arise from multipotential mesenchymal stem cells that give rise to a number of committed and restricted cell lineages including those for osteoblasts, chondroblasts, adipocytes and myoblasts (Fig. 2.1). The fact that stem and primitive osteoprogenitors are neither morphologically nor molecularly well characterized, coupled to their low frequency, has meant that much of what we know about either class of cell has been gained through manipulations in culture. Bone marrow stromal cells grown in vitro form colonies of fibroblastic cells (colony forming unit-fibroblast, CFU-F; or colony forming cell-fibroblastic, CFC-F) that, when placed in diffusion chambers and implanted into rodents, give rise to a range of differentiated cell phenotypes including osteoblasts, chondroblasts, adipocytes and fibroblasts. Many investigators have now also reported the formation of a range of differentiated cell phenotypes in vitro in marrow stromal populations and concluded that they arose from a mesenchymal stem cell or stromal stem cell. It is clear, however, that CFU-F are heterogeneous in size, morphology and potential for

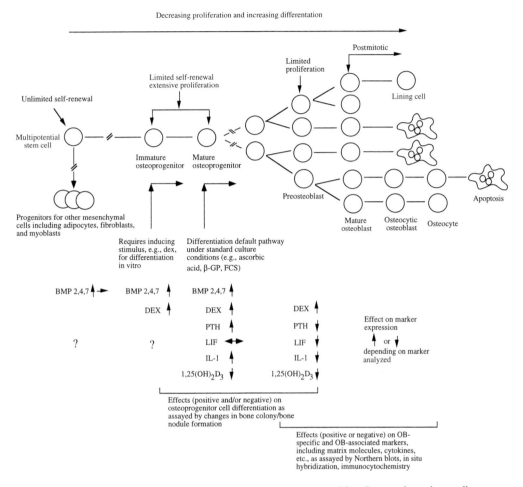

Fig. 2.1   Postulated transitional stages recognizable in the osteoblast lineage based on cell morphology in vivo and colony assays in vitro. Updated from Aubin (1998).

differentiation, consistent with the view that they belong to a lineage hierarchy in which only some of the cells are primitive, and perhaps multipotential stem or progenitor cells, while others are more restricted. This is consistent with data that show that only a proportion of CFU-F are CFU-alkaline phosphatase (CFU-AP) and further that only a proportion of these are CFU-osteogenic (CFU-O, clonogenic bone colonies or bone nodules) (Aubin, 1999) (see below). Critical issues remain in most experiments reported on stromal stem cells, including the identifiable commitment and restriction points in the stromal cell hierarchy, the ratios of stem to other more restricted progenitors in various stromal populations, the clonality of progeny, and demonstration that putative stem cells exhibit genuine stem cell kinetics, i.e., show unlimited self-renewal capacity and ability to recapitulate an entire lineage. Such issues may become increasingly important as work on stromal populations increases in intensity based on their proposed utility for tissue regeneration and gene therapy.

More definitive evidence for the existence of stem or multipotential mesenchymal cells has been obtained by analysis of the differentiation outcomes of clonally derived immortalized (e.g., via large T-antigen expression) or spontaneously immortalized cell lines in vitro, such as the mouse embryonic fibroblast line C3H10T1/2, the rat calvaria-derived cell lines RCJ3.1 and ROB-C26, and the mesodermally derived C1 line. While none of these lines behaves exactly alike and the results of experiments with them differ in detail, they do have some common features, including the ability of the clonal population to give rise, under appropriate culture conditions, to multiple differentiated cell phenotypes including osteoblasts, chondroblasts, myoblasts and adipocytes. Data are consistent with the existence of a lineage hierarchy in which the multipotential cell gives rise to more restricted bi- or tripotential cells, and these ultimately give rise to monopotential progenitors. Both a stochastic process with an expanding hierarchy of increasingly restricted progeny (e.g., RCJ3.1 cells) and a non-random, single step process in which multipotential (i.e., tripotential) progenitors become exclusively restricted to a single lineage by particular culture conditions and inducers (environment) (e.g., C1 cells) have been proposed. While there are caveats influencing interpretation of results on clonal lines, it is interesting to consider that the different cellular systems may recapitulate different pathways to the same developmental endpoints. In this view, culture condition restraints may shift markedly the frequency of apparently random or stochastic commitment/restriction events to favor particular outcomes, as might also be achieved in vivo under particular environmental conditions or at particular developmental times (Aubin, 1998).

Committed osteoprogenitors, i.e., progenitor cells restricted to osteoblast development (CFU-O), can be identified by functional assays of their proliferation and differentiation capacity in vitro, i.e., the bone nodule assay (reviewed in Aubin, 1998). At least some evidence suggests that a majority of the osteoprogenitors present in various bone-derived cell isolates, including calvarial and bone marrow stromal cell cultures, and measured by the bone nodule assay (Fig. 2.1, see also below), have only a limited self-renewal capacity in culture. Evidence documented first in rat calvaria cell populations, and now shown in other bone-derived populations, including those from bone marrow stroma and vertebra, also suggests the existence of at least two distinct populations of osteoprogenitors. One population appears capable of constitutive differentiation in vitro, i.e., in standard differentiation conditions will undergo a series of steps leading to the mature phenotype, while the other population comprises recruitable or inducible osteoprogenitors, i.e., will undergo osteoblastic differentiation in vitro only following the addition of specific inductive stimuli such as glucocorticoids. In the case of gluco-corticoids, there are data to suggest that the progenitors requiring glucocorticoids may be more primitive than those differentiating without added glucocorticoids, a possibility that may also apply to the progenitors responding to at least some of the other stimulators. The number and proportion of more primitive vs. more mature progenitors in different bone-derived populations may vary significantly. For example, in young adult rat bone marrow stroma, the majority of osteoprogenitors appear to belong to the glucocorticoid-requiring or more primitive class although a low number of more mature progenitors is present (Aubin, 1999). Other stimu-lators in addition to glucocorticoids, including other steroids (e.g., progesterone: (Ishida & Heersche, 1997) or other factors such as Bone Morphogenetic Proteins (BMPs, e.g., BMP-6: Boden et al., 1997), increase the number of bone nodules or bone colonies in culture (see also below). Whether all such progenitors belong to the same unidirectional lineage pathway (i.e., immature progenitors induced by a variety of agents to undergo differentiation to mature osteoblasts) or constitute recruitment from other parallel lineages remains to be explicitly established (Aubin, 1998). It should also be noted that significant species variations can be seen, e.g., concentrations of glucocorticoids that are stimulatory to differentiation and increase bone nodule number in rat calvaria and rat bone marrow stromal cul-tures have been reported to be inhibitory in mouse stromal cultures, indicating that some caution is required in extrapolating to the human situation.

In addition to committed osteoprogenitors, several investigators have docu-mented, in both stromal- and other bone-derived cultures including those from calvaria, mixed colony types (e.g., individual colonies in which more than one kind of differentiated cell type is present simultaneously) and/or manipulated cultures such that apparently committed cells expressed alternative differentiation patterns. This has been of particular interest for the relationships between adipocytes and osteoblasts, an issue of significant clinical interest in osteoporosis and the aging or immobilized skeleton (summarized in Aubin & Heersche, 1997; Gimble et al., 1996). A number of studies on human bone- and bone marrow-derived cells have supported observations on rodent marrow stromal populations that a cell exists that appears to be at least bipotential for adipocytes and osteoblasts and that an inverse relationship between the osteoblast and adipocytic phenotypes may reflect the ability of single or combinations of agents to alter the differentiation pathway these bipotential cells will transit. Dedifferentiation has been posited to account for observations in some cultures of stroma in which highly differentiated adipocytes are thought to revert to a less differentiated, more proliferative fibroblastic precur-sor phenotype and then to an osteogenic phenotype. On the other hand, it was recently found that osteoblasts, differentiated to the point of already expressing osteocalcin, were able to undergo rapid alternate differentiation events that led to essentially 100% of the formerly osteoblastic cells expressing adipogenesis (Nuttall et al., 1998). Thus, although osteocalcin is a very late marker of osteoblast maturation (see below), the data are consistent with osteoblasts being able to transdifferentiate to adipocytes. There is some evidence also to support the occurrence of transdifferentiation events or other kinds of interrelationships between chondroblasts and osteoblasts. Taken together, these data suggest that the role of plasticity in development of osteoblasts and cells of related lineages must be considered in more detail (for discussion, see Aubin, 1998).

These observations, together with discrepancies between results in calvaria vs. stromal and other populations and species differences, emphasize the need for a greater molecular understanding, for more markers of differentiation stages and for more rigorous assessment of the functional capacity of individual progenitors from various sites in bone and in the developing and adult skeleton. In the last several years, significant strides have been made towards identification of the molecular mechanisms underlying some aspects of lineage restriction, commitment and/or differentiation within these mesenchymal lineages. The 'master genes', exemplified by the MyoD, myogenin and Myf-5 helix–loop–helix transcription factors in muscle lineages, are one paradigm in which one transcription factor is induced and starts a cascade that leads to sequential expression of other transcription factors and of phenotype specific genes. A factor of a totally different family, the nuclear receptor family member peroxisome proliferator activated receptor $\gamma2$ or PPAR$\gamma2$, plays a key role in adipocyte differentiation and in conversion of mature osteoblasts to adipocyte phenotype. Only recently, Cbfa-1, a member of yet another family of transcription factors, the runt homology domain family, has been found to play a non-redundant role in osteoblast development during embryogenesis (reviewed in Ducy & Karsenty, 1998). While Cbfa-1 has all the characteristics expected of a transcriptional activator of osteoblast differentiation, and clearly plays an obligatory role in osteoblast differentiation in mouse and man, critical questions remain, including, e.g., what genes lie upstream and downstream of Cbfa1 to regulate the osteoblast differentiation process.

Morphological and histochemical criteria for transitional stages in the differentiation of osteoblasts

While different bones of the body arise in different ways (i.e., via intramembranous or endochondral formation) and from different embryonic tissues (i.e., neural crest (from ectoderm) and mesoderm), the mature osteoblast phenotype is defined by the ability of these cells to make a mineralized tissue recognizable as bone. By morphological and histochemical criteria, coupled to analyses of proliferation via

^{3}H-thymidine or more recently BrdU incorporation, four maturational stages in osteoblast development have been identified in bone: the preosteoblast, osteoblast, osteocyte, and bone lining cell. By these definitions, osteoblasts are postproliferative, cuboidal, highly polarized, strongly alkaline phosphatase-positive cells lining bone matrix at sites of active matrix production; they are connected by gap junctions and other junctional complexes including the adherens-type, and form a sheet-like contiguous layer over large areas. Osteoblasts can also now be recognized by their ability to synthesize a number of phenotype-specific or -associated macromolecules, including the collagenous and non-collagenous bone matrix proteins, certain hormone receptors and cytokines and growth factors, as will be discussed later. The preosteoblast is considered the immediate precursor of the osteoblast and is identified in part by its localization in the adjacent one or two cell layers distant from the osteoblasts lining bone formation surfaces. Although preosteoblasts resemble osteoblasts histologically and ultrastructurally, and stain for alkaline phosphatase activity, they have not yet acquired expression of many of the mature osteoblast markers and, unlike osteoblasts, they are thought to possess a limited capacity to divide. Some authors have used the term osteoprogenitor to identify a spindle-shaped cell residing in close proximity to the preosteoblast layer, but further from bone formation surfaces, in the fibrous periosteal layer of bone; these cells may be equivalent to the ^{3}H-thymidine-incorporating undifferentiated mesenchymal cells residing in the stromal tissues of bone marrow and also termed osteoprogenitors. Two recently isolated new markers for these cells, ALCAM, identified by expression cloning with the monoclonal antibody SB-10 (Bruder et al., 1997) and HOP-26 (Joyner et al., 1997), together with the STRO-1 antibody which recognizes these cells amongst others (Gronthos et al., 1994), may help further clarify these relationships. A small proportion (estimated at 10–20%) of osteoblasts incorporate themselves within the newly formed extracellular matrix; these embedded cells, considered the most mature differentiation stage of the osteoblastic lineage, are osteocytes. Osteocytes are also thought to be postproliferative, are smaller than osteoblasts, have lost many of their cytoplasmic organelles, have decreased alkaline phosphatase activity compared to matrix synthesizing osteoblasts, and are often considered to be relatively inactive metabolically. However, while it is true that synthesis of many bone matrix macromolecules and alkaline phosphatase activity are reduced in osteocytes compared with levels expressed in osteoblasts (see below), at least certain markers continue to be highly expressed, e.g., those recognized by other recently isolated monoclonal antibodies (Fig. 2.2) (Aubin & Turksen, 1996). Osteocytes have also been reported to alter expression of certain growth factors or cytokines after mechanical challenge and are now receiving increased attention as the responders and transducers of mechanical stimulation of bone (Mullender &

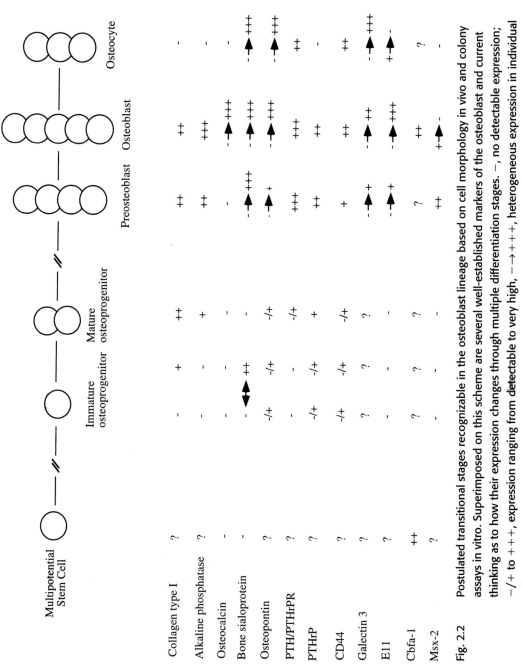

Fig. 2.2 Postulated transitional stages recognizable in the osteoblast lineage based on cell morphology in vivo and colony assays in vitro. Superimposed on this scheme are several well-established markers of the osteoblast and current thinking as to how their expression changes through multiple differentiation stages. −, no detectable expression; −/+ to +++, expression ranging from detectable to very high, −→+++, heterogeneous expression in individual cells.

Huiskes, 1997). Some authors have placed another transitory stage between the osteoblast and osteocyte to depict a cell just becoming embedded in osteoid, the so-called osteocytic osteoblast. Certain biochemical markers suggest that such a transitory cell does exist (summarized in Aubin & Turksen, 1996). Finally, in the adult skeleton, the majority of bone surfaces that are not being remodeled (i.e., undergoing resorption or formation) are covered by flat, thin, elongated, bone-lining cells, which are thought to represent the inactive (in terms of matrix production) form of the osteoblast. These are postproliferative cells, although Turner and colleagues have recently proposed that lining cells can be 'reactivated' to synthetically robust osteoblasts in response to particular stimuli such as challenge with PTH (Dobnig & Turner, 1995). Together, osteocytes and bone lining cells apparently account for only a relatively small proportion of the original osteoblasts, raising the question of what happens to the rest. There is some recent evidence for apoptosis of osteoblasts formed in vitro (Lynch et al., 1998), and in vivo, a process that may be enhanced by certain hormones or other regulators of osteoblast activity (e.g., Jilka et al., 1998; Machwate et al., 1998).

Biochemical and molecular features that characterize differentiation from osteoprogenitor cell to mature osteoblast phenotype

The mature osteoblast phenotype is characterized by the ability of the cells to synthesize membrane-associated alkaline phosphatase, bone matrix molecules including collagen type I (COLL-I) and a variety of non-collagenous proteins such as osteocalcin, BSP, and osteopontin, proteoglycans, and hormone and growth factor receptors, in particular PTH/PTHrP1R (Fig. 2.2). As described in detail later, however, different osteoblasts may express only a subset of molecules from the potential osteoblast repertoire.

While not specific for osteoblast lineage cells, high expression of the bone/liver/kidney (also called tissue non-specific, TN-AP) isoform of alkaline phosphatase is considered an important trait of osteoblastic cells. There is good evidence from experimental manipulations in vitro, and from alkaline phosphatase mutations leading to hypophosphatasia in man, that alkaline phosphatase is involved in the mineralization process. However, alkaline phosphatase expression is already high in preosteoblasts, well before a need for mineralization and prior to expression of the non-collagenous matrix molecules, including osteocalcin and BSP (Fig. 2.2). Alkaline phosphatase has also been suggested to play a role in the regulation of osteoprogenitor/osteoblast adhesion, migration and/or differentiation, functions also ascribed to TN-AP in cell migratory and morphogenetic events in early mouse embryos.

While synthesized in many cell types, COLL-I is a primary product of osteoblasts during bone matrix formation constituting approximately 90% of the total organic matrix in mature bone; by both *in situ* hybridization and immunolabeling, mature osteoblasts express very high levels of COLL-I. COLL-I, however, is also clearly expressed already by the preosteoblast stage, and indeed, upregulation of COLL-1 occurs prior to upregulation of any of the other current matrix molecules and prior to upregulation of alkaline phosphatase (Aubin, 1998; Liu et al., 1994). Of the non-collagenous proteins, osteopontin is a secreted phosphoglycoprotein isolated originally from the extracellular matrix of bone and synthesized by osteoblastic cells. Osteopontin, however, is not exclusive to bone since it is expressed by transformed cells and by many non-skeletal tissues and cells in response to stimulation of proliferation and induction by tumor promoters, growth factors and hormones in vitro (for review, see Denhardt & Noda, 1998). Most analyses now show that osteopontin is already detectable at relatively early differentiation stages in proliferating precursor cells, but that it is upregulated in some preosteoblasts and is high in osteoblasts. Osteopontin shares some structural features with another bone matrix protein, BSP. In contrast to osteopontin, BSP has a very restricted tissue distribution and is almost exclusively produced by skeletal cells, including hypertrophic chondrocytes, osteoblasts, and osteocytes. In bone sections, BSP is highly expressed by osteoblasts, but is also detectable in preosteoblasts in at least some regions of bone and may also be expressed transiently in earlier progenitor cells. Finally, osteocalcin is a major non-collagenous protein of bone highly expressed in mature osteoblasts; of osteoblast markers, osteocalcin is currently considered the most specific and the latest of expressed markers, undetectable in preosteoblasts and abundantly expressed only in postmitotic osteoblasts, and indeed, only in some mature osteoblasts in vitro and in vivo as recently reported (for review, see Aubin, 1998; see also below and Fig. 2.2).

Osteoblasts also respond to, and express, receptors for a growing list of hormones and growth factors, including – as one of the most specific for osteoblasts – PTH/PTHrP1R. They also synthesize and secrete a variety of other proteins into the bone extracellular matrix, including, e.g., osteonectin, BAG-75, fibronectin, biglycan, decorin, CS-PG-II, galectin-3, and CD44, amongst others. These macromolecules are also found in other tissues, but when taken together, their expression by osteoblasts and deposition into the matrix reflects the extensive biosynthetic repertoire of the osteoblast (see below). One challenge now is to determine whether the expression profiles of these and other molecules expressed by osteoblasts provide landmarks for helping to define stages of osteoblast maturation. In this regard, there are still many discrepancies reported in different bone cell models, and in different species (for a recent review, see Aubin et al., 1999).

Progression from the immature progenitor cell to the mature osteoblast and osteocyte: cell culture models

Cellular features

Based on the various criteria summarized, osteoblastic cells in vivo are categorized in a presumed linear sequence progressing from osteoprogenitor to preosteoblasts, osteoblasts, and lining cells or osteocytes (Fig. 2.1, 2.2). To identify cells earlier than the preosteoblast remains problematic, although as raised above, tools such as the STRO-1 antibody, the SB-10 antibody and HOP-26 antibody are beginning to provide further insight. A variety of studies on cell culture models, including primary cultures and normal and transformed cell lines, has augmented the observations on bone tissue *in situ*. Particularly notable are attempts to correlate progressive changes in osteoblast-associated properties with a progression in the state of differentiation of the cells. Based upon the profile of expression of osteoblastic characteristics and morphological features reminiscent of osteoblasts in vivo, the cell lines MC3T3–E1, UMR201 and RCT1 cells have been described as relatively immature, UMR 106 as preosteoblastic cells, and ROS 17/2.8 as more differentiated osteoblasts. However, in at least some of the lines derived from osteosarcoma, including ROS 17/2.8, the regulation between proliferation and expression of differentiated phenotype may be aberrant compared to their normal counterparts. Other examples of marked heterogeneity in a variety of the now numerous reported clonal lines, both in terms of expressed properties and regulation by hormones and growth factors lend ambiguity to attempts to order these lines in a lineage hierarchy.

As already raised, an alternative model is primary osteoblastic cell cultures, from both isolated bone marrow stromal populations and populations derived from fetal rat calvariae or more recently from a variety of other bones and other species. When maintained under suitable culture conditions, these cells form three-dimensional bone-like nodules with the histological, ultrastructural and immunohistochemical appearance of embryonic/woven bone. Cells virtually identical to the same morphological stages described in vivo can be identified, and the nodular matrix contains the major bone matrix proteins summarized above. The nodules represent the end product of the proliferation and differentiation of relatively rare osteoprogenitor cells (also called CFU-O) present in the starting cell population. Estimates of the frequency of these osteoprogenitors by limiting dilution indicated that such cells are present at a measurable but low frequency (i.e., $<1\%$) in rat calvaria populations and rat and mouse bone marrow stromal populations under standard isolation and culture conditions. However, as raised above, the frequency of the progenitors differentiating to bone nodules can be regulated (increased or decreased) by a variety of hormones, growth factors and cytokines (see also below). Osteoprogenitors forming bone nodules appear to have a limited capacity for self-renewal in both calvaria and stromal populations, consistent with their being true committed progenitors with a finite lifespan (Fig. 2.1). Morphologically recognizable osteoblasts associated with bone nodules appear in long-term bone cell cultures at predictable and reproducible periods after plating (2–3 weeks or longer in some cases). Analyses of individual progenitors forming colonies in low density cultures indicated that progenitors undergo approximately eight population doublings prior to overt differentiation, i.e., to achieving cuboidal morphology and matrix deposition consistent with their having reached a mature osteoblast stage; inhibition of proliferation inhibits bone nodule formation.

Molecular features

The process of formation of bone nodules has been subdivided into three developmental stages: (i) proliferation, (ii) extracellular matrix development and maturation, and (iii) mineralization, with characteristic changes in genes associated with proliferative and cell cycling activity and those associated with specific osteoblast activities (for review, see Aubin, 1998). Genes associated with proliferative stages, e.g., histones, proto-oncogenes such as c-*fos* and c-*myc*, characterize the first phase, while certain cyclins, e.g., cyclins B and E, are upregulated postproliferatively. While some variations have been noted which may reflect species or cell model differences, generally, the expression profiles of osteoblast markers in vitro appear largely to recapitulate expression profiles seen by both *in situ* hybridization and immunocytochemistry on bone sections. Thus, alkaline phosphatase is already detected in preosteoblasts and increases to high levels in osteoblasts then decreases when mineralization is well progressed; osteopontin appears prior to certain other matrix proteins including BSP and osteocalcin; BSP is first detected in some precursors but is high in differentiated osteoblasts forming bone; and osteocalcin appears with mineralization. COLL-I, while present from relatively early proliferative stages, peaks at late matrix maturational stages (Fig. 2.2).

The nodule system is increasingly being used to investigate many aspects of osteoprogenitor regulation, proliferation and differentiation. The approach has led to the conclusion that in rat calvaria cultures at least all osteoblast markers summarized above are upregulated prior to the cessation of proliferation except for osteocalcin (Aubin, 1998). Further studies are ongoing to explore the nature of transitional stages that characterize osteoblast development. One approach has combined the use of global amplification poly(A)PCR (which allows entire gene repertoires to be amplified in sample sizes as small as single cells and colonies), immunolabeling (which allows visual or positional cues to be used in tandem), and replica plating (which allows retrospective identification of very early osteoprogenitors). Based on the simultaneous expression patterns of osteoblast-associated genes (COLL-I, alkaline phosphatase, osteopontin, BSP, osteocalcin, PTH/PTHrP1R), and potential regulatory molecules (PTHrP, and growth factor receptors, e.g., FGFR-1 and PDGFRa), at least seven transitional stages can be identified in vitro (Aubin, 1998; Liu & Aubin, 1994], not just the three stages discussed earlier.

Heterogeneity of the mature osteoblast phenotype

One aspect of the osteoblast phenotype that is becoming increasingly well-documented in both studies on cell systems in vitro and bone tissue in vivo is inter-cellular heterogeneity in the osteoblast phenotype, i.e., heterogeneity in gene expression profiles. This was probably first most clearly evident in vitro, where reports of characterization of osteoblastic cell lines are notable as much for the differences amongst lines as for the similarities. More recently, striking heteroeogeneity in the expressed gene repertoires – at both mRNA and protein levels – in mature osteoblasts residing in bone nodules formed in vitro have been documented; the heterogeneity appears not to be related to cell cycle differences and extends to virtually all osteoblast-associated markers analyzed to date (Liu et al., 1997). A few reports have suggested that osteoblasts in different skeletal sites may also be different. For example, differences in expression profiles between younger vs. older rat osteoblasts (osteoblasts of different secretory lifetimes) have been reported for osteocalcin and BSP (for original references and other examples, see Aubin, 1999). In a recent study of osteoblasts in 21-day-old fetal rat calvaria, a bone characterized by well-demarcated maturational zones, it was found that out of nine osteoblast markers analyzed simultaneously, only two, alkaline phosphatase and PTH/PTHrP1R, appeared to be 'global' or 'ubiquitous' markers expressed by all osteoblasts in all zones. Other data suggest that COLL-I also belongs to this category. However, all other markers analyzed, including such markers as osteopontin, BSP, osteocalcin, and PTHrP, were differentially expressed at both mRNA and protein levels in only subsets of osteoblasts, depending on the maturational state of the bone (e.g., nascent vs. remodeling) and the age of the osteoblast, on the environment (endocranium, ectocranium) and on the microenvironment (adjacent cells in particular zones) in which the osteoblasts reside (Candeliere et al., 1997) (Fig. 2.2). These results indicate that histologically identical osteoblasts at different skeletal sites are molecularly heterogeneous and imply that they are also functionally heterogeneous, given (a) that matrix molecule expression is different, and (b) that ligand and hormone receptor expression – and *ergo* their ability to respond to regulatory cues – is different. The nature of the signals leading to diversity of osteoblast gene expression profiles is not known, although cross-talk between cells of different maturational stages or different lineages, variations in the cellular micro-environment including the degree and nature of the crystal structure of deposited mineral, and/or heterogeneous expression of combinations of various transcription factors in different cohorts of osteoblasts, are all possibilities. The fact that the heterogeneity is apparently controlled both transcriptionally and posttranscriptionally implies that the regulation is very complex but, once established, feedback regulatory loops could contribute to maintenance and even amplification of the phenotypic differences (for further discussion, see Aubin et al., 1999).

The true biological or physiological consequence of the observed differences in mRNA and protein expression repertoires is not known, but it supports the notion that not all mature osteoblasts are functionally identical and predicts that the make-up of different parts of bones may be significantly different, as previously suggested by the observations that the presence and amounts of extractable non-collagenous bone proteins are different in trabecular vs. cortical bone and in different parts of the human skeleton, which may also contribute to the heterogeneity in trabecular microarchitecture seen at different sites. The heterogeneous phenotype of mature osteoblasts at different skeletal sites may contribute to site-specific differences in disease manifestation such as seen in osteoporosis and to regional variations in the ability of osteoblasts to respond to therapeutic agents. The proclivity for some osteoblasts within certain bones and certain sites to differentially manifest disease may reside, at least in part, in somatic cell mosaicism, but may also occur, despite the widespread presence of a mutation or environmental factor, because only certain osteoblasts may be capable of response – pathological or normal – based on heterogeneous expression profiles of molecules such as those just summarized. A highly pertinent example of potential site-specific cellular responses concerns the estrogen receptors (ERs). Recent studies support the notion that ERα and ERβ are differentially expressed in different parts of bones, e.g., ERβ was reported to be highly expressed in the cancellous bone of lumbar vertebrae and distal femoral metaphysis but expressed at much lower levels in the cortical bone of the femur (Onoe et al., 1997). These data offer a possible mechanism by which the estrogen deficiency caused by ovariectomy induces bone resorption preferentially in cancellous bone and in vertebrae. Further analysis of differential expression profiles for a variety of receptors in different skeletal sites, and at different maturational age of the cells and skeleton, should provide further insight into site-specific effects of not only estrogen, but other treatments including, e.g., fluoride, calcitonin, PTH, and even calcium.

Osteoprogenitors and osteoblasts in the aging skeleton

Elsewhere in this volume (Chapter 14) the issues of osteoblast number and activity in the aging skeleton are discussed in detail. Studies in vivo are being augmented by attempts to isolate the bone cell populations and assess stem cell/osteo-progenitor/CFU-F number, ability to proliferate and differentiate, and ability to be regulated by a variety of hormones and growth factors in vitro. The published data on changes in stem or progenitor cell number or colony-forming ability are diverse, with data to support increases, decreases or no change in CFU-F, CFU-AP and/ or CFU-O number. For example, an increase in CFU-F number in aged vs. younger mice in the SAM-P (senescence-accelerated) mouse model has been reported (Tsuboi et al., 1991). On the other hand, some investigators (Tsuji et al., 1990) recovered fewer, but comparably sized, CFU-AP and CFU-O from old vs. younger rats, while others (Oreffo et al., 1998) found that CFU-F number was unchanged, but that there was a significant decrease in colony size in cells from aged human control or osteoporotic vs. younger samples. In the latter study, which suggested a generalized proliferation defect with age, there was a significant decrease in CFU-AP as a percentage of CFU-F in samples from osteoporotics compared to controls, suggesting a differentiation defect in these populations. However, in another study, a proportional decrease in both CFU-F and CFU-AP (suggesting no differentiation defect), and an increased proliferation rate in stromal cell cultures from older vs. younger mice, were seen, although the proliferation response to serum was lower in cells from older animals, suggesting a reduced ability to respond to growth factors and/or hormonal cues (Bergman et al., 1996). Consistent with the latter idea, CFU-F from older mice were reported to produce less TGF-β than those from younger mice, interpreted as the mechanism underlying the lower number and size of recovered CFU-F colonies (Gazit et al., 1998). Other examples of putative changes in osteoblastic cell activity or responsiveness include reduced osteocalcin production in response to $1,25(OH)_2D_3$ (Battmann et al., 1997) and loss of ERα regulation and diminution of ligand–receptor signal transduction (Ankrom et al., 1998) in human bone cells of increasing donor age. While it seems likely that differences in the kinds of cells being recovered from bone samples and differences in experimental approaches and conditions account for some of the discrepancies reported, and potential species differences must also be considered, such data are consistent overall with other observations that osteoblasts in the aged skeleton may not be identical to those in the younger organism, an area that deserves further attention.

Stage-specific regulation of osteoprogenitor cell differentiation and bone formation

The patterning of bones, differences in formation of the appendicular vs. axial skeleton, the ultimate size and shape of bones are now known to be influenced by a large number of genes, including, for example, hox genes (e.g., Hoxd-13), the runt family member Cbfa-1, growth factors (e.g., GDF-5), and PTHrP or its receptor,

PTH/PTHrP1R, amongst others. However, the factors that regulate osteoblast recruitment, osteoblast number, the rate and the duration of osteoblast activity in vivo are largely not known. In experimental models, bone marrow injury associated with local bleeding, clotting and neovascularization, recapitulates a process similar to callus formation during fracture repair, with the induction of an environment rich in growth factors (e.g., PDGF, FGF, TGF-β, VEGF) followed by a process of very active bone formation (for review, see Rodan, 1998). To elucidate the target cells responding (stem cells, mesenchymal precursors, committed progenitors) and the precise nature of the responses in bone and non-bone cells in the environment, these and a growing list of other systemic or local growth factors, cytokines and hormones are also being tested in many models in vitro. As outlined above, because of the now well-established proliferation and differentiation stages underlying formation of bone nodules in vitro, this model has provided strong support for several concepts proposed earlier. For example, there is growing evidence that at least some of the actions of growth and differentiation factors are dependent on the relative stage of differentiation (either more or less mature) of the target osteogenic cells, with, e.g., stimulatory/mitogenic or inhibitory responses when test factors are added to proliferative progenitor stages and stimulation or inhibition of sensitive/differentiation stage-specific precursors when the same factors are added later (Fig. 2.1). This is true, for example, for the inflammatory cytokine IL-1, which has potent regulatory activities throughout osteoblast differentiation, but is stimulatory when osteoblastic cell cultures are exposed transiently during proliferative culture stages and inhibitory when cells are exposed transiently during differentiation stages; the inhibitory effects dominate when cells are exposed chronically through proliferation and differentiation stages in culture (Ellies & Aubin, 1990). Another example of clinical significance is that reported for PTH, which has been found to increase bone mass when given intermittently, but decrease it when infused continuously, in various models. In an experiment to analyze possible underlying cellular mechanisms, rat calvaria cells were treated for 1 hour vs. 6-hour pulses in 48-hour cycles during a 2–3 week culture period. Inhibition (1-hour pulse; apparently related to cAMP/PKA pathways) or stimulation (6-hour pulse; apparently related to cAMP/PKA, Ca^{2+}/PKC, and IGF-I) in osteoblast differentiation was seen (Ishizuya et al., 1997); chronic exposure inhibits osteoblast differentiation, in an apparently reversible manner at a relatively late presoteoblast stage. Other factors appear to be without detectable effect during relatively narrow windows of time during osteoblast development, e.g., the inhibitory effects of LIF on late preosteoblastic stages (Malaval et al., 1998). Finally, virtually all agents tested have effects on gene expression in mature osteoblasts that may or may not correlate with effects on the differentiation process itself and may be opposite for different osteoblast genes, e.g., dexamethasone stimulates osteoprogenitor cell differentiation to mature osteoblasts in vitro, while upregulating alkaline phosphatase and BSP expression and downregulating COLL-I and osteocalcin expression, in mature osteoblastic cells. The molecular mechanisms mediating these complex effects are generally poorly understood; however, ability to form particular transcription factor complexes, localization and levels of endogenous expression of cytokine receptors, and expression of other regulatory ligands within specific subgroups of osteogenic cells as they progesss from a less to a more differentiated state may all play roles. For example, changing levels of endogenous expression of BMP family members has been postulated to initiate a cascade of cytokines and growth factors that themselves play stage-specific roles in osteoblast development. Further, it has been suggested that the stimulatory effects of glucocorticoids in bone nodule assays in vitro is mediated, at least in part, via their ability to downregulate endogenous production of inhibitory cytokines such as LIF and upregulate stimulatory factors such as BMP-6.

Acknowledgements

This work was supported by grant number MT-12390 from MRC (Canada). I apologize to all those investigators whose work could not be referred to directly due to space limitations, but many other important references can be found in the reviews quoted.

REFERENCES

Ankrom, M. A., Patterson, J. A., d'Avis, P. Y., Vetter, U. K., Blackman, M. R., Sponseller, P. D., Tayback, M., Robey, P. G., Shapiro, J. R., & Fedarko, N. S. (1998). Age-related changes in human oestrogen receptor alpha function and levels in osteoblasts. *Biochem. J.*, **333**, 787–94.

Aubin, J. E. (1998). Bone stem cells. 25th Anniversary Issue. New directions and dimensions in cellular biochemistry. Invited chapter. *J. Cell. Biochem. Suppl.*, **30/31**, 73–82.

Aubin, J. E. (1999). Osteoprogenitor cell frequency in rat bone marrow stromal cell populations: role for heterotypic cell–cell interactions in osteoblast differentiation. *J. Cell. Biochem.*, **72**, 396–410.

Aubin, J. E. & Turksen, K. (1996). Monoclonal antibodies as tools for studying the osteoblast lineage. *Microsc. Res. Tech.*, **33**, 128–40.

Aubin, J. E. & Heersche, J. M. N. (1997). Vitamin D and osteoblasts. In *Vitamin D*, ed. D. Feldman, F. H. Glorieux & J. W. Pike, pp. 313–28. San Diego, CA: Academic Press.

Aubin, J. E., Candeliere, G. A., & Bonnelye, E. (1999). Heterogeneity of the osteoblast phenotype. *The Endocrinologist*, **9**, 25–31.

Battmann, A., Battmann, A., Jundt, G., & Schulz, A. (1997). Endosteal human bone cells (EBC) show age-related activity in vitro. *Exp. Clin. Endocrinol Diabetes*, **105**, 98–102.

Bellows, C. G., Ishida, H., Aubin, J. E., & Heersche, J. N. M. (1990). Parathyroid hormone reversibly suppresses the differentiation of osteoprogenitor cells into functional osteoblasts. *Endocrinology*, 127, 3111–16.

Bergman, R. J., Gazit, D., Kahn, A. J., Gruber, H., McDougall, S., & Hahn, T. J. (1996). Age-related changes in osteogenic stem cells in mice. *J. Bone Miner. Res.*, 11, 568–77.

Boden, S. D., Hair, G., Titus, L., Racine, M., McCuaig, K., Wozney, J. M., & Nanes, M. S. (1997). Glucocorticoid-induced differentiation of fetal rat calvarial osteoblasts is mediated by bone morphogenetic protein-6. *Endocrinology*, 138, 2820–8.

Bruder, S. P., Horowitz, M. C., Mosca, J. D., & Haynesworth, S. E. (1997). Monoclonal antibodies reactive with human osteogenic cell surface antigens. *Bone*, 21, 223–35.

Candeliere, G. A., Liu, F., & Aubin, J. E. (1997). Heterogeneity of marker expression by osteoblasts in different zones of bone in the 21 day fetal rat calvaria. *J. Bone Miner. Res.*, 12, S187.

Denhardt, D. T. & Noda, M. (1998). Osteopontin expression and function: role in bone remodeling. 25th Anniversary Issue. New directions and dimensions in cellular biochemistry. *J. Cell. Biochem. Suppl.*, 30/31, 92–102.

Dobnig, H. & Turner, R. T. (1995). Evidence that intermittent treatment with parathyroid hormone increases bone formation in adult rats by activation of bone lining cells. *Endocrinology*, 136, 3632–8.

Ducy, P. & Karsenty, G. (1998). Genetic control of cell differentiation in the skeleton. *Curr. Opin. Cell Biol.*, 10, 614–19.

Ellies, L. G. & Aubin, J. E. (1990). Temporal sequence of interleukin 1α-mediated stimulation and inhibition of bone formation by isolated fetal rat calvarial cells *in vitro*. *Cytokine*, 2, 430–7.

Gazit, D., Zilberman, Y., Ebner, R., & Kahn, A. (1998). Bone loss (osteopenia) in old male mice results from diminished activity and availability of TGF-beta. *J. Cell Biochem.*, 70, 478–88.

Gimble, J. M., Robinson, C. E., & Kelly, K. A. (1996). The function of adipocytes in the bone marrow stroma: An update. *Bone*, 19, 421–8.

Gronthos, S., Graves, S. E., Ohta, S., & Simmons, P. J. (1994). The STRO-1+ fraction of adult human bone marrow contains the osteogenic precursors. *Blood*, 84, 4164–73.

Ishida, Y. & Heersche, J. N. (1997). Progesterone stimulates proliferation and differentiation of osteoprogenitor cells in bone cell populations derived from adult female but not from adult male rats. *Bone*, 20, 17–25.

Ishizuya, T., Yokose, S., Hori, M., Noda, T., Suda, T., Yoshiki, S., & Yamaguchi, A. (1997). Parathyroid hormone exerts disparate effects on osteoblast differentiation depending on exposure time in rat osteoblastic cells. *J. Clin. Invest.*, 99, 2961–70.

Jilka, R. L., Weinstein, R. S., Bellido, T., Parfitt, A. M., & Manolagas, S. C. (1998). Osteoblast programmed cell death (apoptosis): modulation by growth factors and cytokines. *J. Bone Miner. Res.*, 13, 793–802.

Joyner, C. J., Bennett, A., & Triffitt, J. T. (1997). Identification and enrichment of human osteoprogenitor cells by using differentiation stage-specific monoclonal antibodies. *Bone*, 21, 1–6.

Liu, F. & Aubin, J. E. (1994). Identification and molecular characterization of preosteoblasts in the osteoblast differentiation sequence. *J. Bone Miner. Res.*, 9, S125.

Liu, F., Malaval, L., & Aubin, J. E. (1997). The mature osteoblast phenotype is characterized by extensive plasticity. *Exp. Cell. Res.*, 232, 97–105.

Liu, F., Malaval, L., Gupta, A., & Aubin, J. E. (1994). Simultaneous detection of multiple bone-related mRNAs and protein expression during osteoblast differentiation: polymerase chain reaction and immunocytochemical studies at the single cell level. *Dev. Biol.*, **166**, 220–34.

Lynch, M. P., Capparelli, C., Stein, J. L., Stein, G. S., & Lian, J. B. (1998). Apoptosis during bone-like tissue development in vitro. *J. Cell. Biochem.*, **68**, 31–49.

Machwate, M., Rodan, S. B., Rodan, G. A., & Harada, S. I. (1998). Sphingosine kinase mediates cyclic AMP suppression of apoptosis in rat periosteal cells. *Mol. Pharmacol.*, **54**, 70–7.

Malaval, L., Gupta, A. K., Liu, F., Delmas, P. D., & Aubin, J. E. (1998). LIF, but not IL-6, regulates osteoprogenitor differentiation: Modulation by dexamethasone. *J. Bone Miner. Res.*, **13**, 175–84.

Mullender, M. G. & Huiskes, R. (1997). Osteocytes and bone lining cells: which are the best candidates for mechano-sensors in cancellous bone? *Bone*, **20**, 527–32.

Nuttall, M. E., Patton, A. J., Olivera, D. L., Nadeau, D. P., & Gowen, M. (1998). Human trabecular bone cells are able to express both osteoblastic and adipocytic phenotype: implications for osteogenic disorders. *J. Bone Miner. Res.*, **13**, 371–82.

Onoe, Y., Miyaura, C., Ohta, H., Nozawa, S., & Suda, T. (1997). Expression of estrogen receptor β in rat bone. *Endocrinology*, **138**, 4509–12.

Oreffo, R. O., Bord, S., & Triffitt, J. T. (1998). Skeletal progenitor cells and ageing human populations. *Clin. Sci. (Colch.)*, **94**, 549–55.

Rodan, G. A. (1998). Control of bone formation and resorption: biological and clinical perspective. 25th Anniversary Issue. New directions and dimensions in cellular biochemistry. *J. Cell. Biochem. Suppl.*, **30/31**, 55–61.

Tsuboi, I., Morimoto, K., Horie, T., & Mori, K. J. (1991). Age-related changes in various hemopoietic progenitor cells in senescence-accelerated (SAM-P) mice. *Exp. Hematol.*, **19**, 874–7.

Tsuji, T., Hughes, F. J., McCulloch, C. A., & Melcher, A. H. (1990). Effects of donor age on osteogenic cells of rat bone marrow in vitro. *Mech. Ageing Dev.*, **51**, 121–32.

3

Osteoclasts: characteristics and regulation of formation and activity

Johan N. M. Heersche and Morris F. Manolson

Introduction

Bone tissue adapts itself continuously to changing demands during development and growth (modeling) and in response to stress or damage (remodeling). The modeling and remodeling processes involve degradation of bone tissue by large multinucleated cells, called osteoclasts, and synthesis and deposition of new bone by mononuclear cuboidal cells lining bone, called osteoblasts. A close anatomical and functional relationship exists between resorptive and formative cells at discrete remodeling sites called 'basic multicellular units of bone remodeling' or BMU (Frost, 1966). This is, in all likelihood, responsible for the phenomenon in which treatments of metabolic bone disease developed to inhibit resorption often result in simultaneous inhibition of formation. The mechanism(s) whereby the actions of the resorbing osteoclasts and the bone forming osteoblasts are co-ordinated are not yet clear. Nevertheless, striking progress has been made in our understanding of osteoblast–osteoclast interaction with regard to regulating osteoclast formation.

This chapter focuses on osteoclasts and osteoclastic bone resorption. Morphological characteristics of osteoclasts, the processes whereby osteoclasts degrade bone, the origin of osteoclasts and the regulation of osteoclast formation and activity will be reviewed here.

Morphological characteristics of osteoclasts

Osteoclasts are easily recognized in histological sections of bone tissue as large multinucleated cells with up to 25 nuclei and are found in close association with bone surfaces (Fig. 3.1). They are often located in slight 'indentations' of the bone surface called Howship's lacunae, which result from osteoclasts having dissolved a small area of bone underneath the cell. Osteoclasts contain large amounts of the enzyme tartrate-resistant acid phosphatase (TRAP), and when stained histochemically for this enzyme become quite conspicuous. What also becomes apparent in histological sections so stained, however, is that not all osteoclasts contain large

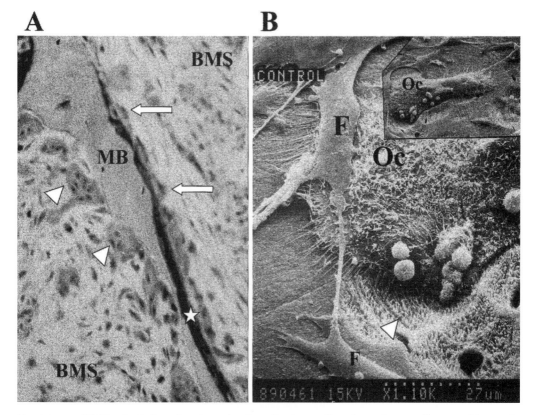

Fig. 3.1   (A) Histological section through mineralized cancellous bone from an iliac crest biopsy of a patient with renal osteodystrophy. Note osteoblasts (arrows), multinucleated osteoclasts in Howship's lacunae (arrrowheads), mineralized bone (MB), unmineralized osteoid (star), and bone marrow stroma (BMS). (B) Scanning electron micrograph of an osteoclast isolated from rabbit long bone and cultured for 24 hours on a thin slice of devitalized bovine cortical bone. *Insert*: low magnification. Note extensive filopodia on the basolateral surface, the fibroblastic cells (F) in close association with the osteoclast (Oc) and the collagen fibers of the bone matrix in the area partially resorbed by the osteoclast (arrowheads).

numbers of nuclei: mononuclear TRAP-positive cells can frequently be seen, and osteoclasts containing from two to four nuclei are not uncommon. Electron microscopic examination of cross-sections through actively resorbing osteoclasts reveal several more morphological features such as an abundance of mitochondria and cytoplasmic vesicular structures. The area where the cells closely adhere to bone, called the clear zone, is characterized by an abundance of microfilaments and the absence of cellular organelles. The area adjacent to the clear zone where the osteoclast plasma membrane exhibits extensive folding is referred to as the 'ruffled border' (Holtrop & King, 1977). When actively resorbing osteoclasts *in situ* are fixed, stained immunohistochemically with antibodies against F-actin, and then viewed under fluorescence microscopy, the clear zone area appears as a ring-like structure surrounding the ruffled border area (Lakkakorpi & Vaananen, 1991). This ring of actin-containing filaments delineates the area where the osteoclast closely adheres to the bone surface, likely via integrin receptors, and forms a sealed-off extracellular compartment between the ruffled border and the bone surface where bone resorption takes place. When *in situ* resorbing osteoclasts are viewed using scanning electron microscopy, they appear as large, bulging cells with a surface covered with numerous filopodia (Fig 3.1). In places where the osteoclast has moved away from an area it has been resorbing previously, exposed collagen fibres can frequently be seen, representing remains of the organic matrix after the osteoclast has removed the mineral component of the bone matrix.

The mechanism of osteoclastic bone resorption

Under normal conditions, osteoclasts are solely responsible for removing approximately 500 mg of calcium per day from the adult human skeleton. The rate of bone remodeling is determined by the number of BMU which are operative at any given time. In the normal human skeleton, activation occurs about once every 10 seconds, and the total number of BMU in operation at any one time has been calculated to be about 35 million (Parfitt, 1983). The H^+ ions required to dissolve the hydroxyapatite crystals comprising the mineral component of the bone matrix during the resorption process are generated by the activity of carbonic anhydrase type II (CAII), an enzyme which uses CO_2 and H_2O to generate H_2CO_3, which subsequently dissociates into H^+ ions and HCO_3^- ions. The protons thus generated are extruded into the extracellular space by a vacuolar-type H^+ATPase (V-ATPase) located on the osteoclast ruffled border membrane and there dissolve the bone mineral by H^+/Ca^{2+} exchange (Blair et al., 1989). It is interesting to note that the osteoclast appears to be essentially self-sufficient in generating the components required to complete this part of the resorptive process: protons generated by CAII activity, using CO_2 produced during the oxidative phosphorylation of glucose in the mitochondria, are extruded by the activity of a V-ATPase requiring ATP, which is similarly generated by mitochondrial oxidative phosphorylation of glucose. The required glucose enters the osteoclast through a GLUT-2 transporter (Williams et al., 1997), and all components of the system (mitochondria, the proton pump, the GLUT-2 transporter and CAII) are abundant in osteoclasts.

Proton extrusion into the extracellular resorption zone is accompanied by Cl^- extrusion via a chloride channel (Schlesinger et al., 1997). The driving force behind Cl^- extrusion is the potential difference that arises from electrogenic proton transport across the ruffled border membrane. In keeping with the self-sufficiency of the osteoclast, the required Cl^- ions enter the cell through a Cl^-/HCO_3^- exchanger located on the basolateral surface of the cell, which is driven by HCO_3 accumulated by CAII activity combined with proton extrusion (Teti et al., 1989).

The degradation of the organic matrix of bone is less well understood, and it is not known which specific enzymes degrade the diverse components of the organic matrix. It is clear, however, that two classes of enzymes, matrix metalloproteinases and cysteine proteinases, play a major role since inhibition of the activity of both classes of enzymes results in the accumulation of collagen fibres in the extracellular resorption zone (Everts et al., 1992). Interestingly, osteoclasts in different parts of the skeleton may differ in terms of the relative importance of matrix metalloproteinases and cysteine proteinases in the resorption process: matrix metalloproteinases have been shown to be responsible for organic matrix degradation by osteoclasts in the skull bone, whereas cysteine proteinases appear to be involved in osteoclastic resorption of both long bones and skull bones (Everts et al., 1999).

How degradation products are removed from the sealed-off resorption space between ruffled border and bone surface has been the subject of extensive speculation. One possibility is that osteoclasts move away from the resorption area temporarily thereby allowing accumulated degradation products to diffuse away. Resorbing osteoclasts have been observed, using time-lapse videomicroscopy, to move back and forth within a clearly delineated resorption space (Gaillard et al., 1979). Recent evidence suggests that matrix degradation products can also be removed from the lacunae by endocytotic vesicles. After endocytosis of degradation products at the ruffled border area, vesicles translocate to the basolateral surface and there release their contents by exocytosis (Nesbitt & Horton, 1997; Salo et al., 1997). Fig. 3.2 summarizes the major pathways involved in the resorptive process. It is of interest to note that osteoclasts seem to be unable to resorb unmineralized osteoid (see also Fig. 3.1) despite the fact that they possess the necessary enzymes to digest organic bone matrix during the process of removing mineralized bone. No satisfactory explanation has been provided thus far for this phenomenon.

The origin of osteoclasts

The origin of cells in bone and other connective tissues has occupied the minds of investigators ever since it was realized that tissues require an influx of new cells to repair structure and restore function after wounding. Cohnheim (1867: see Allgower, 1956, p. 4) was of the opinion that white blood cells are responsible for all the products of wound exudate, and could 'transform' into connective tissue cells. His contemporary, Virchow, did not agree, and stated that connective tissue cells, like other cell types, arise exclusively from local division of similar cells (see

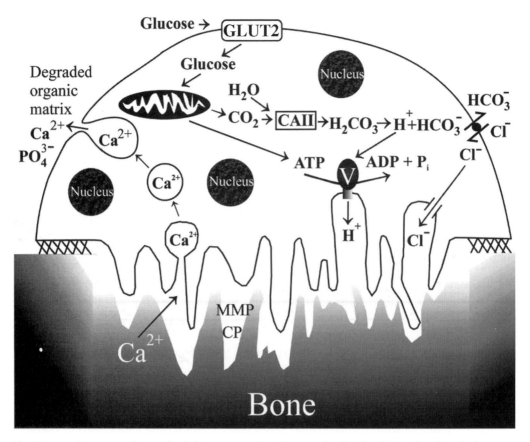

Fig. 3.2   Summary of osteoclastic bone resorption. See text for details. CAII: carbonic anhydrase type II, CP: cysteine proteinases, GLUT-2: Glucose transporter. MMP: matrix metalloproteinases, V: V-ATPase.

Allgower, 1956). It has taken almost a century to resolve this question. Using ^{3}H-thymidine labeling of proliferating precursor cells to trace these cells, Gothlin and Ericsson (1973) found that osteoclasts were derived from a bloodborne precursor belonging to a hemopoietic cell line, while the osteoblasts were derived from a local progenitor cell of connective tissue origin. Subsequent experiments by Walker (1975) made it virtually certain that osteoclasts were cells from the hemopoietic lineage: he transplanted spleen cells or bone marrow cells from normal mice into irradiated osteopetrotic littermates and found that this resulted in the formation of normal osteoclasts. Later experiments by Marks et al. (for review, see Marks, 1989) demonstrated that some osteopetrotic mutations in mice could be cured by transplantation of hemopoietic cells, while others could not. Thus, while some mutations result in intrinsic defects of the osteoclast lineage cells, other osteopetrotic mutations affect a different pathway.

Regulation of osteoclast activity and osteoclast differentiation

Stimulation or inhibition of osteoclastic bone resorption may involve changes in activity of existing osteoclasts, changes in the total number of osteoclasts, or changes in size of the osteoclasts. Previously, most in vitro systems used to evaluate osteoclastic bone resorption used explanted embryonic or newborn rat or mouse long bones or calvariae. With these in vitro systems, direct or indirect effects of agonists on osteoclasts or effects on osteoclast differentiation vs. osteoclast activity could not be distinguished. However, the development by Boyde et al. (1984) and Chambers et al. (1984) of culture systems in which functional osteoclasts could be analyzed on their flat-surfaced natural substratum has allowed separation of effects on osteoclastic resorption from effects on osteoclast formation and direct effects on osteoclasts from indirect effects mediated by other cell types.

When results obtained from studies of the effects of the bone resorbing hormones, parathyroid hormone (PTH) and 1,25-dihydroxyvitamin D$_3$ (1,25-(OH)$_2$D$_3$) in bone organ culture systems and in isolated osteoclast cultures were compared, it became rapidly clear that these hormones did not activate osteoclasts directly, but that the signals were transmitted by other cell types in bone tissue, presumably stromal cells or osteoblasts. As a result, elucidation of the mechanisms whereby osteoblastic cells interact with osteoclast-lineage cells became a major focus of investigation. The first breakthrough towards solving this problem came from studies analyzing the cause of bone defects in the osteopetrotic op/op mouse (Felix et al., 1996). These mice almost completely lack osteoclasts and tissue macrophages as a result of a single point mutation in the gene encoding macrophage colony stimulating factor (M-CSF), while injection of M-CSF partially corrects the defect. Marrow cells from op/op mice co-cultured with osteoblast-like cells or stromal cells from normal littermates (or vice versa) revealed that the defect in osteoclast differentiation in op/op mice resulted from the failure of osteoblastic/stromal cells to produce M-CSF required for osteoclast differentiation.

In mouse bone marrow cultures, formation of osteoclast-like cells is stimulated by the addition of osteotropic hormones (e.g., PTH, 1,25 (OH)$_2$D$_3$,PGE$_2$) or cytokines (e.g., IL-1, IL-6, IL-11, oncostatin M and leukocyte inhibitory factor (LIF) (for review, see Suda et al., 1997). However, since marrow cultures contain both hemopoietic cells and stromal cells, this system is not suitable to distinguish between effects mediated through osteoblastic or stromal cells and direct effects on osteoclast progenitors. This problem was solved by designing a co-culture system consisting of spleen cells and osteoblastic cells from calvariae (or established marrow-derived stromal cell lines). Osteoclast formation in such co-cultures required the presence of 1,25 (OH)$_2$D$_3$, PTH, PGE$_2$ or the cytokines mentioned above. The effects on osteoclast differentiation were mediated through the osteoblastic or stromal cell component of the cultures, and osteoclast differentiation required direct cell–cell contact between the activated osteoblastic/stromal cell population and the hemopoietic cells. The membrane-bound mediator, named osteoclast differentiation factor (ODF), was subsequently cloned and identified (Yasuda et al., 1998), and proved to be identical to the previously identified protein osteoprotegerin ligand (OPGL) (Lacey et al., 1998), which in turn is identical to the ligand for the receptor activator of $NF_\kappa B$ (RANKL). Thus it is likely that the receptor on the osteoclast recognizing ODF ($=$ OPGL $=$ RANKL) is the RANK receptor, and that ligand–receptor interaction induces osteoclast differentiation (Kong et al., 1999). That RANKL (OPGL) is an absolute requirement for osteoclast formation was proven conclusively by the generation of OPGL knockout mice. These mice had severe osteopetrosis due to a complete lack of osteoclasts. The osteoblastic origin of RANKL (OPGL) was confirmed by setting up co-cultures of spleen cells from $OPGL^{-/-}$ mice with normal osteoblasts, which generated functional osteoclasts, and co-cultures of spleen cells from normal mice with osteoblasts from $OPGL^{-/-}$ mice, which did not form osteoclasts. Thus, lack of RANKL (OPGL) production in osteoblastic cells of $OPGL^{-/-}$ mice was the cause of the osteoclast deficiency.

It was discovered virtually simultaneously that osteoclast formation could be inhibited by a soluble receptor for RANKL, osteoprotegerin (OPG), which is secreted by a large variety of cells and organs, including fibroblasts, osteoblasts, lung, heart, kidney and intestine (Simonet et al., 1997). OPG-deficient mice are severely osteoporotic (Bucay et al., 1998), while mice overexpressing OPG have an osteopetrotic phenotype. OPG acts by binding RANKL, thereby preventing interaction of RANKL with its receptor on the osteoclast lineage cells and thus inhibiting osteoclast differentiation. The consensus view now is that osteoclast formation in the bone microenvironment is regulated by the interaction of RANKL and OPG, where the amount of unbound RANKL available to interact with the RANK receptor on osteoclasts or osteoclast precursors determines the rate of osteoclast formation.

Knockout or transgenic mice have also been used extensively to study the consequences on osteoclastic resorption resulting from the deletion or overexpression of other molecules likely involved in osteoclastic activity. One of the molecules tested this way was TRAP. Surprisingly, the TRAP ($acp5^{-/-}$) knockout mice were not osteopetrotic and, besides having some growth plate abnormalities, were virtually normal (Hayman et al., 1996). This raises the question of what the biological function of TRAP activity in osteoclasts really is, or what enzyme can take over its function in the TRAP knockout mice, a question that is not yet answered. Ablation of $NF_\kappa B1$ and $NF_\kappa B2$ had the expected results: the mice were osteopetrotic, did not develop osteoclasts, but had an increased number of macrophages (Iotsova et al., 1997). A more surprising observation was made, however, in c-*fos* knockout mice (Grigoriadis et al., 1994), which had a similar phenotype to the $NF_\kappa B$ knockouts: osteopetrotic, no osteoclasts and an increased number of macrophages. These mice were not generated with bone studies in mind, and the failure of osteoclast formation in c-*fos*$^-$/$^-$ mice uncovered an unsuspected role for c-*fos* in osteoclast formation. Equally surprising was the observation that the major consequence of ablation of another almost universal enzyme, c-*src*, turned out to be osteopetrosis: the mice have normal numbers of osteoclasts, but they appear to be unable to resorb bone due to an inability to generate a ruffled border area (Soriano et al., 1991). No other abnormalities were observed, indicating that the role of c-*src* in every cell but the osteoclast can be assumed by other members of the *src* family of proteins.

In summary, it is now generally accepted that M-CSF produced by stromal cells is required for the generation of osteoclast precursors. Both hormone-induced stimulation of osteoclast activity and osteoclast differentiation are also mediated via effects on stromal or osteoblastic cells, and the predominant factor mediating these responses appears to be RANKL. Combined addition of M-CSF and a soluble form of RANKL to spleen cell cultures overcomes the need for stromal cells to achieve osteoclast formation in this culture system (Lacey et al., 1998). What still remains unknown is what modulates osteoclast formation and what determines the sites where osteoclasts initiate resorption.

A final point of interest with regard to osteoclastic activity: mature osteoclasts with the potential to resorb bone are not always doing so. Individual osteoclasts cycle through different phases of activity: a rapid migratory phase and a relatively stationary resorptive phase (Kanehisa & Heersche, 1988). As discussed previously, a sealed-off resorption zone and a ruffled border area have to be established for resorption to occur, and it is not clear at the present time what signals initiate this event. Single osteoclasts can excavate two different resorption lacunae simultaneously with resorption progressing at different rates in each zone. Furthermore, initiation and termination of resorption in the different resorption zones are independent. This implies that factors in the bone matrix may have a signaling function in addition to signals reaching the osteoclast from the extracellular fluid environment.

REFERENCES

Allgower, M. (1956). *The Cellular Basis of Wound Repair*. Springfield, IL: Charles C. Thomas.

Blair, H. C., Teitelbaum, S. L., Ghiselli, R., & Gluck, S. (1989). Osteoclastic bone resorption by a polarized vacuolar proton pump. *Science*, **245**, 855–7.

Boyde, A., Ali, N. N., & Jones, S. J. (1984). Resorption of dentine by isolated osteoclasts in vitro. *Br. Dent. J.*, **156**, 216–20.

Bucay, N., Sarosi, I., Dunstan, C. R., Morony, S., Tarpley, J., Capparelli, C., Scully, S., Tan, H. L., Xu, W., Lacey, D. L., Boyle, W. J., & Simonet, W. S. (1998). Osteoprotegerin-deficient mice develop early onset osteoporosis and arterial calcification. *Genes Dev.*, **12**, 1260–8.

Chambers, T. J., Revell, P. A., Fuller, K., & Athanasou, N. A. (1984). Resorption of bone by isolated rabbit osteoclasts. *J. Cell. Sci.*, **66**, 383–99.

Everts, V., Delaisse, J. M., Korper, W., Niehof, A., Vaes, G., & Beertsen, W. (1992). Degradation of collagen in the bone-resorbing compartment underlying the osteoclast involves both cysteine-proteinases and matrix metalloproteinases. *J. Cell. Physiol.*, **150**, 221–31.

Everts, V., Korper, W., Jansen, D. C., Steinfort, J., Lammerse, I., Heera, S., Docherty, A. J., & Beertsen, W. (1999). Functional heterogeneity of osteoclasts: matrix metalloproteinases participate in osteoclastic resorption of calvarial bone but not in resorption of long bone. *FASEB. J.*, **13**, 1219–30.

Felix, R., Hofstetter, W., & Cecchini, M. G. (1996). Recent developments in the understanding of the pathophysiology of osteopetrosis. *Eur. J. Endocrinol.*, **134**, 143–56.

Frost, H. M. (1966). *The Bone Dynamics in Osteoporosis and Osteomalacia.* Springfield, IL: Charles C. Thomas.

Gaillard, P. J., Herrmann-Erlee, M. P., Hekkelman, J. W., Burger, E. H., & Nijweide, P. J. (1979). Skeletal tissue in culture. Hormonal regulation of metabolism and development. *Clin. Orthop.*, **142**, 196–214.

Gothlin, G. & Ericsson, J. L. E. (1973). On the osteogenesis of the cells in fracture callus. *Virchow's Arch. Abt. B. Zellpathol.*, **12**, 318.

Grigoriadis, A. E., Wang, Z. Q., Cecchini, M. G., Hofstetter, W., Felix, R., Fleisch, H. A., & Wagner, E. F. (1994). c-Fos: a key regulator of osteoclast–macrophage lineage determination and bone remodeling. *Science*, **266**, 443–8.

Hayman, A. R., Jones, S. J., Boyde, A., Foster, D., Colledge, W. H., Carlton, M. B., Evans, M. J., & Cox, T. M. (1996). Mice lacking tartrate-resistant acid phosphatase (Acp 5) have disrupted endochondral ossification and mild osteopetrosis. *Development*, **122**, 3151–62.

Holtrop, M. E. & King, G. J. (1977). The ultrastructure of the osteoclast and its functional implications. *Clin. Orthop.*, **123**, 177–96.

Iotsova, V., Caamano, J., Loy, J., Yang, Y., Lewin, A., & Bravo, R. (1997). Osteopetrosis in mice lacking NF-kappaB1 and NF-kappaB2. *Nat. Med.*, **3**, 1285–9.

Kanehisa, J. & Heersche, J. N. (1988). Osteoclastic bone resorption: in vitro analysis of the rate of resorption and migration of individual osteoclasts. *Bone*, **9**, 73–9.

Kong, Y. Y., Yoshida, H., Sarosi, I., Tan, H. L., Timms, E., Capparelli, C., Morony, S., Oliveira-dos-Santos, A. J., Van, G., Itie, A., Khoo, W., Wakeham, A., Dunstan, C. R., Lacey, D. L., Mak, T. W., Boyle, W. J., & Penninger, J. M. (1999). OPGL is a key regulator of osteoclastogenesis, lymphocyte development and lymph-node organogenesis. *Nature*, **397**, 315–23.

Lacey, D. L., Timms, E., Tan, H.-L., Kelley, J. M., Dunstan, C. R., Burgess, T., Elliott, R., Colombero, A., Elliott, G., & Scully, S. (1998). Osteoprotegerin ligand is a cytokine that regulates osteoclast differentiation and activation. *Cell*, **93**, 165–76.

Lakkakorpi, P. T. & Vaananen, H. K. (1991). Kinetics of the osteoclast cytoskeleton during the resorption cycle in vitro. *J. Bone Min. Res.*, **6**, 817–26.

Marks, S. C., Jr. (1989). Osteoclast biology: lessons from mammalian mutations. *Am. J. Med. Genet.*, **34**, 43–54.

Nesbitt, S. A. & Horton, M. A. (1997). Trafficking of matrix collagens through bone-resorbing osteoclasts. *Science*, **276**, 266–9.

Parfitt, A. M. (1983). The physiological and clinical significance of bone histomorphometric data. In *Bone Histomorphometry. Techniques and Interpretations*, ed. R. Recker, Boca Raton: CRC Press.

Salo, J., Lehenkari, P., Mulari, M., Metsikko, K., & Vaananen, H. K. (1997). Removal of osteoclast bone resorption products by transcytosis. *Science*, **276**, 270–3.

Schlesinger, P. H., Blair, H. C., Teitelbaum, S. L., & Edwards, J. C. (1997). Characterization of the osteoclast ruffled border chloride channel and its role in bone resorption. *J. Biol. Chem.*, **272**, 18636–43.

Simonet, W. S., Lacey, D. L., Dunstan, C. R., Kelley, M., Chang, M. S., Luthy, R., Nguyen, H. Q., Wooden, S., Bennett, L., Boone, T., Shimamoto, G., DeRose, M., Elliott, R., Colombero, A., Tan, H. L., Trail, G., Sullivan, J., Davy, E., Bucay, N., Renshaw-Gegg, L., Hughes, T. M., Hill, D., Pattison, W., Campbell, P., Boyle, W. J. et al. (1997). Osteoprotegerin: a novel secreted protein involved in the regulation of bone density. *Cell*, **89**, 309–19.

Soriano, P., Montgomery, C., Geske, R., & Bradley, A. (1991). Targeted disruption of the c-src proto-oncogene leads to osteopetrosis in mice. *Cell*, **64**, 693–702.

Suda, T., Nakamura, I., Jimi, E., & Takahashi, N. (1997). Regulation of osteoclast function. *J. Bone Miner. Res.*, **12**, 869–79.

Teti, A., Blair, H. C., Teitelbaum, S. L., Kahn, A. J., Koziol, C., Konsek, J., Zambonin-Zallone, A., & Schlesinger, P. H. (1989). Cytoplasmic pH regulation and chloride/bicarbonate exchange in avian osteoclasts. *J. Clin. Invest.*, **83**, 227–33.

Walker, D. G. (1975). Control of bone resorption by hematopoietic tissue. The induction and reversal of congenital osteopetrosis in mice through use of bone marrow and splenic transplants. *J. Exp. Med.*, **142**, 651.

Williams, J. P., Blair, H. C., McDonald, J. M., McKenna, M. A., Jordan, S. E., Williford, J., & Hardy, R. W. (1997). Regulation of osteoclastic bone resorption by glucose. *Biochem. Biophys. Res. Commun.*, **235**, 646–51.

Yasuda, H., Shima, N., Nakagawa, N., Yamaguchi, K., Kinosaki, M., Mochizuki, S., Tomoyasu, A., Yano, K., Goto, M., Murakami, A., Tsuda, E., Morinaga, T., Higashio, K., Udagawa, N., Takahashi, N., & Suda, T. (1998). Osteoclast differentiation factor is a ligand for osteoprotegerin/osteoclastogenesis-inhibitory factor and is identical to TRANCE/RANKL. *Proc. Natl Acad. Sci., USA*, **95**, 3597–602.

4

Bone matrix proteins

Marc D. McKee and Jaro Sodek

Introduction

Bone represents the largest proportion of the connective tissues in the human body where it functions in the protection of internal organs, as a framework for muscle attachment to generate locomotion, and as an ion reservoir for calcium and other mineral elements. The unique biophysical properties of bone reflect the macromolecular composition and organization of the mineralized extracellular matrix (ECM), which is largely produced and regulated by specialized cells of the osteoblastic lineage. The ECM is formed from a scaffold of collagen fibrils within and between which are found uniform-sized crystals of carbonate-substituted hydroxyapatite. Other proteins, including proteoglycans, sialoproteins and various acidic glycoproteins regulate the formation of the collagen fibrils and apatite crystals and mediate interactions with the osteoblastic cells that generate and maintain the matrix. Characteristically, bone is remodeled continuously during postnatal growth and skeletal maintenance, thus permitting continuous adaptivity for changes in size and structure. Bone mass is maintained through a carefully regulated balance between synthesis and resorption which can be monitored by analysis of metabolized matrix components in body fluids – typically in serum and urine. Loss of regulation, observed in metabolic bone diseases, can lead to increased (osteopetrosis) or decreased (osteoporosis) bone mass, primarily reflecting changes in the amount of mineralized ECM. While the basic components of the bone matrix are similar, their organization can vary quite significantly, generating mineralized tissue with different attributes that have functional importance. Thus, in newly formed 'woven' bone, which is produced rapidly during *de novo* formation of endochondral and intramembranous bone and in fracture repair, the collagen fibrils are relatively loosely packed and somewhat randomly oriented, an organization within which a significant amount of mineral crystals are formed between the fibrils. The woven bone is generally replaced by a more mature 'lamellar' bone in which the collagen scaffold is laid down in alternating sheets (lamellae) of more closely packed and aligned fibrils, within which the mineral crystals are primarily intrafibrillar.

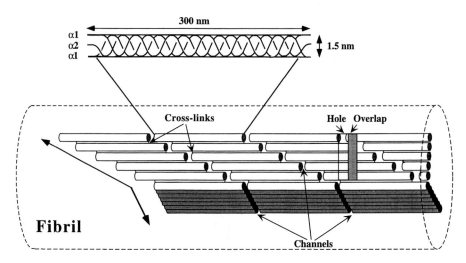

Fig. 4.1   Diagram depicting the structure of a collagen molecule and the arrangement of collagen molecules in a fibril. The type I collagen molecule, as found in bone, consists of two α1(I), and one α2(I), chains that form a triple-helical structure extending ~300 nm in length with short telopeptides involved in cross-link formation at each end. The molecules pack in a quarter-stagger array, with successive molecules separated by a gap (hole) which forms a continuous channel along two dimensions of the fibril. The calcium phosphate crystals (apatite) found in bone are initially formed in these channels. Figure not drawn to scale.

Collagen

The collagen fibrils in bone are formed from type I collagen molecules (>95%) with small amounts of type V collagen (<5%) which can form heterotypic fibres with type I collagen. Some type II, III, IX, X and XIV collagen may also be found in bone, most notably in specialized attachment structures such as osseous tendon and ligament insertion sites. By weight, collagen comprises 85–90% of total bone protein. As shown in Fig. 4.1, type I collagen molecules consist of two α1(I) chains and an α2(I) chain, which intertwine in a specific manner to form a unique, triple-helical structure which is characteristically resistant to proteolytic enzymes. Essentially, all the information required for the formation of the collagen helix, and also for the subsequent assembly of collagen fibrils from collagen molecules, resides in the nucleotide sequence of the individual genes encoding the collagen α chains (Kielty et al., 1992). The gene for the human α1(I) chain is found on chromosome

17, and for α2(I) on chromosome 7 (Vuorio & de Crombrugghe, 1990). Each α chain (~160 kDa) is synthesized as a precursor molecule which contains a central helical region (~100 kDa) flanked at each end by large domains, the extension peptides, required for the assembly of the procollagen molecule within the cell. Assembly begins by the association and covalent cross-linking of two procollagen α1 chains and an α2 chain in the rough endoplasmic reticulum through the carboxy-terminal propeptides (~35 kDa). This is followed by the intertwining of the chains to form the central helical region and then the association of the amino-terminal propeptides (~25 kDa). On secretion, the procollagen peptides are proteolytically removed allowing triple-helical collagen molecules, 300 nm long and 1.5 nm thick, to assemble into fibrils. The propeptides become incorporated into the bone matrix or appear in the serum where they can be measured as a systemic indicator of bone formation (Parfitt et al., 1987).

The formation of the triple-helical structure of collagen is directed by a repetitive Gly–X–Y sequence of amino acids in the central region of each α chain. The amino acid proline and its posttranslationally modified form, hydroxyproline, which together represent ~22% of the amino acids in the helical region, are frequently found in the X and Y positions, respectively. Because the ring structure in the side chain of these amino acids prevents rotation of the peptide bond, twisting of the α chain into a left-handed polyprolyl (minor helix) structure, with three amino acids per turn, is favored. However, stabilization of the minor helix requires all three chains to twist together into a right-handed, triple (major) helix. In turn, the major helix is stabilized by the presence of the hydroxyprolines which mediate extensive hydrogen bond formation with peptide bond $-NH$ and $C=O$ groups. The position of the glycine at every third position in each α chain is crucial for the formation of the major helix since the side chains at this position occupy the central core of the cylindrical structure of the triple helix. When the three α chains are tightly packed together into the triple helix, only the proton of the glycine side chain can fit into the space available. Substitution of glycine by any other amino acid will disrupt and destabilize the helical structure, resulting in impaired fibril formation and mineralization, as observed in many forms of osteogenesis imperfecta (Byers, 1992).

The side chains of the amino acids in the X and Y positions provide the surface characteristics of the collagen molecule and therefore are crucial for the precise assembly of the molecules into fibrils. The fibrils are thin (10–300 nm diameter) rope-like structures, many micrometers in length, that display a characteristic banding pattern when viewed by electron microscopy. This periodicity reflects the properties of the surface amino acids in combination with the organization of the collagen molecules into a quarter-stagger (64–67 nm) array in which successive collagen molecules are separated by a gap (hole) which forms a continuous helical channel running along the fibril (Fig. 4.1). While hierarchical twisting of the α chains, and collagen molecules, in alternating directions provides the rope-like characteristics of the fibril, the high tensile strength that is a characteristic feature of fibrillar collagens is due to covalent cross-link formation between lysines and modified lysines within and between the collagen molecules. Lysines and hydroxy-lysines are modified by lysyl oxidase to aldehydes termed allysines and hydroxy-allysines, which can form aldimines with unmodified lysines and hydroxylysines. The modified lysines are present in short, non-helical extensions (telopeptides) at each end of the collagen molecule. In bone, pairs of allysines can form aldol condensation products within the telopeptide region, whereas intermolecular aldimine bonds are formed between hydroxyallysines juxtaposed with hydroxylysines in the helical region of laterally associated collagen molecules to form the bifunctional hydroxylysino-5-oxo-norleucine cross-link. Maturation of cross-links involves subsequent interactions with additional lysine-derived side chains to form the trifunctional cross-links such as pyridinoline, which is used as a diagnostic marker of bone resorption (Delmas et al., 1991). The precise alignment of collagen molecules is clearly crucial for cross-link formation and, consequently, for the tensile strength of the collagen fibrils.

Although the staggered arrangement of collagen molecules in fibrils is well established, the higher order arrangement of the molecules within the fibrils to form larger fibres is less clear and may be different in various connective tissues. Thus, microfibrils such as the proposed 'pentafibril' structure comprising a five-molecule repeat of staggered collagen molecules could associate laterally either in a continuum of the same staggered alignment of the collagen molecules, or they could align in register to give an identical banding pattern in the fibril. At this level of structure, other collagens, such as type V collagen, and non-collagenous proteins (NCPs) and the proteoglycans, will influence the size of the fibrils and the subsequent formation of collagen fibres. The initial orientation of the fibrils, however, is likely directly regulated by the bone-forming cells, producing either a woven or lamellar bone structure. In both woven and lamellar bone, mineral crystals within the collagen fibrils (intrafibrillar) are believed to form initially within the gap region (Fig. 4.1) such that their c-axes are generally aligned with the long axis of the collagen fibril (Weiner & Traub, 1986). Further mineral crystal formation and growth occurs within the channels created by the gap region as well as in the spaces between the collagen molecules. A critical step in this process is the nucleation of apatitic mineral, although the mechanism(s) of mineral nucleation and regulation still have not been clearly resolved. Thus, while fibrillar collagen alone is capable of heterogeneous nucleation of apatite, the possible involvement of a collagen-binding, mineral-nucleating macromolecule (presumably located in the gap region or at the surface of the fibrils) must also be considered. The involvement of other macromolecules in nucleation is indicated by the formation of crystals between the collagen fibrils (interfibrillar), as typically observed in woven bone. It is likely that multiple mechanisms for nucleation and regulation of crystal growth are involved.

Non-collagenous extracellular matrix proteins

Whereas collagen fibrils in all connective tissues are constructed and organized by cells to provide a flexible and porous, fibrillar scaffolding necessary for cell adhesion, cell signaling and tissue compartmentalization, specialized connective tissues like bone, tooth (dentin and cementum), and sometimes cartilage, must also accommodate a solid, inorganic mineral phase. This unique and intriguing property is generally viewed as requiring a specialized class of proteins rather broadly referred to as the non-collagenous, ECM proteins. Given the importance of the biomineralization process in creating a rigid, supporting skeleton that serves multiple, critical functions in vertebrates, it is evident that this process must be exquisitely controlled. The regulation of the precipitation and growth of something as remarkable as mineral salts within biological tissues is a feature maintained by evolution in many invertebrates as well as in vertebrates, and reflects a wonderful 'symbiosis' between geochemical and geophysical substances and laws, and their 'intelligent' use by biological systems. Whereas calcium and phosphorus are incredibly abundant elements found across the continents and oceans of our planet, it is precisely the use of ionic forms of these elements by cells that remarkably distinguishes many biological systems in their ability to 'sense' and respond to local environmental stimuli. Hard vertebrate tissues have additionally acquired the ability to direct the incorporation of mineral salts into their structure – a process that must be harmonious with all other simultaneously ongoing physiological processes likewise using these same mineral ions, of which there are many. Such a complex system of overlapping pathways involving translocation of soluble mineral ions used in cell signaling and protein modification, vs. the precipitation of an inorganic, solid mineral phase within a pre-established organic framework, requires careful and reliable mineral ion processing. This regulation, at least for calcium handling within the milieu of the ECM, is thought to reside within a class of posttranslationally modified proteins typically being acidic in nature and containing covalently attached phosphate and carbohydrate side chains. There is a general consensus, based on a variety of protein data both from invertebrate and vertebrate experimental studies in vivo and in vitro, that such phosphorylated, acidic glycoproteins first initiate (nucleate), and then regulate (inhibit), the formation and growth of crystals in hard tissues (Gorski, 1992; Hunter, 1996). This process appears not to be a passive one, driven solely by physicochemical forces acting upon the mineral ions, but rather is a genetically controlled, active phenomenon guided by the chemistry of the resident proteins themselves (Schinke et al., 1999).

Most of the major (in terms of abundance) non-collagenous matrix proteins have been isolated from bone over the past several decades (Gehron Robey, 1996; Young et al., 1993), and typically a large percentage of these can be recovered only after exhaustive decalcification of the bone, thus indicating their affinity for mineral and their classification as mineral-binding proteins (Termine et al., 1981). While collectively, NCPs occupy roughly only 10% of the organic matrix by weight (Fig. 4.2), on a molar basis, they are commonly found in similar proportions to collagen, with some variation among tissues and species. However, until recently, the precise function of most proteins in the ECM of bone, except possibly for type I collagen, has generally been unknown. This is, in large part, attributable to the difficulty of isolating these macromolecules and studying their involvement in complex osteogenic events in vitro. However, recent studies (both in vitro and in vivo) have provided substantial insight into the potential roles of the structural, mineral-regulating, and cell-adhesive proteins of the bone ECM – the major ones of which, and those which have been best characterized and/or are unique, are discussed briefly below.

Bone sialoprotein

Bone sialoprotein (BSP) comprises about 10% of the NCPs found in the ECM of bone, and its isolation from bone generally requires extensive, dissociative extraction and decalcifying techniques, thus characterizing it as a mineral-binding protein (Ganss et al., 1999). The primary sequence of the nascent protein comprises approximately 327 amino acids including a 16-residue leader sequence (Chenu et al., 1994). Glu and Gly residues constitute about one-third of the total amino acids, and there are two–three stretches of polyGlu located in the N-terminal half of the protein, which appear to be involved in binding to apatite crystals that form the mineral phase of bone. BSP also contains an Arg–Gly–Asp (RGD) motif near the carboxy-terminus which can mediate cell binding and signaling via integrin receptors. Conservation of the primary sequence is high among mammals, with 45% identity, and a further 10–23% conservative replacements. Structure predictions indicate an open, flexible structure with significant α-helix and some β-sheet regions. However, BSP is extensively modified by posttranslational events that almost double the mass of the protein and which can influence protein structure. Posttranslational modifications include both N-linked and O-linked glycosylation that introduce substantial amounts of glucosamine and galactosamine, and also sialic acid – hence, the term sialoprotein. Phosphorylation occurs mostly at Ser residues within the amino-terminal half of the protein, most likely from the activity

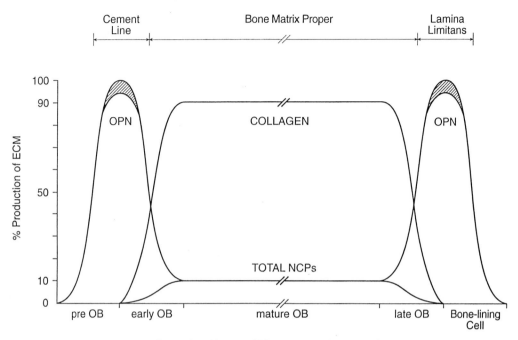

Extracellular Matrix Accumulation During Osteogenesis

Fig. 4.2   Temporal sequence of extracellular matrix deposition in bone by osteoblast lineage cells and its assembly into discrete structural features of the bone matrix. Based on biochemical analyses from a variety of in vitro and in vivo studies, and on immunocytochemical and *in situ* hybridization observations, the following interpretation has evolved for the sequential accumulation and organization of bone proteins into an extracellular matrix. Whereas the bulk of the bone matrix consists primarily of type I collagen fibrils (~90% by weight) produced by fully differentiated osteoblasts, secretion of non-collagenous proteins (primarily OPN) both early (by preosteoblasts) and late (by bone-lining cells) during osteoblast differentiation results in the formation of a collagen-deficient cement line and a lamina limitans, respectively. This unique architectural design allows for intimate apposition, and potentially bonding, of newer bone to the older bone in the case of a cement line, and in the case of the surface-located lamina limitans, provides a proteinaceous substratum 'primed' for future cell adhesion and signaling events. Collectively, these and other elements, together with minerals, constitute the extracellular matrix of bone.

of casein kinase II. Whereas the phosphate groups found within this class of proteins are generally thought to sequester calcium ions and to participate in influencing crystal nucleation and growth, experimental removal of the phosphates in vitro does not affect the ability of BSP to promote crystal formation, thus emphasizing the putative importance of the acidic polyGlu stretch in BSP for crystal nucleating activity (Hunter & Goldberg, 1994). BSP occurs in a sulfated form, with sulfation occurring on Tyr residues. However, the significance of the sulfation, which flanks the RGD sequence and can bind calcium ions, is not known.

The human BSP gene is found on chromosome 4 (in mouse, on chromosome 5), at a locus together with a number of other genes for bone and tooth ECM proteins, and consists of seven exons and six introns. The BSP gene proximal promoter sequence contains a highly conserved 'BSP box', within which inverted TATA and CCAAT sequences, consensus sites for binding AP-1, cAMP (CRE), NF$_\kappa$B, Osf2/Cbfa1 (OSE2) and the homeobox genes *ftz* and *en* (Ganss et al., 1999). Expression of BSP is induced by glucocorticoids and transforming growth factor-β1 (TGF-β1), and suppressed by vitamin D metabolites and phorbol esters.

BSP has a tissue distribution that is generally restricted to bones and teeth. In these tissues, BSP is secreted by the resident matrix-forming cells, and it accumulates in the ECM where mineralization is occurring – a distribution presumably reflecting its participation in the calcification process and its binding to mineral. Its appearance in bone tissue either just prior to, or coincident with, the first indications of mineral deposition, and its ultrastructural co-localization with the initial crystals observed in the osteoid of forming bone (Chen et al., 1994), support the role of BSP in the regulation (possibly nucleation) of calcification. In vitro studies of crystal nucleation and growth in the presence of BSP also support this concept (Hunter and Goldberg, 1994). While a mineral-regulating role may be the major activity of BSP, the presence of the conserved RGD motif suggests that this protein might also be involved in cell adhesion and signaling in bone, and both osteoblast-like cells and osteoclasts have been shown to adhere to BSP in vitro.

Osteopontin

Osteopontin (OPN), like BSP, is a phosphorylated, sialic acid-rich, acidic glycoprotein found not only in the ECM of bones and teeth (Butler et al., 1996), but as a soluble protein in a variety of other soft tissues and biological fluids, most notably urine and milk. It is also typically found at sites of pathologic calcification including kidney stones, atherosclerotic plaques and breast cancer microcalcifications. OPN binds calcium at high capacity ($\sim$50 Ca^{2+}) but with low affinity (mM)(Chen et al., 1992). In mammals, OPN is a single-chain protein of 264–301 amino acids which shows approximately 40% identity across species. The protein is rich in the amino acids Asp, Glu and Ser (the most highly conserved), and contains an acidic 'polyAsp' (9–10 amino acids) region in the amino-terminal half of the molecule that binds to mineral. An Arg–Gly–Asp (RGD) integrin-binding motif is present roughly halfway along the molecule near a thrombin cleavage site. Beyond the thrombin cleavage site, there is little conservation of primary sequence except for the immediate carboxy-terminus. A hydrophobic leader sequence of 16 amino acids is well conserved among species. Secondary structure predictions identify numerous regions of putative α-helix and β-sheet, although the paucity of hydrophobic amino acids indicates an open flexible structure similar to BSP. Posttranslational modifications include extensive phosphorylation at serines and a threonine having consensus sequences for casein kinase II activity, with phosphorylation varying significantly among tissue sources of the protein (Sorensen et al., 1995). O-linked glycosylation of OPN is extensive, and N-linked glycosylation may also occur. OPN is also a substrate for the cross-linking activity of transglutaminases, including factor XIIIa, which can covalently link OPN to other NCPs, and to itself, producing high molecular-weight aggregates of OPN which can be extracted from bone (Prince et al., 1991).

OPN is encoded by a single-copy gene that maps in humans to chromosome 4 (chromosome 5 in the mouse). Of note, the mouse OPN gene maps to the ric^r locus, suggesting a possible involvement in resistance to infection associated with rickettsial immunity and other microbial infections (Patarca et al., 1993). The OPN gene consists of seven exons, although variant forms of OPN may arise from differential RNA splicing. Upstream regulatory sequence in the promoter region includes, among others, a TATA, an inverted CCAAT, and a GC box, AP (PEA/TPA) and Osf2/Cbfa1 (OSE2) binding sites, a vitamin D response element (VDRE) and a Ras activation element (RAE). Expression of OPN is positively regulated at the transcriptional level by TGF-β, vitamin D_3, PDGF, EGF, BMPs and retinoic acid, and negatively regulated by PTH.

Based on the widespread distribution of OPN in various hard (Butler et al., 1996; McKee & Nanci, 1996) and soft tissues (Brown et al., 1992), and its diverse structural motifs, OPN most likely serves as a multifunctional protein in different tissues. In both normal and pathological calcified tissues, OPN typically is intimately associated with the mineral phase. In bone, this consists of small calcification foci in the osteoid, with the highest levels appearing at the so-called 'mineralization front' where calcification becomes pervasive throughout the ECM. Moreover, OPN is typically concentrated in structures termed laminae limitantes – sites where calcification has been temporarily or permanently terminated (McKee & Nanci, 1996). Cement lines deep within the bone – representing interfacial sites where bone formation has occurred following resorptive activity by osteoclasts (i.e., bone remodeling) – also show a substantial accumulation of OPN, possibly reflecting regulation of early calcification events during the deposition of nascent bone subsequent to bone resorption (the reversal phase) (McKee & Nanci, 1995). Extensive in vitro data indicate that bone OPN (and the urinary form) is an extremely potent inhibitor of calcification, and that the phosphate and carboxylate side chains are important in this inhibition activity (Hunter et al., 1994). Following nucleation of mineral by one or more other factors, OPN may serve to inhibit crystal growth over time such that this process occurs in a precisely controlled manner. Such fine control over bone calcification is to be expected considering the vital importance of the skeleton, the complexity of the ECM that must eventually become impregnated with mineral, and the fact that the most abundant bone cells – the osteocytes – are entombed within calcified bone and must maintain viable 'living' quarters by halting the advance of mineral that might otherwise obliterate their lacunae. Equally important is the observation that OPN is concentrated at practically all cell–matrix interfaces in bone (McKee & Nanci, 1996), and it is expected that in these circumstances, integrin binding to the RGD sequence of mineral-bound OPN may be important in cell adhesion and signaling, events that have been demonstrated in vitro. Importantly, soluble OPN has also been shown to act as a cytokine, thereby modulating a wide variety of activities pertaining to the various bone cell lineages (Gerstenfeld, 1999).

Osteonectin/SPARC

One of the first acidic NCPs to be isolated from bone using dissociative extraction techniques and decalcification, osteonectin was obtained primarily from the mineral-binding fraction of bone, comprising roughly 10–15% of the NCPs of bone from large mammals (Termine et al., 1981). However, only low levels of osteo-nectin are found in the bone of rodents. Osteonectin is a highly conserved protein (~90%) that is found in many soft tissues as well (Lane & Sage, 1994), and it is also known to bind to collagen and thrombospondin 1. Osteonectin is transcribed from a single gene on human chromosome 5 (mouse chromosome 11), having 10 exons coding for a mature protein of approximately 300 amino acid residues and a 17-residue signal peptide found in exon 2. The amino-terminal domain I of the protein is rich in glutamic and aspartic acid and binds calcium to low affinity sites such that a conformational transition to α-helix occurs. Domain II is rich in cysteines that participate in disulfide bonds. Domain III contains an α-helical region susceptible to cleavage by trypsin-like proteases, and, an EF-hand-type calcium-binding site. Domain IV contains a high-affinity, EF-hand calcium-binding site. The protein also contains significant β-pleated sheet structure. Posttranslational modifications of osteonectin include approximately 4–5% glycosylation (mostly sialic acid and some fucose) with two potential N-glycosylation sites.

The promoter region of osteonectin contains a purine-rich region with GA repeats (for binding GGA protein) and multiple CCTG repeats. Also included are multiple binding sites for SP1, AP1, cAMP(CRE), growth hormone (GHE), heat shock proteins (HSE) and metal ions (MRE). Factors influencing the expression of osteonectin in bone are not well understood. Although biosynthesis of osteonectin has been studied in a number of in vitro systems, responses to different factors have been variable and often modest in extent depending on the animal species and the culture conditions. In cultured human bone cells, relatively little change in expression is seen after most treatments.

Osteonectin is either transiently or constitutively expressed in a number of tissues during development, maturation and repair (Reed & Sage, 1996), and it is expressed by many cell types in vitro – possibly indicating deregulation by culture conditions and thus its designation as a culture-shock protein. As a mineral-binding protein, osteonectin accumulates in the calcified ECM of bone and may play some as yet undetermined role in this process. While the role of this protein in hard tissues is not yet clear, based on its domain structure and observed activities in vitro, it is likely that it functions in modulating various cell-matrix interactions during osteogenesis.

Bone acidic glycoprotein-75

Bone acidic glycoprotein-75 (BAG-75) is an acidic, $\sim$75 kDa glycoprotein of rat bone ECM (Gorski et al., 1990) that has not yet been cloned. While similar in many ways to other ECM proteins in the various hard tissues, a partial cDNA sequence for BAG-75 indicates that certain homologous regions are non-identical and unique. Interestingly, whereas most other NCPs found in bone matrix are also found in tooth cementum, a hard tissue very similar to bone, BAG-75 immuno-reactivity is absent from cementum, and appears to be primarily abundant in woven bone (compared to mature, lamellar bone). BAG-75 contains elevated levels of sialic acid ($\sim$8% by weight) and a substantial number of phosphate groups ($\sim$44 residues/mole). Like osteopontin and bone sialoprotein, BAG-75 binds calcium electrostatically with high capacity, but low affinity, and contains a polyacidic amino acid stretch consisting of both Glu and Asp.

Several observations indicate that BAG-75 self-associates to form multimeric complexes in vitro and in vivo (Gorski et al., 1997). In vitro, macromolecular assemblies of BAG-75 form spherical meshworks of 10 nm microfibrils that have the capacity to sequester large amounts of phosphate ions. Accordingly, it has been proposed that this feature may be used to compartmentalize mineral ions within the ECM in vivo by acting as an ion barrier, restricting the local diffusion of phosphate ions and thus influencing mineralization. In another direct comparison of acidic phosphoproteins, BAG-75 was found to be a relatively potent inhibitor of bone resorption by rat and chicken osteoclasts in vitro (Sato et al., 1992), and that the recognition of the substratum surface by osteoclasts might require degradation of BAG-75-containing complexes at the surface of, and within, the bone.

Osteocalcin

Osteocalcin (also known as bone Gla protein; BGP) is a member of a family of proteins that includes the blood coagulation factors and which are distinguished by their ability to be posttranslationally modified by vitamin K-dependent enzymes (Ducy & Karsenty, 1996). The action of vitamin K-dependent γ-carboxylase on conserved stretches of sequence creates two Gla residues from glutamic acid (three in mouse osteocalcin) that are required for the protein to be functional and to bind calcium. Osteocalcin production is essentially specific to cells of bone and teeth, and by weight, comprises roughly 15% of the NCPs found in bone. Its plasma concentration has become an important marker for a variety of metabolic bone diseases where its presence in serum generally correlates with the rate of bone turnover (Calvo et al., 1996). The mature, intact osteocalcin molecule is relatively small (6 kDa), having 49 amino acids, and it is neither phosphorylated nor glycosylated, although it does have a single disulfide bond. It is susceptible to tryptic proteolysis at two Arg–Arg sites within its primary structure. The human gene is on chromosome 1 (in mouse, on chromosome 3), having four exons encoding 125 amino acids (prepro-osteocalcin) that includes a signal peptide of 26 residues. The pro-osteocalcin is γ-carboxylated, and then processed to the 6 kDa mature form. Interestingly, in the mouse and rat, three genes with nearly identical coding sequences have been identified, two of which are expressed only in bone and tooth (OG1 and OG2), with the third gene of the cluster, osteocalcin-related gene (ORG), expressed at 100-fold lower levels in the kidney (Desbois et al., 1994).

The promoter region of all osteocalcin genes has a TATA box, but only some species have a CCAAT box (Lian et al., 1998). A group of numerous and overlapping regulatory elements has been referred to as the 'osteocalcin box', a region containing binding sites for AP1, AP2, NF1, viral core enhancer (VCE), vitamin D receptor (VDRE), vitamin A (VA), cAMP (CRE), glucocorticoids (GRE), TNF-α (TNFRE), and MSX (a homeobox gene). The osteocalcin promoter also contains several copies of an osteoblast-specific, *cis*-acting element termed OSE2. OSE2 is the binding site of the only transcriptional activator of osteoblast differentiation identified to date and termed Osf2/Cbfa1 (Ducy et al., 1997). The mouse osteocalcin promoter contains another osteoblast *cis*-acting element named OSE1, and the human and rat osteocalcin promoter contains a vitamin D responsive element that upregulates osteocalcin synthesis, but which is altered and non-functional in the mouse gene.

Immunolocalization studies of osteocalcin indicate that the majority of this protein co-localizes with the mineralized compartments of the bone matrix. Based on secondary structure predictions, on data from circular dichroism, and on knowledge of the γ-carboxylation sites within the protein, it was proposed that osteocalcin contained two antiparallel α-helical domains – one rich in acidic amino acids, and the other containing the Gla residues. Interestingly, calculation of the spacing between Gla residues in the 'Gla helix' was similar to the interatomic spacing of calcium ions in the apatite lattice, and it was suggested that this domain could bind to crystal surfaces and regulate their growth (Hauschka & Wians, 1989). Indeed, in vitro assays for crystal growth have shown that osteocalcin functions as an inhibitor of mineralization. More definitive genetic studies in vivo have recently been performed using transgenic, 'knockout' mice where the osteocalcin genes (OG1 and OG2) have been deleted (Ducy et al., 1996). While the bone mineral in these animals does indeed show some differences from control wild-type mice, the most pronounced phenotypic observation is an increase in bone mass resulting from increased bone formation rates by osteoblasts. Thus, osteocalcin appears to generally function as a regulator of bone formation.

Fibronectin

Fibronectin is one of the most abundant ECM proteins found in connective tissues (Mosher, 1993). It is also a major circulating protein in serum, and thus a significant proportion of this protein extracted from bone could have an extraskeletal origin. Relatively little is known regarding the skeletal form of fibronectin. Virtually all connective tissue cells produce fibronectin, where it is found at the cell surface or is released into the ECM. In bone, it appears to be present in both cellular and ECM compartments, and is most likely involved in specific cell–matrix interactions mediated by integrin ($\alpha_4\beta_1$) binding that occur prior to matrix calcification. Its role in mineralized matrix is less evident, where it is somewhat homogeneously distributed throughout the bone, with no obvious preferential accumulation at specific sites indicative of any particular function. The gene encoding fibronectin is located on human chromosome 7 and is very complex, possessing up to 50 exons that produce a large, dimeric protein composed of two highly homologous subunits joined by disulfide bonds (Potts & Campbell, 1996). Alternative splicing of the mRNA is prevalent and produces multiple variants depending on the tissue, stage of development and species. Each of the subunits has multiple, well-characterized domains with specific functions. The gene and protein domain structure of fibronectin have been extensively studied, and the reader is directed toward several thorough reviews on this molecule (Potts & Campbell, 1994).

Small proteoglycans

Biglycan (BGN) and decorin (DCN) are widely distributed and relatively small proteoglycans found in bone (Bianco et al., 1990). They consist of a protein core and one (DCN) or two (BGN) glycosaminoglycan (GAG) side chains. In soft connective tissues, the GAGs are dermatan sulfate, whereas in bone they are chondroitin-4-sulfate. A third, small chondroitin sulfate-containing proteoglycan, CS-PG-III, which binds to the mineral phase of bone (Nagata et al., 1991), has been isolated from porcine bone, but its core protein is less well characterized to date. Although the core proteins of DCN and BGN are distinct entities, they nevertheless show strong structural homology, with ~55% amino acid identity, with the rest being conservative replacements – a feature indicative of gene duplication. The genes are found on human chromosomes X (BGN)(Geerkens et al., 1995) and 12 (DCN; mouse chromosome 10)(Vetter et al., 1993) and produce proteins each having four readily identifiable domains. The N-terminal domain I contains the GAG binding sites to Ser. Domain II contains 4 cysteines that form disulfide bonds. Domain III contains 10 repeats of similar leucine-rich motifs of 14 amino acids that might be involved in binding to other proteins, and N-linked glycosylation sites. Domain IV has relatively greater sequence divergence, but contains two cysteines for disulfide bonds.

In bone, these PGs may account for up to 10% of the NCPs, but decrease with age of the bone. BGN and DCN are mostly present in uncalcified portions of bone tissue. Whereas DCN intimately associates with ('decorates') the surface of collagen fibrils in the ECM and regulates fibril formation, stability and growth, BGN appears to be preferentially associated with several cell types. BGN is also a prominent component of articular cartilage, and binds to type V collagen – a major collagen in blood vessels. Given the domain structures of these two PGs, it is likely that each does not act alone, but binds to other matrix components to exert their function (Roughley & Lee, 1994). For example, the core protein of DCN binds collagen, fibronectin and TGF-β.

Another small, keratan sulfate-containing proteoglycan expressed by osteoblasts, osteoadherin, has recently been isolated from bone and cloned (Sommarin et al., 1998). Dominant features of the primary structure are the presence of 11 leucine-rich repeats, multiple cysteines for disulfide bonding, six potential sites for N-linked glycosylation, and four putative tyrosine sulfating sites. A characteristic distinguishing property of osteoadherin is a large, acidic C-terminal domain that is not found in other members of the leucine-rich repeat family of proteins and which most likely binds to bone mineral. Despite not having a cell-binding RGD motif, osteoadherin does bind to primary osteoblasts in culture – a binding that can be inhibited by RGD (but not RGE) peptides, and appears to involve the $\alpha_v\beta_3$ integrin receptor possibly utilizing an RID mimic of the classical RGD binding site.

Other proteins found in bone matrix

While the major structural elements that collectively define the ECM of bone have been briefly described above, there exist many additional, extracellular organic constituents too numerous to expound upon here in any great detail. To emphasize this, a partial list of organic molecules is given below – some of which are more completely described in excellent reviews that are available in the literature on each class of molecules, or on the individual molecules themselves (Boskey, 1996; Gehron Robey, 1996; Heinegård et al., 1989; Young et al., 1993). As a word of caution, because many published biochemical studies used whole, intact long bones without a dissection procedure to first separate the cartilaginous component from the true bone matrix, in some cases it is not altogether clear whether a particular molecule is a bona fide constituent of the bone matrix itself, or whether in fact it derives from the ECM of cartilage.

Considering the dimensions and mass of the axial and appendicular vertebrate skeleton, and given its extensive ramifications and associations with virtually every tissue and organ system of the body, and particularly the vascular system, site-specific variation in matrix composition is not surprising. In addition to the local cellular production of secreted organic constituents, bone has long been known to act as a repository for circulating plasma proteins and for heavy-metal ions (e.g., lead) and other substances derived from the diet (e.g., fluoride) or after inadvertent ingestion of toxic substances (Bronner, 1996; Kleerekoper, 1996).

Other non-collagenous, organic molecules reported to exist in the ECM of bone and not described here include: matrix metalloproteinases, cysteine proteinases, serine proteinases, proteinase inhibitors, plasminogen activator, plasminogen activator inhibitor, matrix phosphoprotein kinases, growth factors, TGF, IGFs, FGFs, PDGFs, CSFs, TNF, interleukins, bone morphogenetic proteins, growth factor binding proteins, tetranectin, thrombospondins, fibromodulin, alkaline phosphatase, osteoglycin, protein S, proteolipids, lipids, albumin, α_2HS-glycoprotein (fetuin), immunoglobulin, transferrin, hemoglobin, α_1-antitrypsin, Apo A1 lipoprotein, vitronectin, lysyl oxidase, TRAMP and propeptides of type I and V collagens.

REFERENCES

Bianco, P., Fisher, L. W., Young, M. F., Termine, J. D., & Gehron Robey, P. (1990). Expression and localization of the two small proteoglycans biglycan and decorin in developing human skeletal and non-skeletal tissues. *J. Histochem. Cytochem.*, **38**, 1549–63.

Boskey, A. L. (1996). Matrix proteins and mineralization: an overview. *Connect. Tissue Res.*, **34–5**, 411–17.

Bronner, F. (1996). Metals in bone: Aluminum, boron, cadmium, chromium, lead, silicon, and strontium. In *Principles of Bone Biology*, ed. J. P. Bilezikian, L. G. Raisz, & G. A. Rodan, pp. 295–303. San Diego, CA: Academic Press.

Brown, L. F., Berse, B., Van De Water, L., Papadopoulos-Sergiou, A., Perruzzi, C. A., Manseau, E.

J., Dvorak, H. F., & Senger, D. R. (1992). Expression and distribution of osteopontin in human tissues: widespread association with luminal epithelial surfaces. *Mol. Biol. Cell*, **3**, 1169–80.

Butler, W. T., Ridall, A. L., & McKee, M. D. (1996). Osteopontin. In *Principles of Bone Biology*, ed. J. & P. Bilezikian, L. G. Raisz, & G. A. Rodan, pp. 167–81. San Diego, CA: Academic Press.

Byers, P. H. (1992). Osteogenesis imperfecta. In *Connective Tissue and its Heritable Disorders: Molecular, Genetic and Medical Aspects*, ed. P. P. Royce, & B. Steinman, pp. 317–50. New York, NY: Wiley-Liss.

Calvo, M. S., Eyre D. R., & Gundberg C. M. (1996). Molecular basis and clinical application of biological markers of bone turnover. *Endocr. Rev.*, **17**, 333–68.

Chen, J., McKee, M. D., Nanci, A., & Sodek, J. (1994). Bone sialoprotein mRNA expression and ultrastructural localization in fetal porcine calvarial bone: comparisons with osteopontin. *Histochem. J.*, **26**, 67–78.

Chen, Y., Bal, B. S., & Gorski, J. P. (1992). Calcium and collagen binding properties of osteopontin, bone sialoprotein, and bone acidic glycoprotein-75 from bone. *J. Biol. Chem.*, **267**, 24871–8.

Chenu, C., Ibaraki, K., Robey, P. G., Delmas, P. D., & Young, M. F. (1994). Cloning and sequence analysis of bovine bone sialoprotein cDNA: conservation of acidic domains, tyrosine sulfation consensus repeats, and RGD cell attachment domain. *J. Bone Miner. Res.*, **9**, 417–21.

Delmas, P. D., Schlemmer, A., Gineyts, E., Riis, B., & Christiansen, C. (1991). Urinary excretion of pyrodinoline crosslinks correlates with bone turnover measured on iliac crest biopsy in patients with vertebral therapy. *J. Bone Miner. Res.*, **6**, 639–44.

Desbois, C., Hogue, D. A., & Karsenty, G. (1994). The mouse osteocalcin gene cluster contains three genes with two separate spatial and temporal patterns of expression. *J. Biol. Chem.*, **269**, 1183–90.

Ducy, P. & Karsenty, G. (1996). Skeletal Gla proteins: gene structure, regulation of expression and function. In *Principles of Bone Biology*, ed. J. P. Bilezikian, L. G. Raisz, & G. A. Rodan, pp. 183–95. San Diego, CA: Academic Press.

Ducy, P., Desbois, C., Boyce, B., Pinero, G., Story, B., Dunstan, C., Smith, E., Bonadio, J., Goldstein, S., Gundberg, C., Bradley, A., & Karsenty, G. (1996). Increased bone formation in osteocalcin-deficient mice. *Nature*, **382**, 448–52.

Ducy, P., Zhang, R., Geoffroy, V., Ridall, A. L., & Karsenty, G. (1997). Osf2/Cbfa1: a transcriptional activator of osteoblast differentiation. *Cell*, **89**, 747–54.

Eyre, D. R. (1996). Biochemical markers of bone turnover. In *Primer on the Metabolic Bone Diseases and Disorders of Mineral Metabolism*, ed. M. J . Favus, pp. 114–19. Philadelphia, PA: Lippincott-Raven.

Ganss, B., Kim, R. H., & Sodek, J. (1999). Bone sialoprotein. *Crit. Rev. Oral Biol. Med.*, **10**, 79–98.

Geerkens, C., Vetter U., Just, W., Fedarko, N. S., Fisher, L. W., Young, M. F., Termine, J. D., Robey, P. G., Wohrle, D., & Vogel W. (1995). The X-chromosomal human biglycan gene BGN is subject to X inactivation but is transcribed like an X–Y homologous gene. *Hum. Genet.*, **96**, 44–52.

Gehron Robey, P. (1996). Bone matrix proteoglycans and glycoproteins. In *Principles of Bone Biology*, ed. J. P. Bilezikian, L. G. Raisz, & G. A. Rodan, pp. 155–65. San Diego, CA: Academic Press.

Gerstenfeld, L. C. (1999). Osteopontin in skeletal tissue homeostasis: an emerging picture of the autocrine/paracrine functions of the extracellular matrix. *J. Bone Miner. Res.*, **14**, 850–5.

Gorski, J. P. (1992). Acidic phosphoproteins from bone matrix: a structural rationalization of their role in biomineralization. *Calcif. Tissue Int.*, **50**, 391–6.

Gorski, J. P., Griffin, D., Dudley, G., Stanford, C., Thomas, R., Huang, C., Lai, E., Karr, B., & Solursh, M. (1990). Bone acidic glycoprotein-75 is a major synthetic product of osteoblastic cells and localized as 75- and/or 50-kDa forms in mineralized phases of bone and growth plate and in serum. *J. Biol. Chem.*, **265**, 14956–63.

Gorski, J. P., Kramer, E. A., Chen, Y., Ryan, S., Fullenkamp, C., Delviscio, J., Jensen, K., & McKee, M. D. (1997). Bone acidic glycoprotein-75 self-associates to form macromolecular complexes in vitro and in vivo with the potential to sequester phosphate ions. *J. Cell. Biochem.*, **64**, 547–64.

Hauschka, P. V. & Wians, F. H. (1989). Osteocalcin-hydroxyapatite interaction in the extracellular organic matrix of bone. *Anat. Rec.*, **225**, 180–8.

Heinegård, D., Hultenby, K., Oldberg, Å., Reinholt, F., & Wendel, M. (1989). Macromolecules in bone matrix. *Connect. Tissue Res.*, **21**, 3–14.

Hunter, G. K. (1996). Interfacial aspects of biomineralization. *Curr. Opin. Solid State Mater. Science*, **1**, 430–5.

Hunter, G. K. & Goldberg, H. A. (1994). Modulation of crystal formation by bone phosphoproteins: role of glutamic acid-rich sequences in the nucleation of hydroxyapatite by bone sialoprotein. *Biochem. J.*, **302**, 175–9.

Hunter, G. K., Kyle, C. L., & Goldberg, H. A. (1994). Modulation of crystal formation by bone phosphoproteins: Structural specificity of the osteopontin-mediated inhibition of hydroxyapatite formation. *Biochem. J.*, **300**, 723–8.

Kielty, C. M., Hopkinson, I., & Grant, M. E. (1992). The collagen family: structure, assembly, and organization in the ECM. In *Connective Tissue and its Heritable Disorders: Molecular, Genetic and Medical Aspects*, ed. P. P. Royce, & B. Steinman, pp. 103–47. New York, NY: Wiley-Liss.

Kleerekoper, M. (1996). Fluoride and the skeleton. In *Principles of Bone Biology*, ed. J. P. Bilezikian, L. G. Raisz, & G. A. Rodan, pp. 1053–62. San Diego, CA: Academic Press.

Lane, T. F. & Sage, E. H. (1994). The biology of SPARC, a protein that modulates cell–matrix interactions. *FASEB J.*, **8**, 163–73.

Lian, J. B., Stein, G. S., Stein, J. L., & van Wijnen, A. J. (1998). Osteocalcin gene promoter: unlocking the secrets for regulation of osteoblast growth and differentiation. *J. Cell Biochem.*, Suppl. **30–31**, 62–72.

McKee, M. D. and Nanci, A. (1995). Osteopontin and the bone remodeling sequence: colloidal-gold immunocytochemistry of an interfacial extracellular matrix protein. *Ann. NY Acad. Sci.*, **760**, 177–89.

McKee, M. D. & Nanci, A. (1996). Osteopontin at mineralized tissue interfaces in bone, teeth and osseointegrated implants: ultrastructural distribution and implications for mineralized tissue formation, turnover and repair. *Microsc. Res. Tech.*, **33**, 141–64.

Mosher, D. F. (1993). Assembly of fibronectin into extracellular matrix. *Curr. Opin. Struct. Biol.*, **3**, 214–22.

Nagata, T., Goldberg, H. A., Zhang, Q., Domenicucci, C., & Sodek, J. (1991). Biosynthesis of bone proteins by fetal porcine calvariae in vitro. Rapid association of sulfated sialoproteins (secreted phosphoprotein-1 and bone sialoprotein) and chondroitin sulfate proteoglycan (CS-PGIII) with bone mineral. *Matrix*, 11, 86–100.

Parfitt, A. M., Simon, L. S., Villanueva, A. R., & Krane, S. M. (1987). Procollagen type I carboxy-terminal extension peptide in serum as a marker of collagen biosynthesis in bone. Correlation with iliac bone formation rates and comparison with total alkaline phosphatase. *J. Bone Miner. Res.*, 2, 427–36.

Patarca, R., Saavedra, R. A., & Cantor, H. (1993). Molecular and cellular basis of genetic resistance to bacterial infection: the role of the early T-lymphocyte activation- 1/osteopontin gene. *Crit. Rev. Immunol.*, 13, 225–46.

Potts, J. R. & Campbell, I. D. (1994). Fibronectin structure and assembly. *Curr. Opin. Cell Biol.*, 6, 648–55.

Potts, J. R. & Campbell, I. D. (1996). Structure and function of fibronectin modules. *Matrix Biol.*, 15, 313–20.

Prince, C. W., Dickie, D., & Krumdieck, C. L. (1991). Osteopontin, a substrate for transglutaminase and factor XIII activity. *Biochem. Biophys. Res. Commun.*, 177, 1205–10.

Reed, M. J. & Sage, E. H. (1996). SPARC and the extracellular matrix: implications for cancer and wound repair. *Curr. Top. Microbiol. Immunol.*, 213, 81–94.

Roughley, P. J. & Lee, E. R. (1994). Cartilage proteoglycans: structure and potential functions. *Microsc. Res. Tech.*, 28, 385–97.

Sato, M., Grasser, W., Harms, S., Fullenkamp, C., & Gorski, J. P. (1992). Bone acidic glycoprotein-75 inhibits resorption activity of isolated rat and chicken osteoclasts. *FASEB J.*, 6, 2966–76.

Schinke, T., McKee, M. D., & Karsenty, G. (1999). Extracellular matrix calcification: where is the action? *Nature Genet.*, 21, 150–1.

Sommarin, Y., Wendel, M., Shen, Z., Hellman, U., & Heinegard, D. (1998). Osteoadherin, a cell-binding keratan sulfate proteoglycan in bone, belongs to the family of leucine-rich repeat proteins of the extracellular matrix. *J. Biol. Chem.*, 273, 16723–9.

Sorensen, E. S., Hojrup, P., & Petersen, T. E. (1995). Posttranslational modifications of bovine osteopontin: Identification of twenty-eight phosphorylation and three O-glycosylation sites. *Protein Sci.*, 4, 2040–9.

Termine, J. D., Belcourt, A. B., Conn, K. M., & Kleinman, H. K. (1981). Mineral and collagen-binding proteins of fetal calf bone. *J. Biol. Chem.*, 256, 10403–8.

Vetter, U., Vogel, W., Just, W., Young, M. F., & Fisher, L. W. (1993). Human decorin gene: intron-exon junctions and chromosomal localization. *Genomics*, 15, 161–8.

Vuorio, E. & de Crombrugghe, B. (1990). The family of collagen genes. *Ann. Rev. Biochem.*, 59, 837–72.

Weiner, S. & Traub, W. (1986). Organization of hydroxyapatite crystals within collagen fibrils. *FEBS Lett.*, 206, 262–6.

Young, M. F., Ibaraki, K., Kerr, J. M., & Heegard, A-M. (1993). Molecular and cellular biology of the major non-collagenous proteins in bone. In *Cellular and Molecular Biology of Bone*, ed. M. Noda, pp. 191–234. San Diego, CA: Academic Press.

5

Local regulators of bone turnover

Lawrence J. Fraher and Patricia H. Watson

Introduction

To attempt to understand a disease such as osteoporosis, we must come to a complete elucidation of the nature or pathology of the disorder, the cellular mechanisms whereby the pathology develops and, lastly, what caused the cellular machinery to go awry in the first place (e.g., control by genes, hormones, growth factors, vitamins, minerals, etc.). While many investigators may still disagree on a unified definition of osteoporosis which fully describes its pathology, for a number of years now we have fairly well understood the nature of the disease, and to describe the gross cellular mechanisms which do go awry. That is to say that we can all agree that the end result of undermineralized bone is due to a chronic imbalance of skeletal turnover whereby more mineral is removed than is incorporated into the matrix. It is only recently, however, that we have been able to tackle why the cellular machinery goes wrong, and that has resulted from a clearer understanding of the role(s) of growth factors and cytokines in the skeletal microenvironment. Both bone itself and the bone marrow compartment produce, store, and are influenced by a plethora of cytokines, stem factors and growth factors. However, in this brief chapter we will concentrate on those factors which are known to be both produced and stored within the matrix of bone itself; these are the insulin-like growth factors (IGFs), fibroblast growth factors (FGFs), transforming growth factor-β (TGF-β), and the bone morphogenic proteins (BMPs). These factors appear to have clear functions in regulation of bone modeling/remodeling, and their actions on bone formation have been extensively studied both in vitro and in vivo (Bikfalfi et al., 1997; Canalis et al., 1993; Mohan & Baylink, 1991; Mundy, 1993; Linkhart et al., 1996). A major endocrine/paracrine growth factor in bone, namely parathyroid hormone related peptide (PTHrP) is the subject of another chapter within this volume.

Insulin-like growth factors

The insulin-like growth factor regulatory system comprises; (i) two growth factors (IGF-I and IGF-II); (ii) two receptors, the type I recognizing IGF-I, IGF-II and insulin and the type II receptor being a high affinity receptor for IGF-II preferentially; (iii) six binding proteins which can act as carrier proteins (circulating factors), delivery systems to the receptors (modulators of biological activity) and shields from proteolytic enzymes (enhancing bioavailability); and (iv) IGF binding protein specific proteases (which release free IGFs for target cell association (Hodsman et al., 1999)). Many studies using a variety of model systems have clearly shown that both IGF-I and IGF-II stimulate osteoblastic cell proliferation and differentiated functions such as the production of type I collagen (Dequeker et al., 1993; Johansson & Rosen, 1998; Mohan et al., 1995; Rosen et al., 1994a). Testing the reverse situation, where IGF activities are inhibited by utilizing either neutralizing antibodies, receptor antibodies or exogenous IGF binding proteins, osteoblast proliferation and collagen synthesis are inhibited (Mohan et al., 1995).

The expression of IGF is high in cells of developing periosteum and growth plate, healing fracture callus and developing ectopic bone (Andrew et al., 1993; Lazowski et al., 1994; Prisell et al., 1993). Shown in Fig. 5.1 is the proximal end of the tibia of a 3-month-old female rat visualized by *in situ* hybridization for the mRNA of IGF-I. In this image the intensity of the signal is related to areas of active growth on both the endosteal and periosteal bone surfaces. IGFs are also important in mediating the effects of systemic hormones on bone formation such as the inhibitory effects of glucocorticoids (Chevally et al., 1996), the stimulatory effect of growth hormone (Ernst & Rodan, 1990) and the potent anabolic effects of parathyroid hormone (Watson et al., 1995).

IGF-I has also been reported to be detectable in osteoclasts (Lazowski et al., 1994) and in in vitro experiments, IGF-I can both increase the formation of mature osteoclasts from marrow stem cell precursors (Mochizuki et al., 1992) and prolong the survival of osteoclasts in mixed rabbit osteoclast and stromal cell cultures (Takada et al., 1994). These studies, taken together, might suggest that the IGFs may not only promote bone formation by the proliferation and function of osteoblasts, but may also stimulate cells of the osteoclastic lineage and promote bone resorption.

The IGFs are not only produced and act on bone cells in a paracrine/autocrine fashion, but also become incorporated into the collagen matrix during the formation phase of bone turnover. In fact IGF-I and IGF-II are the most abundant growth factors stored in bone collagen and the activity associated with IGF-II was once termed 'skeletal growth factor' (Mohan et al., 1988). Baylink et al. have proposed

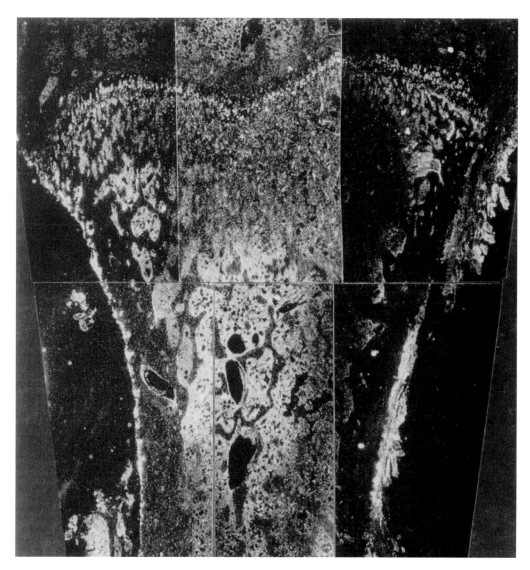

Fig. 5.1   Proximal end of the female rat tibia (at 12 weeks of age) visualized by *in situ* hybridization for the IGF-I messenger RNA.

that this pool of IGFs incorporated in the matrix acts as a reservoir of growth factor which will be released from bone during the osteoclastic resorptive phase of bone turnover and will act to both recruit and stimulate a new population of osteoblasts. This mechanism suggests that we can have a 'bank account' of growth factors which either determine or strongly influence the restoration of the bone that was removed by resorption, thus completing the bone remodeling cycle (Linkhart et al., 1996). From this reasoning it is then but a short leap to suggest that, if our initial 'deposit' into the account is small, or that we get into a situation of deficit accounting, we will be doomed to ultimate bone mineral loss.

Fibroblast growth factors

The fibroblast growth factors (FGFs) are a large family ($\geq$17 members at the present time) of heparin-binding polypeptides that are involved in the promotion of proliferation, migration, differentiation and survival of a wide variety of cell types (Burgess & Maciag, 1989). The prototypic members of this family, namely acidic fibroblast growth factor (aFGF) and basic fibroblast growth factor (bFGF) are now referred to as FGF-1 and FGF-2, respectively. Prior to specific receptor binding, both molecules associate with low affinity heparan sulphate proteogly-cans, which are presumed to facilitate binding to the high affinity target cell surface receptor. Bound receptors then dimerize which leads to intrinsic activation of tyro-sine phosphorylation and activation of kinase cascades which ultimately trigger altered gene expression (Klagsbrun & Baird, 1991). A second activation mechanism has also been proposed whereby FGF-2 can be directly translocated to the nucleus where it activates gene transcription (Baldin et al., 1990).

FGF-2 has been described as a potent agent promoting the development of mes-oderm during embryogenesis (Kimelman & Kirschner, 1987) and mRNAs for the FGF receptors are highly expressed in developing bones (Wanaka et al., 1991; Peters et al., 1993). Cultured bovine calvarial osteoblasts were the first bone cells shown to produce, secrete and store FGF-2 in bone matrix (Globus et al., 1989). FGF-2 appears to act on cultured bone cells in a different way from the IGFs in as much that, while FGF-2 promotes proliferation of the cells, it also inhibits alkaline phos-phatase activity and reduces the expression of the collagen type I and osteocalcin genes (Debiais et al., 1998). The results of a large of number of studies of the effects of FGFs on osteoblastic cells in vitro have been conflicting as both positive and neg-ative effects have been reported in about equal amounts. Most recent studies have drawn the conclusion that the FGFs can have markedly differing effects on bone cells depending upon the distinct stage of differentiation of the target cell (Debiais et al., 1998). Some studies have also suggested that the effects of FGF-2 may be via its effects on the expression of transforming growth factor-β in osteoblastic cells both in vitro and in vivo (Nakamura et al., 1995; Noda & Vogel, 1989).

An important role for FGF-2 that is now well described is in endochondral devel-opment at the stage of chondrocyte hypertrophy. FGF-2, which acts as an inhibitor of chondrocyte maturation to hypertrophy, does so via induction of expression of PTHrP, and in doing so abrogates the action of the bone morphogenic proteins present at the same site which tend to inhibit PTHrP (Terkeltaub et al., 1998). Opposing effects of FGF-2 (inhibits) and the stimulatory BMPs are also exerted on the elaboration of inorganic pyrophosphatase (PPI), which regulates the ability of hypertrophic chondrocytes to mineralize the matrix (Terkeltamb et al., 1998).

Transforming growth factor-β

Transforming growth factor-β (TGF-β) belongs to a large family of polypeptide molecules that share a number of structural and functional properties (Massague, 1996). Other members of the family include the bone morphogenic proteins (BMPs), the activins, the inhibins, Mullerian inhibiting substance (MIS) and the *Drosophila* decapentaplegic gene product (DPP-C). To date, there have been some nine different isoforms of TGF-β described and five different receptors. Of the receptors, the type II is expressed on most target cells and is a transmembrane serine/threonine kinase that, upon occupation, phosphorylates a second trans-membrane kinase the TGF-β type I receptor, and this is an absolute requirement for signal transduction (Massague, 1996; Wieser et al., 1995).

The TGF-β isoforms are involved in a variety of cellular events which regulate bone growth and turnover (Bonewald & Dallas, 1994; Hill & Logan, 1992). A large amount of latent TGF-β is incorporated into the bone matrix during formation and is stored for future release and activation during osteoclastic bone resorption, when it may well act as a stimulatory factor for osteoblast recruitment, thus becoming a coupling factor (Maiti & Singh, 1996; Mundy, 1991). Results of the effects of TGF-β on osteoblasts in vitro have been conflicting for the most part, due to the use of many different heterologous assay systems. In general, exposure to TGF-β leads to the induction of matrix synthesis by osteoblasts, while it tends to inhibit mineralization of the matrix and also inhibits osteoclast recruitment and differentiation thus restricting bone resorption (Dieudonne et al., 1994; Massague, 1996; Tashjian et al., 1985). When exogenous TGF-β was administered to experimental animals, it was generally stimulatory for bone growth, it could also ameliorate the bone loss due to estrogen deficiency, and has been implicated in the stimulation of bone formation due to mechanical loading (Beaudreuil et al., 1995; Klein-Nulend et al., 1995; Rosen et al., 1994b).

In recent studies the skeletal system has been investigated in mice lacking the TGF-β1 gene (Geiser et al., 1998). In these animals, tibial metaphyses showed a significant decrease in bone mineral content, but not bone mineral density, when compared with normal animals or their heterozygous littermates. No differences in cortical bone were found. By histomorphometric analysis there was no apparent detriment in either trabecular bone volume, number, thickness or connectivity. However, the width of the tibial growth plate and the longitudinal growth were both significantly decreased in the knockout mice. Acoustic velocity measurements made on demineralized bone suggested that the elastic properties of the bone matrix were compromised, suggesting that TGF-β contributes to the relative stiffness of bone.

Bone morphogenic proteins

The bone morphogenic proteins (BMPs) are members of the transforming growth factor superfamily. Like the transforming growth factors, they are normally present as homodimers of approximately 100 to 140 amino acids, although heterodimers with equal, if not greater, biological activity have been noted (Mehler et al., 1997). Unlike TGF-β, latent forms (proforms complexed to mature counterparts which require proteolytic cleavage for activation) are not normally present. The biological activity of the BMPs have been noted for many years with the observation that ectopic bone formation occurs in certain transplanted connective tissues. This 'osteoinductive' activity was termed osteogenic protein in the 1960s, and it could be isolated from a number of connective tissues (Urist, 1965). There are now some 20 or so members of the BMP family and, while they are potent inducers of bone formation, the name is somewhat misleading as they also play vital roles in vertebrate embryogenesis and the development of the CNS, kidney, heart, tooth bud, prostate oocytes, hair follicles and the eye, as well as the skeletal system through effects on both patterning and chondrogenesis (Dudley et al., 1995; Linkhart et al., 1996; Mehler et al., 1997). In a manner parallel to that of the TGFs, the BMPs signal target cells via association with heterodimeric receptors consisting of specific type I and type II proteins.

While the BMPs induce bone formation in both in vivo and in vitro systems, the most abundant member of the family, osteogenic protein-1/BMP-7, stimulates a number of biochemical markers which are characteristic of osteoblastic differentiation. These effects are likely to be due to positive regulation of the IGF system by the BMPs in osteoblasts (Knutsen et al., 1995; Yeh et al., 1996). Thus OP-1/BMP-7 increases IGF type II receptors, increases the expression of IGFBP-3 and IGFBP-5, while decreasing IGFBP-4 in human osteoblasts (Linkhart et al., 1996). BMP-7 also promotes the growth of chondrocytes, is chemotactic and induces adhesion molecule synthesis in nerve cells (Perides et al., 1993). Of other members of the family, BMP-2 increases rat osteoblast IGF-I and IGF-II expression, and can also increase TGF-β and interleukin-6 (IL-6) expression in human osteoblasts (HOBIT cells), while BMP-4 can upregulate TGF-β expression in monocytes (Linkhart et al., 1996).

As noted above under discussion of the FGFs, the BMPs have a vital role to play in regulating chondrogenesis and the transition from proliferating to hypertrophic chondrocytes, and plays an opposing and balancing role with FGF-2 on the expression of the PTHrP system (Terkeltaub et al., 1998).

REFERENCES

Andrew, J. G., Hoyland, J., Freemont, A. J., & Marsh, D. (1993). Insulin-like growth factor gene expression in human fracture callus. *Calcif. Tiss. Int.*, **53**, 97–102.

Baldin, V., Roman, A-M., Bosc-Bierne, I., Amarlic, F., & Bouche, G. (1990). Translocation of bFGF to the nucleus is G1 phase cell specific in bovine aortic endothelial cells. *EMBO J.*, **9**, 1511–17.

Beaudreuil, J., Mbalaviele, G., Cohensolal, M., Morieux, C., Devernejoul, M. C., & Orcel, P. (1995). Short-term local injections of transforming growth factor beta (I) decrease ovariectomy-stimulated osteoclastic resorption in vivo in rats. *J. Bone Miner. Res.*, **10**, 971–7.

Bikfalfi, A., Klein, S., Pintucci, G., & Rifkin, D. (1997). Biological roles of fibroblast growth factor-2. *Endocrine Rev.*, **18**, 26–45.

Bonewald, L. F. & Dallas, S. L. (1994). Role of active and latent transforming growth factor- in bone formation. *J. Cell Biochem.*, **55**, 350–7.

Burgess, W. H. & Maciag, T. (1989). The heparin binding (fibroblast) growth factor family of proteins. *Am. Rev. Biochem.*, **58**, 575–606.

Canalis, E., Pash, J., & Varghese, S. (1993). Skeletal growth factors. *Crit. Rev. Eukaryotic Gene Expression*, **3**, 155–66.

Chevally, T., Kanzaki, S., Strong, D. D., Mohan, S., Baylink, D. J., & Linkhart, T. A. (1996). Glucocorticoid inhibition of bone formation may in part be mediated by alterations in stimulatory IGF binding protein synthesis. *Eur. J. Endocrinol.*, **134**, 591–601.

Debiais, F., Hott, M., Graulet, A. M,. & Marie, P. J. (1998). The effects of fibroblast growth factor-2 on human neonatal calvaria osteoblastic cells are differentiation stage specific. *J. Bone Miner. Res.*, **13**, 645–54.

Dequeker, J., Mohan, S., Finkelman, R. D., Aerssens, J., & Baylink, D. J. (1993). Generalized osteoarthritis associated with increased insulin-like growth factor types I and II and transforming growth factor β in cortical bone from the iliac crest. Possible mechanism of increased bone density and protection against osteoporosis. *Arth. Rheumat.*, **36**, 1702–8.

Dieudonne, S. C., Semeins, C. M., Goei, S. W., Vukicevic, S., Nulend, J. K., Sampath, T. K., Helder, M., & Berger, E. H. (1994). Opposite effects of osteogenic protein and transforming growth factor beta on chondrogenesis in cultured long bone rudiments. *J. Bone Miner. Res.*, **9**, 771–80.

Dudley, A. T., Lyons, K. M., & Robertson, E. J. (1995). A requirement for bone morphogenic protein-7 during development of mammalian kidney and eye. *Genes Dev.*, **9**, 2795–807.

Ernst, M. & Rodan, G. A. (1990). Increased activity of insulin-like growth factor (IGF) in osteoblastic cells in the presence of growth hormone (GH): positive correlation with the presence of the GH-induced IGF-binding protein BP-3. *Endocrinology*, **127**, 807–14.

Geiser, A. G., Zeng, Q. Q., Sato, M., Helvering, L. M., Hirano, T., & Turner, C. H. (1998). Decreased bone mass and bone elasticity in mice lacking the transforming growth factor-β1 gene. *Bone*, **23**, 87–93.

Globus, R. K., Plouet, J., & Gospodarowicz, D. (1989). Cultured bovine bone cells synthesize basic fibroblast growth factor and store it in their extracellular matrix. *Endocrinology*, **124**, 1539–47.

Hill, D. J. & Logan, A. (1992). Peptide growth factors and their interactions during chondrogenesis. *Pro. Growth Factor Res.*, **4**, 45–68.

Hodsman, A. B., Fraher, L. J., & Watson, P. H. (1999). Therapeutics: parathyroid hormone. In *The Aging Skeleton*, ed. J. Marcovic, C. Rosen et al. San Diego, CA: Academic Press.

Johansson, A. & Rosen, C. J. (1998). The insulin-like growth factors: potential anabolic agents for the skeleton. In *Anabolic Treatments for Osteoporosis*, ed. J. E. Whitfield & P. Morley, pp. 185–205. Boca Raton, FA: CRC.

Kimelman, D. & Kirschner, M. (1987). Synergistic induction of mesoderm by FGF and TGF-β and the identification of an mRNA coding for FGF in the *Xenopus* embryo. *Cell*, **51**, 869–77.

Klagsbrun, M. & Baird, A. (1991). A dual receptor system is required for basic fibroblast growth factor activity. *Cell*, **67**, 229–31.

Klein-Nulend, J., Roelofson, J., Sterck, J. G. H., Semeins, C. M., & Berger, E. H. (1995). Mechanical loading stimulates the release of transforming growth-factor-beta activity by cultured mouse calvariae and periosteal cells. *J. Cell Physiol.*, **163**, 115–19.

Knutsen, R., Honda, Y., Strong, D. D., Sampath, T. K., Baylink, D. J., & Mohan, S. (1995). Regulation of insulin-like growth factor components by osteogenic protein-1 in human bone cells. *Endocrinology*, **136**, 857–65.

Lazowski, D. A., Fraher, L. J., Hodsman, A. B., Steer, B., Modrowski, D., & Han, V. K. M. (1994). Regional variation of insulin-like growth factor gene expression in mature rat bone and cartilage. *Bone*, **15**, 563–76.

Linkhart, T. A., Mohan, S., & Baylink, D. J. (1996). Growth factors for bone growth and repair: IGF, TGFβ and BMP. *Bone*, **19**, 1s-12s.

Maiti, S. K. & Singh, G. R. (1996). Transforming growth factor beta (TGF-beta) in bone remodeling, *Curr Sci.*, **71**, 613–17.

Massague, J. (1996) TGF-β signaling: receptors, transducers, and Mad proteins. *Cell*, **85**, 947–50.

Mehler, M. F., Mabie, P. C., Zhang, D., & Kessler, J. A. (1997). Bone morphogenic proteins in the nervous system. *Trends Neurosci.*, **20**, 309–17.

Mochizuki, H., Hakeda, Y., Wakatsuki, N., Usui, N., Akashi, S., Sato, T., Tanake, K., & Kumegawa, M. (1992). Insulin-like growth factor-I supports formation and activation of osteoclasts. *Endocrinology*, **131**, 1075–80.

Mohan, S. & Baylink, D. J. (1991). Bone growth factors. *Clin. Orthop. Rel. Res.*, **263**, 30–48.

Mohan, S., Jennings, J. C., Linkhart, T. A., & Baylink, D. J. (1988). Primary structure of human skeletal growth factor: homology with human insulin-like growth factor-II. *Biochim. Biophys. Acta*, **14**, 44–55.

Mohan, S., Nakao, Y., Honda, Y., Landale, E., Lesser, U., Dony, C., Lang, K., & Baylink, D. J. (1995). Studies on the mechanism by which insulin-like growth factor (IGF) binding protein -4 (IGFBP-4) and IGFBP-5 modulate IGF actions on bone cells. *J. Biol. Chem.*, **270**, 20424– 31.

Mundy, G. R. (1991). The effects of TGF-beta on bone, *Ciba Found. Symp.*, **157**, 137–43.

Mundy, G. R. (1993). Factors which stimulate bone growth in vivo. *Growth Regul.*, **3**, 124–8.

Nakamura, T., Hanada, K., Tamura, M., Shibanushi, T., Nigi, H., Tagawa, M., Fukumoto, S., & Matsumoto. T. (1995). Stimulation of endosteal bone formation by systemic injections of recombinant basic growth factor in rats. *Endocrinology*, **136**, 1276–84.

Noda, M. & Vogel, L. (1989). Fibroblast growth factor enhances type 1 transforming growth factor gene expression in osteoblast-like cells. *J. Cell Biol.*, **109**, 2529–35.

Perides, G., Hu, G., Rueger, D. C., & Charness, M. E. (1993). Osteogenic protein-1 regulates L1 and neural cell adhesion molecule gene expression in neural cells. *J. Biol. Chem.*, **268**, 25197–205.

Peters, K., Ornitz, D., Werner, S., & William, L. (1993). Unique expression pattern of FGF receptor-3 gene during mouse organogenesis. *Dev. Biol.*, **155**, 423–30.

Prisell, P. T., Edwall, D., Lindblad, J. B., Levinovitz, A., & Norstedt, G. (1993). Expression of insulin-like growth factors during bone induction in the rat. *Calcif. Tiss. Int.*, **53**, 201–5.

Rosen, C. J., Donahue, L. R., & Hunter, S. (1994a). Insulin-like growth factors and bone: The osteoporosis connection. *Proc. Soc. Exptl. Biol. Med.*, **206**, 83–102.

Rosen, D., Miller, S. C., DeLeon, E., Thompson, A. Y., Bentz, H., Mathews, M., & Adams, S. (1994b). Systemic administration of recombinant transforming growth factor beta 2 (rTGF-β2) stimulates parameters of cancellous bone formation in juvenile and adult rats. *Bone*, **15**, 355–9.

Takada, Y., Baylink, D. J., Linkhart, T. A., Edwall, E., Kumegawa, M., & Mohan, S. (1994). Calcitrophic hormones and growth factors regulate osteoclast survival in vitro. *J. Bone Miner. Res.*, **9**, S311.

Tashjian, A. J., Voelkel, E. F., Lazzaro, M., Singer, F. R., Roberts, A. B., Derynck, R., Winkler, M. E., & Levine, L. (1985). Alpha and human transforming growth factors stimulate prostaglandin production and bone resorption in cultured mouse calvaria. *Proc. Natl Acad. Sci., USA*, **82**, 4535–8.

Terkeltaub, R. A., Johnson, K., Rohnow, D., Goomer, R., Burton, D., & Deftos, L. J. (1998). Bone morphogenic proteins and bFGF exert opposing regulatory effects on PTHrP expression and inorganic pyrophosphate elaboration in immortalized murine endochondral hypertrophic chondrocytes (MCT cells). *J. Bone Miner. Res.*, **13**, 931–41.

Urist, M. R. (1965). Bone: formation by autoinduction. *Science*, **150**, 893–9.

Wanaka, A., Milbrandt, J., & Johnson, E. M. (1991). Expression of FGF receptor gene in rat development. *Development*, **111**, 455–68.

Watson, P. H., Lazowski, D. A., Han, V. K. M., Fraher, L. J., Steer, B. M., & Hodsman, A. B. (1995). Parathyroid hormone restores bone mass and enhances osteoblast insulin-like growth factor-I gene expression in ovariectomized rats. *Bone*, **16**, 1–9.

Wieser, R., Wrana, J. L., & Massague, J. (1995). GS domain mutations that constitutively activate TβR-I, the downstream signaling component in the TGF-β receptor complex. *EMBO J.*, **14**, 2199–208.

Yeh, L. C. C., Adamo, M. L., Kitten, A. M., Olson, M. S., & Lee, J. C. (1996). Osteogenic protein-1-mediated insulin-like growth factor gene expression in primary cultures of rat osteoblastic cells. *Endocrinology*, **137**, 1921–31.

6

The PTH/PTHrP system and calcium homeostasis

Geoffrey N. Hendy

Introduction

The genetic and physiological relationships between the two calciotropic hormones, parathyroid hormone (PTH) and parathyroid hormone-related protein (PTHrP), and their roles in bone growth and calcium homeostasis will be reviewed. Present understanding of the regulation of calcium homeostasis and skeletal development at the molecular level has been derived in part from an analysis of the effects of disruption or overexpression of particular genes in humans or animals. Such loss of function or gain of function may be either naturally occurring or experimentally induced. The ongoing elucidation of the roles of the calcium-sensing receptor (CaSR) in calcium homeostasis and of PTHrP and the PTH/PTHrP receptor in skeletogenesis provides a good example of this.

Overview of calcium homeostasis

Keeping the concentration of the extracellular fluid calcium concentration within a narrow normal range is critical for many physiological processes, including neuromuscular activity, and normal skeletal development and maintenance. The parathyroid gland plays a central role in calcium homeostasis by sensing a decrease in the blood calcium concentration and responding by synthesizing and secreting more PTH (Fig. 6.1). PTH acts on the kidney to enhance renal calcium reabsorption and to promote the conversion of 25-hydroxyvitamin D to 1,25-dihydroxyvitamin D [$1,25\text{-}(OH)_2D$]. This hormonally active metabolite of vitamin D increases gastrointestinal absorption of calcium and, with PTH, induces skeletal resorption, causing an increase in the circulating calcium concentration. The parathyroid gland senses the restoration of the ambient calcium concentration to normal and reduces PTH release. Alterations in extracellular fluid calcium levels are transmitted through a parathyroid plasma membrane CaSR (Brown & Hebert, 1997) that couples through a G-protein complex to phospholipase C. Increases in extracellular calcium lead to increases in inositol 1,4,5-trisphosphate (IP_3) and mobilization of intracellular calcium stores. The manner in which this inhibits

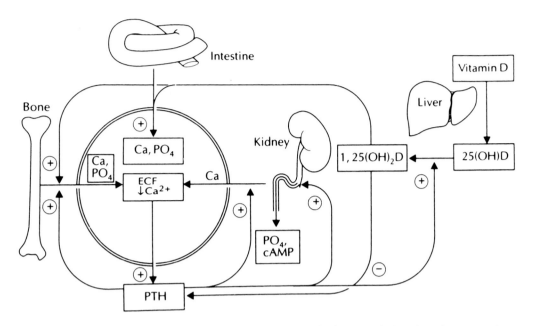

Fig. 6.1   Parathyroid hormone (PTH) and vitamin D control calcium and phosphate homeostasis. A fall in extracellular fluid (ECF) calcium concentration triggers PTH secretion. PTH directly acts on the kidney to promote renal calcium reabsorption and conversion of 25-hydroxyvitamin D [25(OH)D] to 1,25-dihydroxyvitamin D [1,25(OH)$_2$D]. 1,25(OH)$_2$D increases intestinal absorption of calcium (and phosphate) and, with PTH, mobilizes calcium (and phosphate) from bone. Thus extracellular fluid (ECF) calcium is restored to normal neutralizing the signal initiating PTH release. PTH inhibits renal phosphate reabsorption promoting phosphaturia. Reproduced with permission from Brown, E.M. (1995).

hormone secretion is not understood. PTH also modulates the extracellular concentration of the phosphate ion. PTH-induced skeletal lysis increases extracellular phosphate as well as calcium levels. A compensatory decrease in blood phosphate levels occurs by the inhibitory action of PTH on renal phosphate reabsorption, thereby producing phosphaturia.

Inherited abnormalities of the CaSR gene located on chromosome 3p13.3–21 can lead to either hypercalcemia or hypocalcemia depending upon whether they are inactivating or activating, respectively. Heterozygous loss-of-function mutations give rise to familial (benign) hypocalciuric hypercalcemia (FHH) in which the lifelong hypercalcemia is asymptomatic. The homozygous condition manifests itself as neonatal severe hyperparathyroidism (NSHPT), a rare disorder characterized by extreme hypercalcemia and the bony changes of hyperparathyroidism which occur in infancy. The disorder autosomal dominant hypocalcemia (ADH) is due to gain-of-function mutations in the CaSR gene. ADH may be asymptomatic or present with neonatal or childhood seizures. Because of the overactive CaSR in the nephron, these patients are at greater risk of developing renal complications during vitamin D therapy than patients with idiopathic hypoparathyroidism. A common polymorphism in the intracellular tail of the CaSR, Ala to Ser at position 986, has a modest effect on the serum calcium concentration in healthy individuals (Cole et al., 1999). The CaSR is a target for phenylalkylamine compounds – so-called calcimimetics – which are allosteric stimulators of the CaSR's affinity for cations (Nemeth et al., 1998). These orally active compounds are presently being evaluated for treatment of primary and secondary hyperparathyroidism and parathyroid carcinoma (Silverberg et al., 1997).

Parathyroid hormone

PTH is the product of a single-copy gene located on chromosome 11p15 and, in mammals, has 84 amino acids. The gene, which encodes a larger precursor molecule of 115 amino acids, preproPTH, is organized into three exons. Exon 1 encodes the 5′-untranslated region of the messenger RNA, exon 2 encodes the NH_2-terminal pre- or signal peptide and part of the short propeptide, and exon III encodes the $Lys^{-2}-Arg^{-1}$ of the prohormone cleavage site, the 84 amino acids of the mature hormone, and the 3′-untranslated region of the mRNA.

Transcription of the PTH gene occurs almost exclusively in the endocrine cells of the parathyroid gland, and is subject to strong repressor activity in all other cells. Activation of genes in a particular tissue is often related to demethylation of cytosine residues, and the PTH gene in parathyroid cells is hypomethylated at CpG residues relative to other tissues. The human PTH gene has two functional TATA box-controlled transcriptional start sites, a cyclic AMP response element (CRE), and a vitamin D response element (VDRE) in its proximal promoter. Distally, several kilobase pairs upstream of the transcription start site a calcium response element (CaRE), and the sequences that function to repress transcription in non-parathyroid cells are present. PTH gene transcription is negatively regulated by both extracellular calcium and the hormonally active metabolite of vitamin D, $1,25(OH)_2D$.

The primary structure of the major glandular form of PTH, PTH (1–84), has been determined in several mammalian species, including human, bovine, porcine, canine, mouse and rat (Fig. 6.2). In the chicken, the PTH polypeptide contains 88 rather than 84 amino acids. The NH_2-terminal 34 amino acids are the most well-conserved portion of the molecule, and structure and function studies have emphasized the importance of the NH_2-terminal region to bioactivity in all species. Considerable deletion of the middle and COOH-terminal region of the intact polypeptide can be tolerated without apparent loss of biological activity.

Humans have two pairs of parathyroid glands lying in the anterior cervical

PARATHYROID HORMONE

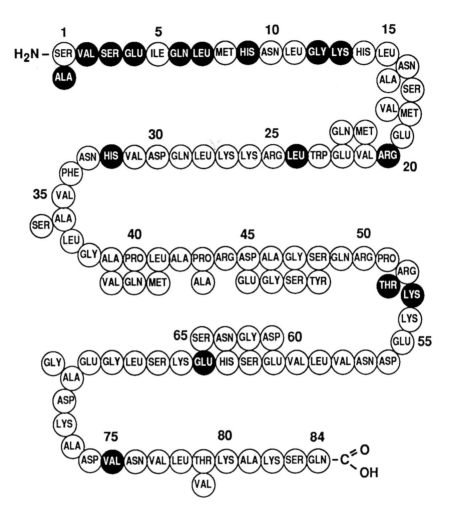

Fig. 6.2   Primary structure of PTH. The backbone sequence is that of the human with substitutions in the rat hormone shown at specific sites. The solid circles show identical amino acids in the human and rat PTH and PTHrP molecules.

region, which are derived from the third and fourth pharyngeal pouches. Rats have a single pair of glands embedded in the cranial part of the thyroid. The chief cell is the predominant cell type in human with some oxyphil cells, which have an acidophilic cytoplasm and mitochondria, also present. Parathyroid cells normally divide at an extremely slow rate – mitoses are rarely observed. Parathyroid cells have limited numbers of secretory granules containing PTH, indicating that relatively little hormone is stored in the gland.

Hyperparathyroidism and hypoparathyroidism

Primary hyperparathyroidism is one of the most common causes of hypercalcemia. The approximate incidence is 1 in 1000, and it is now usually diagnosed in non-symptomatic patients found to be hypercalcemic by multichannel screening (Silverberg & Bilezikian, 1997). However, the classical manifestations of primary hyperparathyroidism still appear. Hypercalciuria and nephrolithiasis occur in about 15% of patients. Skeletal manifestations are relatively mild in the present-day patient, with osteitis fibrosa cystica, brown tumors, cystic lesions, and symptomatic fractures, being rare. However, increased bone turnover can be inferred by increased markers of bone formation and bone resorption. For the underlying etiology of the parathyroid neoplasia the reader is referred elsewhere (Hendy & Arnold, 1996).

Secondary hyperparathyroidism as occurs in chronic renal failure is caused directly or indirectly by decreased $1,25(OH)_2D$ production by the kidney and increased serum phosphate. This leads to hypocalcemia. Thus, the parathyroid gland is subjected to a combination of proliferative signals resulting in hyperplasia. The subsequent renal osteodystrophy is a complex skeletal disorder having several components. There is osteitis fibrosa cystica due to the PTH excess, osteomalacia due to the vitamin D deficiency, extraskeletal calcification due to elevated circulating phosphate levels and adynamic bone disease which is brought on by skeletal resistance to PTH action. For further details of the manner in which primary and secondary hyperparathyroidism influence bone and mineral metabolism (and their relationship to osteoporosis) (see Chapter 15, this volume).

There are several causes of hypoparathyroidism presenting as hypocalcemia and hyperphosphatemia, with removal or damage to the parathyroid glands during neck surgery being the most common. The reader is referred elsewhere (Hendy & Goltzman, 2000) for a fuller description of this and other causes of hypoparathyroidism and its treatment.

Effect of PTH on bone

The best-documented effect of PTH on bone is a catabolic one, which results in the breakdown of mineral constituents and bone matrix, as manifested by the release of calcium and phosphate, by increases in plasma and urinary hydroxyproline, and other indices of bone resorption. This process is mediated by osteoclastic osteolysis, but the mechanism is indirect, since PTH does not bind directly to multinucleated osteoclasts. However, the PTH/PTHrP receptor is expressed on osteoblasts, and osteoblast precursors (so-called parathyroid hormone target or 'PT' cells) (Rouleau et al., 1988) and PTH stimulates second messenger accumulation in osteoblast-enriched populations of cells from skeletal tissues and in osteosarcoma cells of the osteoblast lineage. It is suggested that PTH-induced stimulation of multinucleated osteoclasts occurs through the action of PTH-stimulated osteoblast activity via intermediary factors.

One of these intermediary factors is osteoclast differentiation factor (ODF), also known as osteoprotegerin ligand (OPGL) (Lacey et al., 1998), which is expressed in the bone lining cells or osteoblast precursors which support osteoclast recruitment. ODF/OPGL, which is a member of the tumor necrosis factor (TNF) family, is identical to the molecule TRANCE/RANKL which is expressed in T-cells and previously identified as a dendritic cell survival factor in vitro. Several bone resorbing factors such as PTH, PTHrP, PGE$_2$, some of the interleukins, and 1,25(OH)$_2$D$_3$ upregulate ODF/OPGL gene expression in osteoblasts and bone stromal cells. Interaction of ODF/OPGL with its receptor on osteoclast progenitors and osteoclasts then stimulates their recruitment and activation and delays their degradation. The ablation of the ODF/OPGL gene in mice has confirmed it to be a key regulator of osteoclastogenesis, as well as lymphocyte development and lymphnode organogenesis (Kong et al., 1999). Osteoprotegerin (OPG)/osteoclastogenesis inhibitory factor (OCIF) (Simonet et al., 1997) inhibits osteoclastic bone resorption. OPG/OCIF, although a soluble factor, is a member of the TNF receptor family and it inhibits recruitment, activation and survival of osteoclasts. OPG/OCIF acts as a natural decoy receptor that disrupts the interaction of ODF/OPGL, released by osteoblast-related cells, and its receptor on osteoclast progenitors. OPG/OCIF has therapeutic potential for the treatment of osteoporosis and hypercalcemic conditions such as malignancy-associated hypercalcemia.

The consequences of the effects of PTH on osteoblast activity are complex. The examination of bone after in vivo PTH administration has demonstrated an increase in osteoblasts and new formation, indicating that PTH may also play an anabolic role under some circumstances. This might occur by PTH's ability to stimulate IGF-I production by osteoblasts. PTH (and PTHrP) regulate cellular differentiation, proliferation, and development, and are now considered to be anabolic skeletal agents when made available periodically rather than continuously in vivo. Low and intermittent doses of PTH(1–34) – and PTHrP(1–34) and related analogues – promote bone formation. In clinical studies, daily PTH(1–34) injections increased hip and spine bone mineral density (BMD) (see Chapter 24, this volume).

PTH's bone forming activity may depend more on promoting differentiation of precursor cells into secretory osteoblasts than on an action on mature osteoblasts (Corral et al., 1998). It may suppress osteogenic activity of mature osteoblasts. The anabolic and catabolic effects of PTH on osteoblasts may represent a combination of direct and indirect effects, effects of different domains of the PTH molecule, discrete functions of morphologically similar, but functionally distinct osteoblasts, or differences in hormonal effects based on different times of exposure or different hormone concentrations.

Parathyroid hormone-related protein

In 1941, Fuller Albright reviewed a patient with renal carcinoma (and a single skeletal metastasis) with hypercalcemia accompanied by hypophosphatemia. He speculated that the tumor was secreting a circulating factor that was identical or similar to PTH. It is now appreciated that PTHrP is the responsible causal factor in the majority of cases of hypercalcemia associated with malignancy (Goltzman & Henderson, 1996; Philbrick et al., 1996). In only a handful of cases has the rare occurrence of ectopic PTH synthesis in such tumors been documented. The PTHrP polypeptide shares significant homology with PTH at the NH_2-terminus, and thereby these two distinct ligands can bind and activate the PTH/PTHrP receptor.

The PTHrP gene has the same general organization as the PTH gene in which the same functional domains – the 5'-untranslated region, prepro-sequence of the precursor peptide, and the prohormone cleavage site and most or all of the mature peptide – are encoded by single exons. However, it is a more complex transcriptional unit with additional exons encoding alternative 5'-untranslated regions, carboxyl-terminal peptides, and 3'-untranslated regions being present in some species. The human PTHrP gene maps to chromosome 12p12.1–11.2, whereas the PTH gene is on the short arm of chromosome 11. These two human chromosomes are thought to have been derived by an ancient duplication of a single chromosome, and the PTH and PTHrP genes and their respective gene clusters have been maintained as syntenic groups in the human, rat and mouse genomes. Because of the similarity in NH_2-terminal sequence of their mature peptides, their gene organization, and chromosomal locations, it is likely that the PTH and PTHrP genes evolved from a single ancestral gene and form part of a single gene family. The PTHrP gene is considered to be the more ancient member, phylogenetically.

In contrast to the very limited expression of the PTH gene, the PTHrP gene is widely expressed in both endocrine and non-endocrine tissues. Although initially discovered in malignancies, mRNA encoding PTHrP has been identified in both normal (fetal and adult) and adenomatous tissue as well as in cancers of several species. The list of normal tissues includes adrenal gland, amnion, bone, brain, endothelium, epidermis, heart, kidney, lung, mammary gland, ovary, pancreatic islets, parathyroid gland, pituitary, placenta, prostate, skeletal muscle, small intestine, smooth muscle, spleen, stomach mucosa, testis, thyroid, thymus, urothelium, and uterus. High concentrations of PTHrP are also found in milk. Several fetal tissues express PTHrP, including brain, chorioallantoic membrane, heart, intestine, liver, lung, parathyroid gland, skeletal muscle, skeleton, and yolk sac. Localization has also been demonstrated in adenomatous islet cell tumors, pituitary and para-thyroid tumors. The widespread expression of PTHrP in many tissues during development, with or without continued expression in the adult, suggests that PTHrP expression in tumors need not be viewed as 'ectopic'. Despite the wide-spread expression of PTHrP, circulating levels in healthy individuals are low or undetectable, and passive immunization studies have provided no evidence for it playing any role in normal calcium homeostasis.

PTHrP synthesis and secretion are regulated in a variety of cells by several different agents, including calcium, cyclic AMP, phorbol esters, growth factors (like epidermal growth factor (EGF) and transforming growth factor-beta (TGF-β)), peptide hormones (such as angiotensin II, prolactin and calcitonin) and members of the steroid hormone/nuclear receptor family, such as glucocorticoids, estrogen, retinoic acid, testosterone and 1,25(OH)$_2$D. Tumor cells like adult T-cell leukemia (ATL) cells transformed with human T-cell lymphotrophic virus I (HTLV-1) increase PTHrP expression via the HTLV-1-derived transcription factor Tax$_1$. Cells transformed by EJ-Ha-ras and v-*src* oncogenes have markedly elevated PTHrP expression. In several human and rat cell lines, inhibition of protein synthesis, for example, by cycloheximide, leads to the superinduction of PTHrP mRNA levels. This is the result of both an increase in the gene transcription rate and stabilization of the mRNA. It is suggested that a labile repressor protein regulates transcription and that in the human gene this occurs preferentially at the downstream or proxi-mal promoter.

The complete primary structure of the PTHrP polypeptide is known for several species, including human, rat, and mouse. In each case the PTHrP mRNA encodes a precursor with a 36-amino-acid prepro-sequence at the NH$_2$-terminus. The human PTHrP gene encodes three mature polypeptide isoforms of 139, 141 and 173 amino acids, whereas in rat and mouse single forms of 141 and 139 amino acids, respectively, are found (Fig. 6.3). Strict homology with the corresponding PTH molecules is only found within the first 13 amino acids, thereafter the PTHrP and PTH sequences diverge, although a functional homology in terms of receptor binding extends up to residue 34. Several biologically active peptides can poten-tially be released from PTHrP(1–141). These peptide have distinct activities, sug-gesting they act through different receptors. PTHrP(1–36) mediates hypercalcemia and growth-regulating effects. PTHrP(38–94) promotes placental calcium transfer, and peptides within PTHrP(109–141) inhibit osteoclast function. PTHrP has a bipartite nuclear targeting sequence (NTS) at residues 87–107 and within this domain a nucleolar localizing sequence (NLS) (Henderson et al., 1995). PTHrP localizes to the nucleolus at the G$_1$ phase of the cell cycle, and is translocated to the cytoplasm as cells begin DNA synthesis (Lam et al., 1997). The function of PTHrP's nucleolar localization remains unclear.

PARATHYROID HORMONE-RELATED PROTEIN

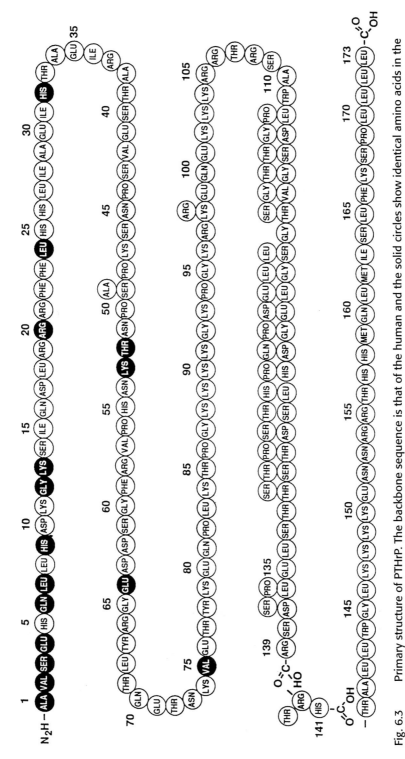

Fig. 6.3   Primary structure of PTHrP. The backbone sequence is that of the human and the solid circles show identical amino acids in the human and rat PTHrP and PTH molecules. Substitutions in rat PTHrP are shown at specific sites. The three alternative COOH-terminal sequences of the human PTHrP isoforms of 139, 141 and 173 amino acids are shown. There is a single 141 amino acid form of rat PTHrP.

PTH/PTHrP receptor

Like other peptide hormones, PTH and PTHrP bind receptors on the plasma membrane of target cells. A related receptor, PTH2R, which also binds PTH weakly but not PTHrP has been identified (Usdin et al., 1995). In contrast to the PTH/PTHrP receptor PTH2R has a very limited tissue expression profile, and its involvement in any disease is unknown. Binding of ligand by these receptors results in stimulation of the enzyme adenylate cyclase on the inner surface of the plasma membrane, and the same receptors can couple to phosphatidylinositol turnover as well. Increased adenylate cyclase activity stimulates cyclic AMP production which activates protein kinase A (PKA) and the products of phospholipase C activity, inositol-(1,4,5)-trisphosphate (IP$_3$) and diacylglycerol (DAG), mobilize intracellular calcium, [Ca^{2+}]i, stores and activate protein kinase C (PKC) activity, respectively. The cascade of events thus initiated lead to the final cellular response to PTH and PTHrP. For these two ligands, whereas the first two NH$_2$-terminal amino acids are critical for signaling the PKA pathway, amino acids 28–34 mediate signaling through the PKC pathway.

PTHrP and PTH/PTHrP receptor in skeletal development

Vertebrate limb development occurs through endochondral bone formation. Proper morphogenesis requires growth plate chondrocytes to undergo temporally and spatially coordinated differentiation. Endochondral bone formation initiates with mesenchymal cell condensation; these core cells differentiate into chondrocytes and peripheral cells become the perichondrium. The central chondrocytes undergo several rounds of proliferation, differentiate into prehypertrophic and then hypertrophic chondrocytes which mineralize the surrounding matrix, and undergo apoptosis. The perichondrium neighboring the prehypertrophic and hypertrophic chondrocytes forms a bone collar and blood vessels invade the mineralized cartilage. Osteoblasts and hematopoietic cells replace the mineralized cartilage with bone and bone marrow.

Mice homozygous for PTHrP gene deletion exhibit a form of chondrodysplasia and die at or soon after birth (Karaplis et al., 1994). The mice display domed and foreshortened cranium, a narrowed thorax and shortened limbs (Fig. 6.4). The long bone epiphyses are shortened because of a reduced number of resting and proliferating chondrocytes and in the normally homogeneous hypertrophic zone clusters of non-hypertrophic chondrocytes persist (Amizuka et al., 1994) . This then distorts the longitudinal columns of hypertrophic chondrocytes resulting in less developed metaphyseal bony spicules. A mouse model in which the PTH/PTHrP receptor gene was deleted has a similar phenotype to that of the PTHrP-deficient mice (Lanske et al., 1996). Thus deletion of either ligand or receptor results in the

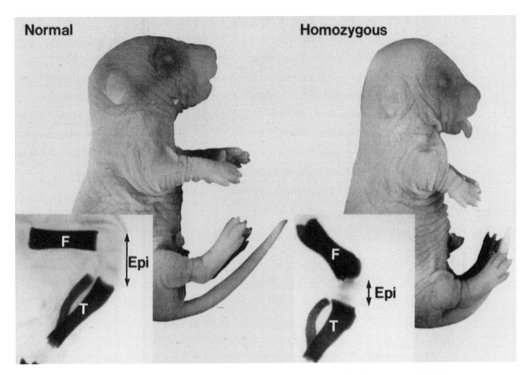

Fig. 6.4   A wild-type 18.5-day-old mouse fetus (normal, left) and a littermate (right) homozygous for PTHrP gene deletion. The characteristic abnormalities of the homozygote include a domed and foreshortened calvarium as demonstrated by the protruding tongue, and shortened limbs. Insets show alizarin red staining of femur (F) and tibia (T) and demonstrate the less developed epiphyseal cartilage of the homozygote. Adapted and reproduced with permission from Karaplis, A.C. et al. (1994).

same abnormalities in epiphyseal cartilage organization and endochondral bone formation.

In these mouse models the basic defect was one of inappropriately rapid ossification of the cartilage template. Not only was there acceleration of the normal ossification process, but there was ossification of the hyaline rib cartilage that normally does not ossify. This led to the rigidity of the thorax most likely accounting for respiratory failure with death occurring immediately after birth.

Haploinsufficient PTHrP mice have skeletal abnormalities

Mice heterozygous for PTHrP gene ablation display no obvious abnormalities at birth. However, at 3 months of age skeletal alterations are evident (Amizuka et al., 1996). The heterozygous mice have shorter blunter snouts relative to their wild-type littermates and exhibit incisal malocclusion due to reduced protrusion of the maxilla. In the epiphyseal growth plate, the normally well-formed longitudinal cartilaginous columns are poorly developed. There are fewer metaphyseal bony spicules and they are abnormally orientated. However, in the diaphysis the cortical bone is normal, as are the serum calcium and PTH concentrations. Therefore, haploinsufficiency of the PTHrP gene leads to some skeletal abnormalities showing that the relative expression of PTHrP clearly plays an important role in osteoblast biology in the adult. Altered expression of PTHrP in osteogenic precursor cells may contribute to the osteopenia in those forms of osteoporosis in which there is reduced bone formation relative to bone resorption. This can be studied further in the haploinsufficient mouse model system.

Targeted overexpression of PTHrP in chondrocytes

Mice with targeted overexpression of PTHrP in chondrocytes exhibit skeletal dysplasia and delayed osteogenesis (Weir et al., 1996). The transgenic animals have markedly shortened limbs and tail. There is enhanced chondrocyte proliferation, delayed maturation of chondrocytes, and inhibition of endochondral bone formation. Thus, the histological abnormalities are the reverse of those in the PTHrP-deficient animals. Therefore, the combined data from these transgenic models of underexpression or overexpression of PTHrP and its receptor indicate that PTHrP by acting at the PTH/PTHrP receptor in chondrocytes plays a critical role in orchestrating endochondral bone formation and ensuring that it takes place at the appropriate rate.

Like PTHrP, Indian hedgehog (IHH) a member of a conserved family of secreted molecules that are critical for embryonic patterning in many organisms, slows the rate of chondrocyte differentiation. IHH is expressed in a layer of maturing prehypertrophic chondrocytes lying immediately distal to the layer of proliferating chondrocytes expressing the PTH/PTHrP receptor. IHH is thought to signal perichondral cells surrounding the prehypertrophic chondrocytes and which will form the bone collar, and also acts either directly or indirectly on proliferating chondrocytes, to upregulate PTHrP in the periarticular region and in proliferating chondrocytes. This then activates PTH/PTHrP receptors in the layer of proliferating chondrocytes slowing their differentiation. The exact details of this pathway remain to be worked out. Thus, PTHrP normally maintains chondrocytic cells in a differentiated state and protects them from apoptosis. The latter property may be the result in part of PTHrP's ability to localize to the nucleolus, which is mediated by the functional nucleolar targeting signal sequence located in the midregion of the molecule. Also, PTHrP stimulates expression of Bcl-2, which retards programmed cell death, in chondrocytes, and ablation of the Bcl-2 gene leads to accelerated maturation of chondrocytes and shortening of the long bones (Amling et al., 1997).

Human chondrodysplasias and PTH/PTHrP receptor mutations

Direct evidence that the PTH/PTHrP receptor mediates the calcium homeostatic actions of PTH and the growth plate actions of PTHrP in humans has come from the study of rare genetic disorders. Jansen's metaphyseal chondrodysplasia (JMC) is inherited in an autosomal dominant fashion although most reported cases are sporadic. The disorder comprises short-limbed dwarfism secondary to severe growth plate abnormalities, asymptomatic hypercalcemia and hypophosphatemia. There is increased bone resorption similar to that in primary hyperparathyroidism and urinary cyclic AMP levels are elevated, but circulating PTH and PTHrP levels are low or undetectable. Although the PTH/PTHrP receptor is found widely in fetal and adult tissues, it is most abundant in three major organs, the kidney, bone and metaphyseal growth plate. It has now been shown that the changes in mineral ion homeostasis and the growth plate in JMC are caused by heterozygous gain-of-function mutations in the PTH/PTHrP receptor gene giving rise to constitutively active receptors (Schipani et al., 1996).

Recently, inactivating or loss-of-function mutations in the PTH/PTHrP receptor have been implicated in the molecular pathogenesis of Blomstrand lethal chondrodysplasia which was first described as a disease entity just under 15 years ago. This rare disease is characterized by advanced endochondral bone maturation, short-limbed dwarfism, and fetal death, thus mimicking the phenotype of PTH/PTHrP receptor-less mice. The majority of BLC cases were born to phenotypically normal, consanguineous parents, suggesting an autosomal recessive mode of inheritance. Mutant PTH/PTHrP receptors identified in BLC fetuses fail to bind ligand or stimulate cAMP or inositol phosphate production (Jobert et al., 1998; Zhang et al., 1998).

REFERENCES

Amizuka, N., Karaplis, A. C., Henderson, J. E., Warshawsky, H., Lipman, M. L., Matsuki, Y., Ejiri, S., Tanaka, M., Izumi, N., Ozawa, H., & Goltzman, D. (1996). Haploinsufficiency of parathyroid hormone-related peptide (PTHrP) results in abnormal postnatal bone development. *Dev. Biol.*, **175**, 166–76.

Amizuka, N., Warshawsky, H., Henderson, J. E., Goltzman, D., & Karaplis, A. C. (1994). Parathyroid hormone-related peptide-depleted mice show abnormal epiphyseal cartilage development and altered endochondral bone formation. *J. Cell Biol.*, **126**, 1611–23.

Amling, M., Neff, L., Tanaka, S., Inoue, D., Kuida, K., Weir, E., Philbrick, W. M., Broadus, A. E., & Baron, R. (1997). Bcl-2 lies downstream of parathyroid hormone-related peptide in a signalling pathway that regulates chondrocyte maturation during skeletal development. *J. Cell Biol.*, **136**, 205–13.

Brown, E. M. (1995). Physiology of calcium metabolism. In *Principles and Practice of Endocrinology and Metabolism*, ed. K. L. Becker, pp. 437–47. Philadelphia, PA: J. B. Lippincott Company.

Brown, E. M. & Hebert, S. C. (1997). Calcium-receptor-regulated parathyroid and renal function. *Bone*, **20**, 303–9.

Cole, D. E. C., Peltekova, V. D., Rubin, L. A., Hawker, G. A., Vieth, R., Liew, C. C., Hwang, D., Evrovski, J., & Hendy, G. N. (1999). A986S polymorphism of the calcium-sensing receptor and circulating calcium concentrations. *Lancet*, **353**, 112–15.

Corral, D. A., Amling, M., Priemel, M., Loyer, E., Fuchs, S., Ducy, P., Baron, R., & Karsenty, G. (1998). Dissociation between bone resorption and bone formation in osteopenic transgenic mice. *Proc. Natl Acad. Sci., USA*, **95**, 13835–40.

Goltzman, D. & Henderson, J. E. (1996). Expression of PTHrP in disease. In *Principles of Bone Biology*, ed. J. P. Bilezikian, L. G. Raisz, & G. A. Rodan, pp. 809–26. San Diego, CA: Academic Press.

Henderson, J. E., Amizuka, N., Warshawsky, H., Biasotto, D., Lanske, B. M. K., Goltzman, D., & Karaplis, A. C. (1995). Nucleolar targeting of PTHrP enhances survival of chondrocytes under conditions that promote cell death by apoptosis. *Mol. Cell. Biol.*, **15**, 4064–75.

Hendy, G. N. & Arnold, A. (1996). Molecular basis of PTH overexpression. In *Principles of Bone Biology*, ed. J. P. Bilezikian, L. G. Raisz, & G. A. Rodan, pp. 757–67. San Diego, CA: Academic Press.

Hendy, G. N. & Goltzman, D. (2000). Hypoparathyroidism and pseudohypoparathyroidism. In *McGraw-Hill Series of Clinical Medicine – Endocrinology. Calcium and Bone Metabolism Section*, ed.-in-chief, A. Pinchera; section ed. J. A. Fischer. Italia. McGraw-Hill Libri. Milano: In Press.

Jobert, A-S., Zhang, P., Couvineau, A., Bonaventure, J., Roume, J., Le Merrer, M., & Silve, C. (1998). Absence of functional receptors for parathyroid hormone and parathyroid hormone-related peptide in Blomstrand chondrodysplasia. *J. Clin. Invest.*, **102**, 34–40.

Karaplis, A. C., Luz, A., Glowacki, J., Bronson, R. T., Tybulewicz, V. L. J., Kronenberg, H. M., & Mulligan, R. C. (1994). Lethal skeletal dysplasia from targeted disruption of the parathyroid hormone-related peptide gene. *Genes Dev.*, **8**, 277–89.

Kong, Y-Y., Yoshida, H., Sarosi, I., Tan, H.L., Timms, E., Capparelli, C., Morony, S., Oliveira-dos-Santos, A., Van, G., Itie, A., Khoo, W., Wakeham, A., Dunstan, C.R., Lacey, D.L., Mak, T.W., Boyle, W.J., & Penninger, J.M. (1999). OPGL is a key regulator of osteoclastogenesis, lymphocyte development and lymph-node organogenesis. *Nature*, **397**, 315–32.

Lacey, D. L., Timms, E., Tan, H. L., Kelley, M. J., Dunstan, C. R., Burgess T., Elliott, R., Colombero, A., Elliott, G., Scully, S., Hsu, H., Sullivan, J., Hawkins, N., Davy, E., Capparelli, C., Eli, A., Qian, Y. X., Kaufman, S., Sarosi, I., Shalhoub, V., Senaldi, G., Guo, J., Delaney, J., & Boyle, W. J. (1998). Osteoprotegerin ligand is a cytokine that regulates osteoclast differentiation and activation. *Cell*, **93**, 165–76.

Lam, M. H., Olsen, S. L., Rankin, W. A., Ho, P. W., Martin, T. J., Gillespie, M. T., & Moseley, J. M. (1997). PTHrP and cell division: expression and localization of PTHrP in a keratinocyte cell line (HaCaT) during the cell cycle. *J. Cell Physiol.*, **173**, 433–46.

Lanske, B., Karaplis, A. C., Lee, K., Luz, A., Vortkamp, A., Pirro, A., Karperien, M., Defize, L. H.

K., Ho, C., Mulligan, R. C., Abou-Samra, A-B., Juppner, H., Segre, G. V., and Kronenberg, H. M. (1996). PTH/PTHrP receptor in early development and Indian Hedgehog-regulated bone growth. *Science*, **273**, 663–6.

Nemeth, E. F., Steffey, M. E., Hammerland, L. G., Hung, B. C. P., Van Wagenen, B. C., DelMar, E. G., and Balandrin, M. F. (1998). Calcimimetics with potent and selective activity on the parathyroid calcium receptor. *Proc. Natl Acad. Sci., USA*, **95**, 4040–5.

Philbrick, W. M., Wysolmerski, J. J., Galbraith, S., Holt, E., Orloff, J. J., Yang, K. H., Vasavada, R. C., Weir, E. C., Broadus, A. E., & Stewart, A. E. (1996). Defining the roles of parathyroid hormone-related protein in normal physiology. *Physiol. Rev.*, **76**, 127–73.

Rouleau, M. F., Mitchell, J., & Goltzman, D. (1988). In vivo distribution of parathyroid hormone receptors in bone: evidence that a predominant osseous target cell is not the mature osteoblast. *Endocrinology*, **123**, 187–91.

Schipani, E., Langman, C. B., Parfitt, A. M., Jensen, G. S., Kikuchi, S., Kooh, S. W., Cole, W. G., & Juppner, H. (1996). Constitutively activated receptors for parathyroid hormone and parathyroid hormone-related peptide in Jansen's metaphyseal chondrodysplasia. *New Engl. J. Med.*, **335**, 708–14.

Silverberg, S. J. & Bilezikian, J.P. (1997). Primary hyperparathyroidism: still evolving? *J. Bone Miner. Res.*, **12**, 856–62.

Silverberg, S. J., Bone, H. G. III, Marriott, T. B., Locker, F. G., Thys-Jacobs, S., Dziem, G., Kaatz, S., Sanguinetti, E. L., & Bilezikian, J. P. (1997). Short-term inhibition of parathyroid hormone secretion by a calcium-receptor agonist in patients with primary hyperparathyroidism. *N. Engl. J. Med.*, **337**, 1506–10.

Simonet, W. S., Lacey, D. L., Dunstan, C. R., Kelley, M., Chang, M. S., Luthy, R., Nguyen, H. Q., Wooden, S., Bennet, L., Boone, T., Shimamoto, G., DeRose, M., Elliott, R., Colombero, A., Tan, H. L., Trail, G., Sullivan, J., Davy, E., Bucay, N., Renshaw-Gegg, L., Hughes, T. M., Hill, D., Pattison, W., Campbell, P., Sander, S., Van, G., Tarpley, J., Derby, P., Lee, R., & Boyle, W. J. (1997). Amgen EST program. Osteoprotegerin: a novel secreted protein involved in the regulation of bone density. *Cell*, **89**, 309–19.

Usdin, T. B., Gruber, C., & Bonner, T. I. (1995). Identification and functional expression of a receptor selectively recognizing parathyroid hormone, the PTH2 receptor. *J. Biol. Chem.*, **270**, 15455–8.

Weir, E. C., Philbrick, W. M., Amling, M., Neff, L. A., Baron, R., & Broadus, A. E. (1996). Targeted overexpression of parathyroid hormone-related peptide in chondrocytes causes chondrodysplasia and delayed endochondral bone formation. *Proc. Natl Acad. Sci., USA*, **93**, 10240–5.

Zhang, P., Jobert, A-S., Couvineau, A., & Silve, C. (1998) A homozygous inactivating mutation in the parathyroid hormone/ parathyroid hormone-related peptide receptor causing Blomstrand chondrodysplasia. *J. Clin. Endocr. Metab.*, **83**, 3365–8.

7

Vitamin D metabolism

Marielle Gascon-Barré

Introduction

Although rickets and osteomalacia were described in England as early as the middle of the seventeenth century, it is only at the beginning of the twentieth century that vitamin D (D) (D refers to both D_3 or cholecalciferol and D_2 or ergocalciferol) was discovered by Mellanby and McCollum who, in their studies on experimental rickets, were able to show that cod liver oil contained antirickets activity. Although genetically determined forms of the disease still exist, nutritionally induced rickets has largely disappeared in North America due to the enrichment of several foods in D_2 or D_3. However, studies in institutionalized and elderly populations indicate that depletion is still quite prevalent in these groups.

Normal vitamin D physiology

Vitamin D metabolism

D_3 is an endogenous secosteroid synthesized in the skin plasma membrane where the ultraviolet B rays of the sun induce a photochemical reaction and a rearrangement of 7-dehydrocholesterol or provitamin D_3 to give rise to the secosteroid previtamin D_3 structure. Under the influence of body heat, previtamin D_3 undergoes a slow and reversible isomerization accompanied by a change in the structure configuration of the molecule leading to the production of vitamin D_3 of endogenous origin. D_3 is then exported to the systemic circulation where, with D of dietary sources, it circulates in serum bound to the vitamin D binding protein (DBP), or is stocked in fat or muscle. In human, 80% of the antirickets activity is stocked in adipose tissue (40%) and muscle (40%), and blood contains only 10% of the antirickets activity (Mawer et al., 1972). D is not active, however, and must be hydroxylated at positions C-25 in the liver, and C-1α in the kidney to acquire its full biological properties (Fig. 7.1).

Kodicek and his group were the first to put forward the hypothesis that D_3 had to be metabolized to be activated. DeLuca's group was the first to demonstrate that

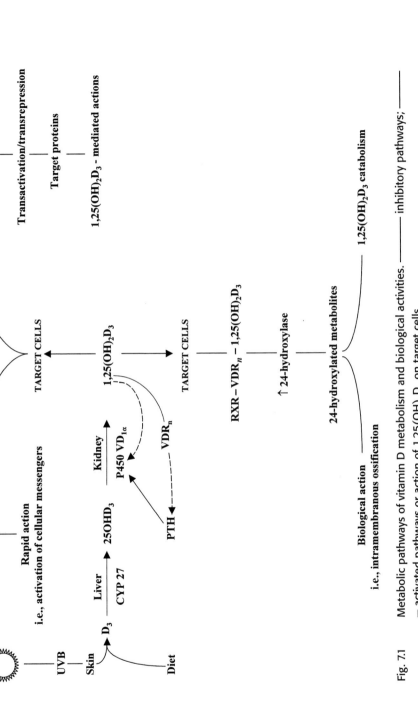

Fig. 7.1   Metabolic pathways of vitamin D metabolism and biological activities. —— inhibitory pathways; —— activated pathways or action of $1,25(OH)_2D_3$ on target cells.

D_3 was indeed metabolized into an active metabolite, which was identified as 25-hydroxyvitamin D_3 ($25OHD_3$ or calcidiol). $25OHD_3$ is almost exclusively produced in liver by a mitochondrial and/or a microsomal mixed-function oxidase system. The mitochondrial D_3 25-hydroxylase has been cloned and found to be a non-selective cytochrome P450 (CYP27) involved mainly in the C-27 hydroxylation of bile acids. $25OHD_3$ is not stocked in liver but is rapidly exported into the systemic circulation where it circulates bound to DBP (with only 0.04% found in the free form) at concentrations ranging from 38–125 nmol/l in normal individuals. However, the 25-hydroxylase is not a tightly regulated enzyme and the serum 25OHD concentrations are markedly elevated in hypervitaminosis D. In circulation, it has a long half-life which is estimated in human to be in the order of 3–4 weeks. Circulating 25OHD concentrations are considered one of the best indicators of the vitamin D nutritional status (Gascon-Barré, 1997).

In 1970, Fraser and Kodicek reported the exclusive production by the kidney of a metabolite more polar than $25OHD_3$. A year later, DeLuca's group as well as Kodicek's group independently identified this new metabolite as $1\alpha,25$-dihydroxyvitamin D_3 ($1,25(OH)_2D_3$ or calcitriol), the hormone of the vitamin D endocrine system. The enzyme 1α-hydroxylase is located in the mitochondrial inner membrane of the nephron proximal tubule. It is tightly regulated and the renal production of $1,25(OH)_2D_3$ depends on the need for calcium and phosphorus. The best characterized regulators of the renal 1α-hydroxylase are: PTH ($\Uparrow$), calcium restriction ($\Uparrow$)/supplementation ($\Downarrow$), phosphorus restriction ($\Uparrow$)/supplementation ($\Downarrow$), growth hormone ($\Uparrow$), and IGF ($\Uparrow$). It is also known that the enzyme is under a negative feedback by $1,25(OH)_2D_3$ itself (Henry, 1997). The 1α-hydroxylase gene has been cloned and identified as a member of the cytochrome P450 family ($P450_{VD1\alpha}$) (Takeyama et al., 1997) and its chromosomal location has been mapped to region 12q13.1–q13.3. Using mice null for the nuclear vitamin D receptor (VDR_n) gene ($VDR_n^{-/-}$), it was shown that regulation of the $P450_{VD1}$ α was dependent on the presence of a functional VDR_n (Takeyama et al., 1997). It is also known that extrarenal (monocytes/macrophages, intestine, bone, decidua, placenta, melanoma and vascular endothelial cells) synthesis of $1,25(OH)_2D_3$ is present in several physiopathological situations (Adams, 1997). However, regulation of the extrarenal 1α-hydroxylase, most particularly in macrophages, has been reported to be under the influence of second messengers, cytokines, hormones, or drugs such as NO, INFγ, dexamethasone or chloroquine/hydroxychloroquine. In normal human, $1,25(OH)_2D_3$ circulates at concentrations of 72 to 120 pmol/l while concentrations below 30 pmol/l are usually observed in chronic renal failure.

Vitamin D dependency rickets type I is an autosomal recessive disorder associated with a dysfunctional 1α-hydroxylase. The disease locus also maps to the chromosomal region containing the 1α-hydroxylase gene (St-Arnaud et al.,

1997b). As expected, D_3 or $25OHD_3$ supplementation is not effective in the treatment of the disorder whereas physiological doses of $1,25(OH)_2D_3$ are associated with a cure of the disease.

The C-24-hydroxylase is a mitochondrial mixed-function oxidase (CYP24) which, in human, is located on chromosome 20q13.2. The enzyme is largely expressed in $1,25(OH)_2$D-responsive cells. The C-24 hydroxylation of either $25OHD_3$ or $1,25(OH)_2D_3$ seems to be the initial and most important pathway for D metabolite elimination, although some 24-hydroxylated D metabolites are now suspected to harbor important biological properties. The 24-hydroxylase is highly enhanced by $1,25(OH)_2D_3$ through a VDR_n-dependent mechanism. Extremely low levels of 24-hydroxylated metabolites are found in VDR_n-null mice. In addition, reduced $1,25(OH)_2D_3$ clearance accompanied by signs of D intoxication and abnormal intramembranous ossification are observed in these animals as well as in those null for the 24-hydroxylase gene (St-Arnaud et al., 1997a).

Vitamin D action

$1,25(OH)_2D_3$, like other steroid hormones, exerts most of its actions through a specific nuclear receptor. VDR_n is a member of the steroid superfamily of receptors belonging to the subfamily shared by the thyroid hormone and retinoic acid receptors (DeLuca & Zierold, 1998). The gene encoding $hVDR_n$ has been shown to be localized to chromosome 12q13–q14 (Haussler et al., 1998). Lately, however, it has become increasingly evident that some actions of the vitamin can also be attributed to a non-genomic mechanism, presumably through a putative membrane receptor (VDR_m) although cloning of the VDR_m has not yet been achieved (Nemere et al., 1998).

Action mediated by the nuclear receptor

The classical actions of the hormone are mediated by the nuclear receptor. VDR_n mediates its action by specifically binding to a nuclear binding site of target genes, the vitamin D response elements (VDRE), following heterodimerization with the retinoid X receptor (RXR). When the two receptors are bound to VDRE, only the VDR binds its ligand and RXR, thus serves as a cofactor in the transcription complex. TFIIB also appears to be required for formation of the transcription complex. VDRE can be described by two direct repeats of GGTTCA (consensus) separated by three non-specific nucleotides (DR-3) (DeLuca & Zierold, 1998).

The action of the $1,25(OH)_2D_3$-VDR_n complex results in an increased intestinal absorption of calcium and phosphorus which, in turn, influences bone formation, mineralization and remodeling (Fig. 7.2). The $1,25(OH)_2D_3$-VDR_n complex is also known to elicit biological effects in several cell systems other than the classical organs involved in calcium and phosphorus metabolism. Indeed, VDR_n is also

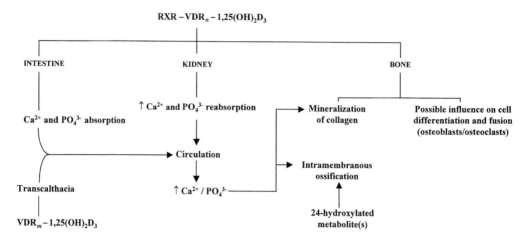

Fig. 7.2   Action of $1,25(OH)_2D_3$ in intestine, kidney and bone.

found in the parathyroid glands, islet cells of the pancreas, hematopoietic cells, promyelocytes, activated lymphocytes, T-cells of the thymus, keratinocytes of skin and reproductive organs, and in the central nervous system (DeLuca & Zierold, 1998). In target cells, VDR_n is able to mediate both transactivation (rat and human osteocalcin, mouse osteopontin, avian β_3 integrin, rat 24-hydroxylase, mouse $CaBP_{28K}$, NPT2, p21) and transrepression (avian and human PTH, rat osteocalcin, rat bone sialoprotein, PKA inhibitor, rat PTHrP- proximal and distal) (Haussler et al., 1998). Amongst the $1,25(OH)_2D_3$-responsive genes, the most tightly regulated is the 24-hydroxylase as its promoter region contains two separate VDR_n binding sites. VDR_n, at both the protein and gene level, has been shown to be regulated in an homologous as well as in an heterologous manner. In non-classical targets, $1,25(OH)_2D_3$ has been shown to influence cell growth and differentiation in normal and malignant tissues, act as an immunosuppressor, and play a role in reproduction and lactation (Feldman et al., 1996).

The disease known as vitamin D-dependency rickets type II is an autosomal recessive disorder, characterized by high circulating concentrations of $1,25(OH)_2D_3$. The disease is associated with a defective VDR_n which prevents its normal transactivating/transrepressing function. Children suffering from type II rickets seem to develop normally until approximately 9 months of age, at which time they develop severe rickets, alopecia and, in subsequent months, a large variety of disorders including dysfunction of the immune system (DeLuca & Zierold, 1998). VDR_n null mice are also born phenotypically normal and exhibit symptoms of rickets/osteomalacia and secondary hyperparathyroidism primarily after weaning (Haussler et al., 1998). Both type II rickets and the $VDR_n^{-/-}$ mouse model illustrate that VDR_n is essential for the normal function of the D_3 endocrine system.

VDR$_n$ polymorphisms

The hVDR$_n$ gene locus is composed of 11 exons (1a, 1b, 1c and 2 to 9) spanning approximately 70–75 kb of DNA. The mRNA transcript contains approximately 4800 nucleotides encoding a protein of 427 amino acids, the so-called M1 isoform of the receptor. The 5′ end of the hVDR$_n$ exhibits, however, alternate splice and/or translation start sites. In exon 2, the absence of a *Fok-1* restriction site (*F*) results in the initiation of translation at a site 3 amino acids downstream and in the production of a gene product 3 amino acids shorter thus giving rise to a neomorph hVDR$_n$ of 424 amino acids or M4 isoform (for initiation of translation at the fourth codon). Haussler et al. (1998) report that the M4 neomorph contributes approximately 65% of hVDR$_n$ alleles intimating an evolutionary advantage in humans. They also report that the M4 isoform is transcriptionally more active than the M1 isoform in a VDRE reporter construct. Moreover, it has now become apparent in the last few years, that VDR$_n$ exhibits several other allelic variations which have been reported in population studies to be linked to diseases such as osteoporosis (see p. 97), breast and prostate cancer, as well as primary hyperparathyroidism.

Markers of the *hVDR$_n$* gene locus are characterized by single diallelic restriction fragment polymorphisms (RFLP). The *Bsm-1* and *Apa-1* restriction endonuclease sites are located in the last intron, whereas a *Taq-1* RFLP in the form of a silent mutation is present within codon 352 of the ninth exon. A strong linkage disequilibrium has been observed between *Bsm-1* and *Taq-1*. Thus, the *B* allele (*BB* genotype represents homozygous absence of the *Bsm-1* restriction site) is mostly associated with the *Taq-1 t* allele (*tt* represents homozygous presence of the *Taq-1* restriction site). In nearly all studies reported to date, the *BB* genotype seems to be equivalent to the *tt* genotype so that, in homozygous form, genotypes for these markers present as either *BBtt* or *bbTT*.

Recently, an additional genetic variation in the hVDR$_n$ gene was found in the form of a microsatellite poly(A) repeat in the 3′UTR, approximately 1kb upstream of the poly(A) tail. Multiple allelic variants of this microsatellite were detected and classified into two groupings, long (L) and short (S), based on the length of the repeat. It has not been established, however, whether this poly (A) microsatellite is a functionally related locus (Haussler et al., 1998).

Interestingly, none of the observed polymorphisms reported to date are located in regions of the gene that affect the structure of the hVDR$_n$ protein.

Non-genomic action of 1,25(OH)$_2$D$_3$

1,25(OH)$_2$D$_3$ also mediates rapid non-genomic actions associated with a putative VDR$_m$ (Norman, 1998). A candidate 66 kDa 1,25(OH)$_2$D$_3$-binding protein has been partially purified from basal–lateral membrane preparations of chick intestine and also shown to be present and to be linked to biological activities in rat chondrocytes (Nemere et al., 1998). The non-genomic effects of $1,25(OH)_2D_3$ are thought to be mediated by a direct action of the hormone on target cell membranes to stimulate signal transduction pathways involving a rapid cellular response. It has been linked to the rapid translocation of calcium in the intestine (transcalthacia), elevation of intracellular calcium, opening of voltage-sensitive Ca^{2+} channels, the production of second messengers, alteration in phospholipid metabolism, phosphate transport, changes in alkaline phosphatase, adenylate cyclase activity, activation of protein kinase C and MAP kinase (Norman, 1998). Interestingly, it has also been shown that the effect of $1,25(OH)_2D_3$ on transcalthacia occurs in D replete but not in D-deficient animals. This observation, therefore, raises the hypothesis that a pre-existing condition to transcalthacia may be dependent on a VDR_n-mediated mechanism.

Effect of aging on vitamin D status, metabolism and action

Aging is suspected to harbor progressive abnormalities in the D endocrine system which are often compounded by a lifestyle where sun exposure is suboptimal and food intake below the recommended dietary allowances for several nutrients including D and calcium. Vitamin D and/or calcium deficiency, abnormal production of active D metabolites, or altered D responsiveness are key factors in the induction of a negative calcium balance. They, therefore, stand to significantly increase the risk of an imbalance in the dynamic interplay between bone formation and bone resorption due to the resulting alterations in calcium homeostasis which will trigger compensatory adaptation mechanisms in the calcium endocrine system most particularly in the calcium-D-PTH axis. Loss of bone mass could, therefore, result if these adaptive responses are inadequate or if they themselves promote an increase in the number of remodeling foci across the surface of trabecular bone (Silverberg et al., 1996).

Nutritional and hormonal status
Vitamin D

Several studies have reported that D depletion is quite prevalent in elderly subjects including postmenopausal women (Gloth et al., 1995; Thomas et al., 1998; Reid, 1996). Several investigators have reported that the cutaneous production of D_3 decreases with aging. Holick et al. (1989) have reported close to a 75% reduction in whole body production of D_3 in the elderly with synthesis of 20.8 nmol/l compared with 78.1 nmol/l in young individuals following whole body exposition to a single minimal erythemal dose of ultraviolet B radiation. This is compounded by changes in lifestyle in elderly subjects who, as mentioned above, often spend little time outdoors most particularly in the winter-time. In addition, sunscreen products which are now highly recommended as protective agents against skin cancer also decrease the cutaneous production of D_3 (Matsuoka et al., 1988).

Numerous studies have also reported decreases in calcium as well as in D intake despite the enrichment of food products such as milk with D. Others, on the other hand, have stressed that D intake does not change with aging if one considers availability of the vitamin through supplementation (Halloran & Portale, 1997). In addition, it has been reported that, in the absence of gastrointestinal diseases, there seems to be no significant change in D absorption with age until the eighth or ninth decade, a notion which is important when considering the efficacy of D supplementation regimens.

25OHD

Considering the reported prevalence of a suboptimal D nutritional status of both dietary and endogenous origin in aging subjects, it is not surprising to observe an accompanying decrease in the circulating 25OHD concentrations in this population. The observed decline in the serum concentrations of 25OHD seems to be due to the combined effect of decreased sun exposure and reduced dietary D intake as it has been observed that, in elderly subjects, 25OHD is positively influenced by wintertime travel, D intake and time spent outdoors and negatively related to weight and age. In addition, in elderly subjects, serum 25OHD concentrations have been reported to be inversely correlated with both serum PTH and markers of bone turnover (Halloran & Portale, 1997). In fact, serum PTH has been shown to rise slowly as the 25OHD concentrations declined below 110 nmol/l (with one study indicating that more than 90% of their cohort exhibited values below 110 nmol/l 25OHD in winter-time (Dawson-Hughes et al., 1997) although Chapuy and Meunier (1997) report that the lower limits of circulating 25OHD which initiate a frank PTH response range between 30 and 50 nmol/l. It is thus postulated that the high prevalence of low winter-time 25OHD may increase the risk of bone loss in elderly men and women. In most cases, D supplementation has been reported to increase serum 25OHD, decrease serum PTH, and also to normalize bone turnover (Halloran & Portale, 1997).

The decrease in circulating 25OHD concentrations observed in elderly subjects does not seem to be due to a decrease in the activity of the D 25-hydroxylase as there does not seem to be a decrease in CYP27 with aging in the absence of liver disease. In support of this observation, assessment of the serum $25OHD_3$ in response to ultraviolet irradiation has shown that there is no difference between young and old subjects including those suffering from osteoporosis. When plasma volume was taken into consideration, it was calculated that the increase in the circulating $25OHD_3$ following UV B irradiation was 0.024 nmol/cm^2 skin irradiated with no age or sex differences over a 17-day irradiation period (Davie & Lawson, 1980).

1,25(OH)$_2$D

It is still not clear whether the serum 1,25(OH)$_2$D concentrations significantly change with advancing age. In men and women, both decreased, unchanged or increased values have been reported. The majority of data reported in women, however, suggest that serum 1,25(OH)$_2$D concentrations in healthy women remain stable or tend to gradually increase through the eighth decade and that menopause has little effect on serum 1,25(OH)$_2$D concentrations. In contrast, others have shown that estrogen deficiency leads to a decreased serum 1,25(OH)$_2$D regardless of age, and that estrogen replacement in postmenopausal women increases both total and free 1,25(OH)$_2$D (Halloran & Portale, 1997).

Animal studies have revealed that, when comparing animals of similar renal function (normal or near normal glomerular filtration rate (GFR)), the levels of 1,25(OH)$_2$D do not seem to decrease with aging and the reported low serum 1,25(OH)$_2$D reflects in large part the age-related fall in GFR (Halloran & Portale, 1997). It is postulated that this observation may well be relevant to the pathogenesis of senile (type 2) osteoporosis (Reid, 1996). In addition, despite increased PTH concentrations with advancing age and a normal response to exogenous PTH (implying a normal 1α-hydroxylase activity), it has been proposed that the serum 1,25(OH)$_2$D concentrations do not change because the levels of GH and IGF-I decrease with aging, an observation which is well illustrated by the fact that serum 1,25(OH)$_2$D concentrations have been reported to increase in elderly subjects treated with GH (Halloran & Portale, 1997). In younger groups of patients with vertebral (type 1) osteoporosis, however, a tendency for 1,25(OH)$_2$D concentrations to be lower has been reported quite often in association with a decrease in serum PTH. This observation supports the hypothesis that circulating PTH tends to be lower in subjects with type 1 osteoporosis than in age-matched subjects due to an increase in the rate of bone resorption. These findings suggest that the changes in 1,25(OH)$_2$D synthesis found in type 1 osteoporosis may represent an appropriate physiological response to increased bone resorption rather than a primary contributor to the osteoporotic process (Reid, 1996).

Vitamin D action

End-organ responsiveness

It has been suggested that the decrease in calcium absorption with age may be related to a decreased intestinal responsiveness to 1,25(OH)$_2$D$_3$ although controversy still exists on that subject. Animal studies have tended to show a decline with age in intestinal calcium uptake, the number of intestinal VDR$_n$, the calbindin response, and the effect of 1,25(OH)$_2$D$_3$ administration on calcium absorption. In a human study, direct measurements of duodenal VDR$_n$ content have shown an age- related decrease of about 30% between the ages of 20 and 80 (Eastell & Riggs,

1997). However, another study has shown that the calcium absorption response to a low calcium diet-induced increase in endogenous $1,25(OH)_2D_3$ was not affected by age. In addition, the reported reduced intestinal calcium absorption observed in some osteoporotic subjects may be related to a physiologically relevant lowering of the $1,25(OH)_2D_3$ concentrations rather than to an altered intestinal responsiveness particularly in type 1 osteoporosis where bone resorption is increased (Reid, 1996).

hVDR$_n$ polymorphisms and bone

Bone mineral density, size and turnover have been proposed to be under genetic regulation. In fact, allelic variations in the hVDR$_n$ have been reported in several studies to correlate with bone mineral density (BMD) as well as with body size in early childhood (Eisman, 1998). Other genetic, hormonal and/or environmental factors are also suspected to interact in the determination of peak bone mass and its subsequent age-related decline. However, the effect of the presently identified hVDR$_n$ polymorphisms on BMD has not been reported in all ethnic groups and the intensity of the effect of certain allelic patterns also varies considerably between studies.

In 1994, Morrison et al. (1994) presented data indicating that hVDR$_n$ alleles could predict BMD. The authors reported that the *bb* genotype was associated with enhanced lumbar spine BMD while the *BB* genotype was correlated with low BMD. However, subsequent studies in other populations have found either modest or no association between the *B* or the *b* alleles and BMD. Lately, Cooper & Umbach (1996) in a meta-analysis compiling 16 hVDR$_n$ polymorphic studies revealed the presence of only a 1.5–2.5% decrease in BMD associated with the *BB* genotype compared with the 12% effect proposed in the original Australian study (Morrison et al., 1994). It has now become clear that other confounding factors such as allelic differences in the estrogen receptor, the TGFβ and collagen IIα genes, age, estrogen status, ethnicity, lifestyle, and D and calcium intake must be accounted for to reveal the true impact of the VDR$_n$ polymorphisms on body size, bone size, BMD and the subsequent development of osteoporosis (Eisman, 1998).

As mentioned by Haussler et al. (1998), the importance of the poly(A) microsatellite as a functionally related locus in the determination of BMD has not yet been established, although by analogy to short tandem repeats in other genes, the length of the repeat may affect crucial parameters, such as mRNA stability. Alternatively, the poly(A) microsatellite may also be tightly linked to another (still unidentified) site which is the true functional locus. In addition, despite its reported increase in in vitro transcriptional activity (Haussler et al., 1998), the importance of the M4 VDR$_n$ isoform as a potential protective variable against an accelerated loss of bone mass has not either yet been established.

Therapeutic intervention

As mentioned above, D deficiency is quite prevalent in the elderly population. Moreover, D deficiency has been reported by several investigators to be correlated with BMD in both the lumbar spine and, in older women, in the femur as well. D depletion is, therefore, of particular concern because it is known to lead to compensatory hyperparathyroidism with its accompanying increased bone turnover which increases the risk of accelerated loss of BMD and of subsequent fractures in this vulnerable population (Chapuy & Meunier, 1997).

However, D supplementation or D metabolite therapy in normal elderly subjects and in those suffering from osteoporosis is still an area of substantial controversy.

Supplementation with D_3

Most studies to date indicate beneficial effects of D supplementation on mineral balance and bone mass in elderly presenting a subnormal D status, but not in those receiving an adequate supply of calcium and D.

In institutionalized or marginally deficient elderly individuals living in the community, daily supplementation regimens with 500 to 800 IU D_3 in association with 500 to 1200 mg of calcium have been shown to maintain normal circulating 25OHD and PTH concentrations. It has also been shown to lead to positive changes in biochemical markers of bone turnover, to reduce bone loss at several sites, and to significantly reduce the incidence of non-vertebral fracture in subjects receiving the intervention than in those receiving a placebo regimen (Chapuy & Meunier, 1997; O'Brien, 1998; Reid, 1998). In fact, Chapuy et al. (1992, 1994) estimated that D_3 and calcium supplementation in elderly women significantly reduced the probability of non-vertebral and hip fractures after 18 to 36 months of treatment. These observations suggest that an optimal intake of both calcium and D may be an easy, cost-effective and safe strategy to implement in order to maintain existing bone mass and reduce the risk of fractures in older men and women (Chapuy & Meunier, 1997; O'Brien, 1998). Supplementation with pharmacological doses of D is not, however, considered beneficial and may lead to serious side effects such as hypercalcemia, calcification of vascular atheromatous plaques, as well as hypercalciuria (Reid, 1998).

$1,25(OH)_2D_3$ or $1\alpha OHD_3$ therapy

There seems to be a consensus on an absence of beneficial effects of $1,25(OH)_2D_3$ administration in normal postmenopausal women between the ages of 50 and 79 (Reid, 1996). However, $1\alpha OHD_3$ has been reported to be beneficial in women whose habitual diet is low in calcium. It is hypothesized that $1\alpha OHD_3$ (which is readily converted to $1,25(OH)_2D_3$ by the hepatic 25-hydroxylase) most likely improves calcium absorption and hence protects against the loss of BMD.

In osteoporotic women receiving the higher calcium intake, $1,25(OH)_2D_3$ in doses 0.5 μg/d or above has also been reported to exhibit beneficial effects on bone density. The hormone seems to achieve this end by increasing intestinal calcium absorption and suppressing PTH stimulation of bone turnover, thus, acting as an antiresorptive agent. However, estrogen replacement therapy and second and third generation bisphosphonates produce severalfold greater increases in spinal bone density than the D hormone. Thus, the use of $1,25(OH)_2D_3$ or of D_3 analogs is an attractive adjunctive therapy rather than a first or second line therapy in situations where intestinal calcium absorption seems to be a factor limiting the overall efficacy of an osteoporosis treatment regimen (Reid, 1996).

In conclusion, in elderly men and women at risk for D deficiency, the evidence suggests significant reductions in non-vertebral fracture rates with physiological replacement regimen particularly when D is combined with calcium supplementation. As mentioned by Reid (1998), it is not yet clear, however, which compound is the principal active agent as calcium monotherapy has also been shown to exhibit beneficial effects at several skeletal sites as well as on fracture incidence (particularly in the first year of treatment in subjects with low calcium intake), or whether the D-calcium combination therapy is necessary for optimal antifracture efficacy.

Note added in proof

$P450_{VD1\alpha}$ has now been named cyp27B1.

REFERENCES

Adams, J. S. (1997). Extrarenal production and action of active vitamin D metabolites in human lymphoproliferative diseases. In *Vitamin D*, ed. D. Feldman, F. H. Glorieux, & J.W. Pike, pp. 903–21. San Diego, CA: Academic Press.

Chapuy, M. C. & Meunier, P. J. (1997). Vitamin D insufficiency in adults and the elderly. In *Vitamin D*, ed. D. Feldman, F. H. Glorieux, & J. W. Pike, pp. 679–93. San Diego, CA: Academic Press.

Chapuy, M. C., Arlot, M., Duboeuf, F., Brun, J., Crouzet, B., Arnaud, S., Delmas, P., & Meunier, P. (1992). Vitamin D_3 and calcium to prevent hip fractures in elderly women. *N. Engl. J. Med.*, **327**, 1637–42.

Chapuy, M. C., Arlot, M. E., Delmas, P. D., & Meunier, P. J. (1994). Effect of calcium and cholecalciferol treatment for three years on hip fractures in elderly women. *Br. Med. J.*, **308**, 1081–2.

Cooper, G. S. & Umbach, D. M. (1996). Are vitamin D receptor polymorphisms associated with bone mineral density? A meta-analysis. *J. Bone Miner. Res.*, **11**, 1841–9.

Davie, M. & Lawson, D. E. M. (1980). Assessment of plasma 25-hydroxyvitamin D response to ultraviolet irradiation over a controlled area in young and elderly subjects. *Clin. Sci.*, **58**, 235–42.

Dawson-Hughes, B., Harris, S. S., Krall, E. A., & Dallal, G. E. (1997). Effect of calcium and vitamin D supplementation on bone density in men and women 65 years of age or older. *N. Engl. J. Med.*, **337**, 670–6.

DeLuca, H. F. & Zierold, C. (1998). Mechanisms and functions of vitamin D. *Nutr. Rev.*, **56**, S4–S10.

Eastell, R. & Riggs, B. L. (1997). Vitamin D and osteoporosis. In *Vitamin D*, ed. D. Feldman, F. H. Glorieux, & J. W. Pike, pp. 695–711. San Diego, CA: Academic Press.

Eisman, J. A. (1998). Vitamin D polymorphisms and calcium homeostasis: a new concept of normal gene variants and physiologic variation. *Nutr. Rev.*, **56**, S22–9.

Feldman, D., Malloy, P. J., & Gross, C. (1996). Vitamin D: Metabolism and Action. In *Osteoporosis*, ed. R. Marcus, D. Feldman, & J. Kelsey, pp. 205–35. San Diego, CA: Academic Press.

Gascon-Barré, M. (1997). The vitamin D 25-hydroxylase. In *Vitamin D*, ed. D. Feldman, F. H. Glorieux, & J.W. Pike, pp. 41–55. San Diego, CA: Academic Press.

Gloth, F. M., Gundberg, C. M., Hollis, B. W., Haddad, J. G., & Tobin, J. D. (1995). Vitamin D deficiency in homebound elderly persons. *J. Am. Med. Ass.*, **274**, 1683–6.

Halloran, B. P. & Portale, A. A. (1997). Vitamin D metabolism: The effects of aging. In *Vitamin D*, ed. D. Feldman, F. H. Glorieux, & J. W. Pike, pp. 541–54. San Diego, CA: Academic Press.

Haussler, M. R., Witfield, G. K., Haussler, C. A., Hsieh, J. C., Thompson, P .D., Selznick, S. H., Dominguez, C. E., & Jurutka, P. W. (1998). The nuclear vitamin D receptor: biological and molecular regulatory properties revealed. *J. Bone Miner. Res.*, **13**, 325–49.

Henry, H. L. (1997). The 25-hydroxyvitamin D 1α-hydroxylase. In *Vitamin D*, ed. D. Feldman, F. H. Glorieux, & J. W. Pike, pp. 57–68. San Diego, CA: Academic Press.

Holick, M. F., Matsuoka, L. Y., & Wortsman, J. (1989). Age, vitamin D and solar ultraviolet. *Lancet*, **ii**, 1104–5.

Matsuoka, L. Y., Wortsman, J., Hanifan, N., & Holick, M. F. (1988). Chronic sunscreen use decreases circulating concentrations of 25-hydroxyvitamin D. *Arch. Dermatol.*, **124**, 1802–4.

Mawer, E. B., Backhouse, J., Holman, C. A., Lumb, G. A., & Stanbury, S. W. (1972). The distribution and storage of vitamin D and its metabolites in human tissues. *Clin. Sci.*, **43**, 413–31.

Morrison, N. A., Qi, J. C., Tokita, A., Kelly, P. J., Crofts, L., Nguyen, T. V., Sambrook, P. N., & Eisman, J.A. (1994). Prediction of bone density from vitamin D receptor alleles. *Nature*, **367**, 284–7.

Nemere, I., Schwartz, Z., Pedrozo, H., Sylvia, V. L., Dean, D. D., & Boyan, B. D. (1998). Identification of a membrane receptor for 1,25-dihydroxyvitamin D_3 which mediates rapid activation of protein kinase C. *J. Bone Miner. Res.*, **13**, 1353–9.

Norman, A. W. (1998). Receptors for 1,25(OH)$_2$D$_3$: past, present, and future. *J. Bone Miner. Res.*, **13**, 1360–9.

O'Brien, K. O. (1998). Combined calcium and vitamin D supplementation reduces bone loss and fracture incidence in older men and women. *Nutr. Rev.*, **1**, 148–58.

Reid, I. R. (1996). Vitamin D and its metabolites in the management of osteoporosis. In *Osteoporosis*, ed. R. Marcus, D. Feldman, and J. Kelsey, pp. 1169–90. San Diego, CA: Academic Press.

Reid, I. R. (1998). The roles of calcium and vitamin D in the prevention of osteoporosis. In *Endocrinology and Metabolism Clinics of North America*, ed. N. B. Watts, pp. 389–98. WB Saunders Co.

Silverberg, S. J., Fitzpatrick, L. A., & Bilezikian, J. P. (1996). The role of parathyroid hormone and vitamin D in the pathogenesis of osteoporosis. In *Osteoporosis*, ed. R. Marcus, D. Feldman, and J. Kelsey, pp. 715–26. San Diego, CA: Academic Press.

St-Arnaud, R., Arabian, A., Travers, R., & Glorieux, F. H. (1997a). Partial rescue of abnormal bone formation in 24-hydroxylase knock-out mice supports a role for $24,25(OH)_2D_3$ in intramembranous ossification. *J. Bone Miner. Res.*, **12**, S111(Abstract).

St-Arnaud, R., Messerlian, S., Moir, J. M., Omdahl, J. L., & Glorieux, F. H. (1997b). The 25-hydroxyvitamin D 1-alpha-hydroxylase gene maps to the pseudovitamin D-deficiency rickets (PDDR) disease locus. *J. Bone Miner. Res.*, **12**, 1552–9.

Takeyama, K. I., Kitanaka, S., Sato, T., Kobori, M., Yanagisawa, J., & Kato, S. (1997). 25-hydroxyvitamin D_3 1-hydroxylase and vitamin D synthesis. *Science*, **277**, 1827–30.

Thomas, M. K., Lloyd-Jones, D. M., Thadhani, R. I., Shaw, A. C., Deraska, D. J., Kitch, B. T., Vamvakas, E. C., Dick, I. M., Prince, R. L., & Finkelstein, J. S. (1998). Hypovitaminosis D in medical in patients. *N. Engl. J. Med.*, **338**, 777–83.

8

Sodium-dependent phosphate transport in kidney, bone and intestine

Harriet S. Tenenhouse

Introduction

Inorganic phosphate (Pi) is a nutrient that is essential for cell function and skeletal mineralization. To accommodate these needs, transport systems have evolved to permit the efficient transfer of Pi anions across hydrophobic membrane barriers. Dietary Pi intake in North America is generally above the RDA and, except for the elderly where low Pi intakes are relatively common, Pi deficiency is unlikely to occur. The major proportion of ingested Pi is absorbed in the small intestine. Hormonal regulation of this process plays only a minor role in the maintenance of Pi homeostasis. Absorbed Pi is either incorporated into organic forms in cells, deposited into bone, or filtered by the kidney. Under normal conditions, only a small percentage of ingested Pi is retained and most of the absorbed Pi is excreted in the urine. The kidney is a major determinant of Pi homeostasis and tubular handling of Pi is subject to regulation by Pi intake and metabolic requirement. The molecular mechanisms involved in these processes are complex and are currently being investigated.

The present chapter will summarize our current knowledge of the cellular and molecular mechanisms involved in the transport of Pi by kidney, bone and intestine. Citations to review articles will be provided where possible.

Renal phosphate transport

Pi transport in the kidney has been the subject of intense investigation and much of the material discussed below is covered in more detail in review articles (see Berndt & Knox, 1992; Gmaj & Murer, 1986; Levi et al., 1997; Mizgala & Quamme, 1985; Murer, 1992; Murer & Biber, 1996a, 1996b, 1997; Murer et al., 1991, 1998; Tenenhouse, 1997, 1999; Wehrle & Pedersen, 1989).

The proximal tubule is the major site of Pi reabsorption, with approximately 60% of the filtered load reclaimed in the proximal convoluted tubule and 15–20% in the proximal straight tubule. In addition, a small but variable portion ($<10\%$)

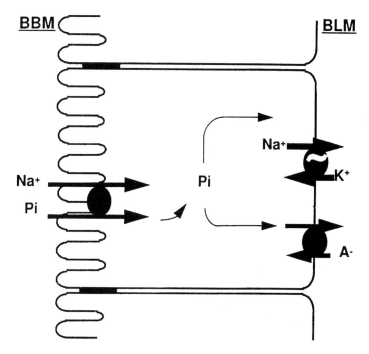

Fig. 8.1   Renal proximal tubular transepithelial Pi transport. Pi entry across the brush border
membrane (BBM) occurs against an electrochemical gradient. The driving force is the Na^+
gradient (outside>inside) maintained by the Na^+,K^+-ATPase at the basolateral membrane
(BLM). It is postulated that Pi is transported out of the cell at the BLM via an anion (A^-)
exchange system.

of filtered Pi is reabsorbed in more distal segments of the nephron. A wide variety
of experimental approaches have been used to characterize renal Pi transport
systems and to elucidate the mechanisms involved in their regulation. These range
from in vivo studies in intact animal models to in vitro studies using purified membrane preparations.

Transepithelial Pi transport is essentially unidirectional and involves uptake
across the brush border membrane (BBM), translocation across the cell and efflux
at the basolateral membrane (Fig. 8.1). Pi uptake at the apical cell surface is the rate-
limiting step in the overall Pi reabsorptive process and the major site of its regulation. It is mediated by Na^+-dependent Pi transporters that reside in the BBM and
depends on the basolateral membrane-associated Na^+,K^+-ATPase to maintain the
Na^+ gradient (outside>inside) that drives the transport process (Fig. 8.1). Na^+/Pi
stoichiometries of both 2:1 and 3:1 have been documented and, given that at
physiological pH both divalent and monovalent anions are present (HPO_4^{2-}/
$H_2PO_4^{1-}$=4/1 at pH 7.4), the transport is both electroneutral and electrogenic.

Na$^+$–Pi co-transport across the BBM is sensitive to changes in pH and is increased 10- to 20-fold when the pH is raised from 6 to 8.5.

Two kinetically distinct Na$^+$-Pi cotransport systems have been identified in the BBM: (i) a high capacity, low affinity system in the proximal convoluted tubule in a position to reabsorb the bulk of filtered Pi, and (ii) a low capacity, high affinity system in the proximal convoluted and straight tubules in a position to reclaim residual Pi (Walker et al., 1987). This topological arrangement of Na$^+$–Pi co-transport systems in series permits highly efficient reabsorption of Pi in the proximal tubule.

Little is known about the translocation of Pi across the cell except that Pi anions rapidly equilibrate with intracellular inorganic and organic phosphate pools. There is also a paucity of data regarding the mechanisms involved in the efflux of Pi at the basolateral cell surface. The latter appears to be a passive process that is driven by the electrical gradient existing across the membrane and occurs via an anion exchange mechanism (Fig. 8.1).

Structural identification of renal Na$^+$-phosphate cotransport systems

cDNAs encoding renal-specific Na$^+$-Pi co-transporters have been identified in several species, first by expression cloning in *Xenopus laevis* oocytes and then by homology screening. The cDNAs, designated NPT1 (type I) and NPT2 (type II), encode two classes of Na$^+$–Pi co-transporters that share only 20% identity. The NPT1 transporters are approximately 465 amino acids in length with seven to nine membrane spanning segments whereas the NPT2 transporters are composed of approximately 635 amino acids and are predicted to span the membrane eight times. The NPT1 and NPT2 genes have been mapped to human chromosomes 6p22 (Chong et al., 1993) and 5q35 (Kos et al., 1994), respectively, by fluorescence *in situ* hybridization. The human and murine NPT2/*Npt2* genes have recently been cloned and characterized (Hartmann et al., 1996).

NPT1 and NPT2 transcripts have been localized to the proximal tubule and NPT1 and NPT2 immunoreactive proteins to the BBM of proximal tubular cells. While NPT1 is uniformly expressed in all segments of the proximal nephron, NPT2 expression is highest in the S1 segments of the proximal tubule.

Functional studies of NPT1 and NPT2 have been conducted in cRNA-injected oocytes and in cDNA-transfected renal cell lines. Both NPT1 and NPT2 mediate high affinity Na$^+$–Pi co-transport. However, their pH profiles differ significantly, with that of NPT2 bearing closer resemblance to the pH-dependence of Na$^+$–Pi co-transport in renal BBM vesicles. Moreover, NPT1 appears to exhibit a broader substrate specificity than NPT2. For example, NPT1 can induce a Cl$^-$ conductance that is inhibited by Cl$^-$ channel blockers and organic anions. On the basis of these findings it was suggested that NPT1 not only mediates BBM Na$^+$-dependent Pi transport but also serves as an apical channel for Cl^- transport and the excretion of anionic xenobiotics. The precise physiological role of NPT1 will thus require further study.

Two novel Pi transporters have been identified in the kidney. Both are cell surface viral receptors (gibbon ape leukemia virus (Glvr-1) and murine amphotropic virus (Ram-1)) that mediate high affinity, electrogenic Na^+-dependent Pi transport when expressed in oocytes and in mammalian cells (Kavanaugh et al., 1994). Although Glvr-1 and Ram-1 show no sequence similarity to NPT1 or NPT2, they share 60% sequence identity with a putative Pi permease of *Neurospora crassa*. Glvr-1 and Ram-1 are widely expressed in mammalian tissues and may serve as 'housekeeping' Na^+–Pi co-transporters. Additional studies are necessary to define the localization of Glvr-1 and Ram-1 in the kidney and determine whether they play a significant role in renal Pi reabsorption.

Hormonal regulation

PTH is the major hormonal regulator of renal Pi reabsorption. PTH acts directly on proximal tubular cells and inhibits Na^+-dependent Pi transport by mechanisms which are dependent on both the cAMP-protein kinase A and protein kinase C (PKC)-phosphoinositide signaling pathways (Cole et al., 1987). PTH decreases the V_{max} of both high capacity, low affinity and low capacity, high affinity BBM Na^+–Pi co-transport systems. Direct evidence for internalization of cell surface NPT2 protein in response to PTH was obtained by immunohistochemistry (Kempson et al., 1995) and, furthermore, agents that interfere with the endocytic pathway disrupt the action of PTH on Na^+–Pi co-transport. Additionally, a recent study provided evidence for PTH-mediated degradation of NPT2 protein in the lysosomal/endosomal fraction of proximal tubular cells (Pfister et al., 1998b).

Other hormones also contribute to the regulation of proximal tubular Pi transport. Growth hormone, insulin-like growth factor-I, insulin, thyroid hormone and 1,25-dihydroxyvitamin D_3 all stimulate Pi reabsorption, whereas PTH-related peptide, calcitonin, atrial natriuretic factor, epidermal growth factor, transforming growth factor-α and glucocorticoids inhibit Pi reclamation. The increase in BBM Na^+–Pi co-transport by thyroid hormone is associated with an increase in NPT2 mRNA, whereas both dexamethasone and epidermal growth factor decreased NPT2 mRNA abundance. Because thyroid hormone and glucocorticoids exert their effects on gene transcription, via ligand activated receptors that bind to response elements in the promoter region of target genes, it was suggested that these hormones exert their effects by modulating NPT2 gene transcription. However, neither thyroid hormone nor dexamethasone have an effect on NPT2 promoter–reporter gene expression (see Hilfiker et al., 1998), suggesting that transcriptional mechanisms are not involved. Moreover, recent studies have been unable to detect a thyroid hormone-mediated increase in NPT2 mRNA (see Hilfiker et al., 1998).

Stanniocalcin, a peptide hormone that counteracts hypercalcemia and stimulates Pi reabsorption in bony fish, is also produced by humans. The infusion of human stanniocalcin in rats elicits a stimulation in renal Pi reabsorption which is associated with an increase in BBM Na^+–Pi co-transport (Wagner et al., 1997). These findings suggest that stanniocalcin may contribute to the overall maintenance of Pi homeostasis in mammals as well as in fish.

5-Hydroxytryptamine (5-HT) is synthesized in the kidney and locally generated 5-HT was shown to interfere with PTH-mediated inhibition of renal Na^+–Pi co-transport (Hafdi et al., 1996). On the basis of these findings, it was suggested that 5-HT is a paracrine modulator of renal Pi transport.

Regulation by dietary phosphate

Dietary Pi intake is a major regulator of renal Pi handling. Pi deprivation elicits an increase in Pi reabsorption which is attributable to an adaptive increase in BBM Na^+–Pi co-transport. Both acute and chronic exposure to low Pi elicit an increase in transport V_{max} that is associated with an increase in NPT2 protein but not NPT2 mRNA (Pfister et al., 1998a). This finding is consistent with recent data demonstrating that low Pi has no effect on NPT2 promoter activity (Hilfiker et al., 1998). The acute response to low Pi is mediated by microtubule-dependent recruitment of existing Na^+–Pi co-transporter protein to the apical membrane (Lotscher et al., 1997). In contrast, exposure to high Pi leads to the internalization of cell surface NPT2 protein into the endosomal compartment by a microtubule-independent mechanism (Lotscher et al., 1997). Internalized NPT2 protein is then subject to lysosomal degradation (Pfister et al., 1998a).

While NPT1 gene expression is not markedly increased by Pi restriction, Glvr-1 and Ram-1 are regulated by extracellular Pi at both the mRNA and functional level (Kavanaugh et al., 1994). The signal for the adaptive response to Pi deprivation is not known. However, it has been suggested that a fall in the cellular Pi concentration plays a role in initiating the Pi transport response.

A new gene product, diphor-1, which is upregulated by dietary Pi restriction was recently identified in kidney by differential display–polymerase chain reaction (Custer et al., 1997). It is a 52-kDa protein that exhibits a high degree of identity with the Na/H exchanger regulatory protein and a tyrosine kinase activating protein. It is highly expressed in the proximal tubule and intestine and specifically increases Na^+–Pi co-transport in oocytes co-injected with NPT2 cRNA. Further work is necessary to determine the precise role of diphor-1 in the renal adaptive response to low Pi.

Inherited disorders of renal phosphate handling

Three Mendelian disorders of Pi homeostasis, X-linked hypophosphatemia (XLH) (Rasmussen & Tenenhouse, 1995), autosomal dominant hypophosphatemic rickets (ADHR) (Econs et al., 1997) and hereditary hypophosphatemic rickets with hypercalciuria (HHRH) (Rasmussen & Tenenhouse, 1995), have received considerable attention. All are characterized by rachitic bone disease, decreased growth rate and short stature, hypophosphatemia and impaired renal Pi reabsorption. Features that distinguish XLH, ADHR and HHRH are their mode of inheritance (X-linked for XLH and autosomal for ADHR and HHRH), and the presence of an associated defect in renal vitamin D metabolism in XLH and ADHR but not in HHRH.

The mutant gene in patients with XLH was identified by positional cloning and designated PHEX (formerly PEX) to signify a Pi-regulating gene with homology to endopeptidases that maps to the X chromosome (The HYP Consortium, 1995). Furthermore, 5′ and 3′ deletions in the Phex gene have been demonstrated in the Hyp and Gy murine homologues of XLH (Beck et al., 1997; Strom et al., 1997). ADHR was recently mapped to human chromosome 12q13 by linkage analysis (Econs et al., 1997), and efforts to identify the gene by positional cloning are in progress. The gene responsible for HHRH has not yet been identified. However, the similarity of the biochemical phenotype in HHRH patients and mice homozygous for the disrupted NPt2 gene (Beck et al., 1998) suggests that NPT2 may be a candidate gene for HHRH. However, linkage analysis with polymorphic markers that flank the NPT2 on human chromosome 5q35, as well as sequence analysis of NPT2 exons in HHRH patients have established that mutations in NPT2 are not responsible for HHRH (Jones et al., 1999).

Phosphate transport in bone

Osteoblasts and matrix vesicles

Because Pi is essential for the mineralization of extracellular matrix and is a vital element for osteogenic cell function, a considerable effort has been devoted to the characterization of Pi transport in osteoblasts (see Caverzasio and Bonjour, 1996). These studies have relied primarily on osteoblast cell lines such as human osteosarcoma-derived SaOS-2 cells, rat osteosarcoma-derived UMR-106 and ROS 17/2.8 cells, and murine- and rat-calvarial-derived MC3T3–E1 and PyMS cells, respectively. To what extent data generated from these in vitro studies reflect the in vivo situation remains to be determined.

Pi transport in osteoblast cell cultures, like that in many other cell types, is Na^+-dependent and regulated by extracellular Pi concentration, with transport activity increasing as the Pi concentration in the culture medium is decreased. Regulation of Na^+-dependent Pi transport in osteoblasts is also achieved by a variety of hormones and other agents, all of which are of interest because of their potential therapeutic applications. PTH and PTHrP stimulate Na^+-dependent Pi uptake by a mechanism that is cAMP dependent. The basis for the differential PTH and PTHrP effects on Na^+–Pi co-transport in osteoblasts and renal proximal tubular cells, where an inhibition in Pi transport is elicited, is not clear. IGF-I, PDGF (platelet-derived growth factor), and fluoride increase Na^+–Pi co-transport by mechanisms that depend on tyrosine phosphorylation. Prostaglandin E_2 also stimulates Na^+–Pi co-transport but, in this case, protein kinase C plays a crucial role in mediating the response (Veldman et al., 1998).

Recently, it was demonstrated that Glvr-1, the ubiquitously expressed cell surface gibbon ape leukemia viral receptor that mediates high affinity, Na^+-dependent Pi transport, is expressed in SaOS-2 cells (Palmer et al., 1997). Moreover, it was demonstrated that the increase in Na^+–Pi co-transport elicited by IGF-I in SaOS-2 cells is associated with a comparable increase in the relative abundance of Glvr-1 mRNA. Further studies are necessary to determine the relative contribution of Glvr-1 to Pi transport in osteoblasts and to identify other Na^+–Pi co-transporters that participate in this process.

Pi transport has also been examined in matrix vesicles, structures derived from osteoblasts, by budding from elongated tubular extensions that project from the plasma membrane of these cells (Caverzasio & Bonjour, 1996). Pi transport in matrix vesicles is Na^+-dependent and reflects the transport activity of the cells from which they originated. It has been proposed that Pi accumulation inside the matrix vesicles is involved in the formation of nucleation sites that are necessary for initiation of the calcification process.

Osteoclasts

Osteoclasts are polarized cells that are involved in bone resorption. They exhibit Na^+-dependent Pi transport which is believed to mediate the transcellular movement of Pi that is released from bone into the resorption cavity (Gupta et al., 1996). Na^+–Pi co-transport in enriched osteoclast preparations is stimulated by the addition of bone particles and is inhibited by the RGDS (arg–gly–asp–ser) motif, suggesting that integrins and cell–matrix interactions are involved in the regulation of the transport process (Gupta et al., 1996). Recent evidence suggests that an NPT2-like Na^+–Pi co-transporter is expressed in osteoclasts. The transporter is localized to discrete vesicles in unpolarized osteoclasts whereas in actively resorbing cells it is associated with the basolateral membrane (Gupta et al., 1997). These data suggest that an NPT2-related Na^+–Pi co-transporter in osteoclasts functions to clear Pi from the resorption cavity. Furthermore, since agents that inhibit Na^+–Pi co-transport also inhibit bone resorption, it has been suggested that Pi transport in the osteoclast plays a key role in the bone resorptive process.

Intestinal phosphate transport

Pi absorption by the small intestine has been investigated by a variety of approaches, ranging from in vivo methods, where the appearance of labeled Pi in the blood is monitored as a function of time after its oral administration, to in vitro studies where the measurement of Pi fluxes across purified mucosal or serosal membrane vesicle preparations are assayed. The studies demonstrate that there are numerous similarities between intestinal and renal transepithelial Pi transport (see Danisi & Murer, 1991). Pi ingested in the diet is transported from the small intestinal lumen across the mucosal brush border membrane against an electrochemical gradient. Mucosal Pi transport is saturable, Na^+-dependent, and is driven by a Na^+–gradient (outside$>$inside), that is maintained by the basolateral membrane-associated Na^+,K^+-ATPase, as described for the renal proximal tubule (Fig. 8.1). The exit of Pi at the serosal surface occurs down an electrochemical gradient and has not been well characterized. However, evidence suggests that the process is carrier mediated, Na^+ independent and electrogenic.

Mucosal Na^+–Pi co-transport is pH-dependent, but unlike the kidney, transport activity is stimulated by lowering the pH from 7.4 to 6. Pi transport across the mucosal membrane is regulated by $1,25(OH)_2D$ and dietary intake of Pi (Cross et al., 1990; Danisi & Murer, 1991). Administration of the vitamin D hormone to either vitamin D deficient or replete animals results in a significant increase in net Pi absorption which is asscoiated with a corresponding increase in Na^+–Pi co-transport V_{max} across the mucosal brush border membrane. These findings, combined with the demonstration that Na^+-dependent Pi transport across the mucosal brush border membrane correlates with intestinal transepithelial Pi transport, uphold the notion that apical Pi uptake is the rate limiting step in Pi absorption by the instestine.

The response of intestinal Pi transport to $1,25(OH)_2D$ is dependent on protein synthesis and occurs several hours after administration. Moreover, it is only apparent after weaning. Recent studies in a pig model with defective renal synthesis of $1,25(OH)_2D$ demonstrated that intestinal brush border membrane Na^+–Pi co-transport V_{max} is similar in mutant and wild-type newborns, but is significantly reduced in mutant weanlings relative to normal weanlings (Schroder et al., 1998). Moreover, while $1,25(OH)_2D$ had no effect on apical Pi transport in mutant newborns, correction of the Pi transport in mutant weanlings was achieved by the administration of $1,25(OH)_2D$. The same study also showed that intestinal Na^+-dependent Pi transport is highly age dependent and decreases significantly in the first 7 days postpartum in both normal and mutant piglets.

Low Pi diet also elicits an increase in mucosal Na^+-dependent Pi transport. However, the response to Pi restriction is likely mediated by $1,25(OH)_2D$. It is well known that the renal synthesis of the vitamin D hormone is stimulated by hypophosphatemic states (Gray & Napoli, 1983) and that the adaptive intestinal response to Pi restriction is blunted in vitamin D deficient animals (Danisi & Murer, 1991).

In an effort to identify intestinal Na^+–Pi co-transporters by expression cloning, a 2 to 3 kv mRNA fraction, isolated from intestine of $1,25(OH)_2D$-treated rabbits, was shown to stimulate Na^+–Pi co-transport in *Xenopus* oocytes (Yagci et al., 1992). More recently, a Pi uptake stimulator (PiUS) that increases Na^+–Pi co-transport in *Xenopus* oocytes was cloned from rabbit intestine (Norbis et al., 1997). However, since hydropathy analysis of the 425-amino acid PiUS protein suggested that it lacks transmembrane segments, it is likely that PiUS is not a Pi transporter itself. Moreover, because PiUS is also expressed in kidney, liver and heart and also stimulated Na^+-independent Pi transport when injected in oocytes, it was suggested that PiUS may not be a specific activator of intrinsic Na^+–Pi co-transport but rather that it may function as a regulator of cellular Pi metabolism (Norbis et al., 1997). A Na^+–Pi co-transporter exhibiting considerable amino acid homology with NPT2 was recently cloned from mouse small intestine and designated type IIb (Hilfiker et al., 1998). The transporter was expressed predominantly in the intestine and was localized to the BBM. Functional studies in cRNA-injected oocytes demonstrated that type IIb-mediated transport has all the features of intestinal Na^+-dependent Pi transport. This work represents a significant advance in our understanding of intestinal Pi transport and has provided tools to investigate the molecular mechanisms involved in its regulation.

REFERENCES

Beck, L., Karrapalis, A. C., Amizuka, N., hewson, A. S., Ozawa, H., & Tenenhouse, H. S. (1998). Targeted inactivation of *Npt2* in mice leads to severe renal phosphate wasting, hypercalciuria and skeletal abnormalities. *Proc. Natl Acad. Sci., USA*, **95**, 5372–77.

Beck. L., Soumounou, Y., Martel, J., Krishnamurthy, G., Gauthier, C., Goodyer, C., & Tenenhouse, H. S. (1997). *Pex/PEX* tissue distribution and evidence for a deletion in the 3′ region of the *Pex* gene in X-linked hypophosphatemic mice. *J. Clin. Invest.*, **99**, 1200–9.

Berndt, T. J. & Knox, F. G. (1992). Renal regulation of phosphate excretion. In *The Kidney, Physiology and Pathophysiology*, ed. D. W. Seldin & G. Giebisch, pp. 2511–32. New York: Raven Press.

Caverzasio, J. & Bonjour, J. (1996). Characteristics and regulation of Pi transport in osteogenic cells for bone metabolism. *Kid. Int.*, **49**, 975–80.

Chong, S. S., Krisatjansson, K., Zoghbi, H. Y., & Hughes, M. R. (1993). Molecular cloning of the cDNA encoding a human renal sodium phosphate transport protein and its assignment to chromosome 6p21.3–p23. *Genomics*, **18**, 355–9.

Cole, J. A., Eber, A. L., Poelling, R. E., Thorne, P. K., & Forte L. R. (1987). A dual mechanism for regulation of kidney phosphate transport by parathyroid hormone. *Am. J. Physiol.*, **253**, E221–7.

Cross, H. S., Debiec, H., & Peterlik, M. (1990). Mechanism and regulation of intestinal phosphate absorption. *Miner. Electrolyte Metab.*, **16**, 115–24.

Custer, M., Spindler, B., Verrey, F., Murer, H., & Biber, J. (1997). Identification of a new gene product (diphor-1) regulated by dietary phosphate. *Am. J. Physiol.*, **273**, F806.

Danisi, G. & Murer, H. (1991). Inorganic phosphate absorption in small intestine. In *Handbook of Physiology – The Gastrointestinal System IV*, ed. M. Field & R. A. Frizzel, pp. 323–36. New York: Oxford University Press.

Econs, M. J., McEnery, P. T., Lennon, F., & Speer, M. C. (1997). Autosomal dominant hypophosphatemic rickets is linked to chromosome 12p13. *J. Clin, Invest.*, **100**, 2653–7.

Gmaj, P. & Murer, H. (1986). Cellular mechanisms of inorganic phosphate transport in kidney. *Physiol. Rev.*, **66**, 36–70.

Gray, R. W. & Napoli, J. L. (1983). Dietary phosphate deprivation increases 1,25-dihydroxyvitamin D$_3$ synthesis in rat kidney in vitro. *J. Biol. Chem.*, **258**, 1152–5.

Gupta, A., Guo, X., Alvarez, U. M., & Hruska, K. A. (1997). Regulation of sodium-dependent phosphate transport in osteoclasts. *J. Clin. Invest.*, **100**, 538–49.

Gupta, A., Miyauchi, A., Fujimori, A., & Hruska, K. A. (1996). Phosphate transport in osteoclasts: a functional and immunochemical characterization. *Kid. Int.*, **49**, 968–74.

Hafdi, Z., Couette, S., Comoy, E., Prie, D., Amiel, C., & Friedlander, G. (1996). Locally formed 5-hydroxytryptamine stimulates phosphate transport in cultured opossum kidney cells and in rat kidney. *Biochem. J.*, **320**, 615–21.

Hartmann, C. M., Hewson, A. S., Kos, C. H., Hilfiker, H., Soumoumou, Y., Murer, H., & Tenenhouse, H. S. (1996). Structure of murine and human renal type II Na$^+$-phosphate co-transporter genes (*Npt2* and NPT2). *Proc. Natl Acad. Sci., USA*, **93**, 7409–14.

Hilfiker, H., Hartmann, C. M., Stange, G., & Murer, H. (1998a). Characterization of the 5′-flanking region of OK cell type II Na-Pi co-transporter gene. *Am. J. Physiol.*, **274**, F197–204.

Hilfiker, H., Hattenhauer, O., Traebert, M., Forster, I., Murer, H., & Biber, J. (1998b). Characterization of a murine type II sodium-phosphate co-transporter expressed in mammalian small intestine. *Proc. Natl Acad. Sci., USA*, **95**, 14564–9.

Jones, A. O., Tzenova, J., Fujiwara, T. M., Frappier, D., Tieder, M., Morgan, K., & Tenenhouse H. S. (1999). NPT2 is not the gene responsible for hereditary hypophosphatemic rickets with hypercalciuria (HHRH) in a Bedouin kindred. *J. Am. Soc. Nephrol.*, **10**, 435A.

Kavanaugh, M. P., Miller, D. G., Zhang, W., Law, W., Kozak, S. L., Kabat, D., & Miller A. D. (1994). Cell-surface receptors for gibbon ape leukemia virus and amphotropic murine retrovirus are inducible sodium-phosphate symporters. *Proc. Natl Acad. Sci., USA*, **91**, 7071–5.

Kempson, S. A., Lotscher, M., Kaissling, B., Biber, J., Murer, H., & Levi, M. (1995). Parathyroid hormone action on phosphate transporter mRNA and protein in rat renal proximal tubules. *Am. J. Physiol.*, **268**, F784–91.

Kos, C. H., Tihy, F., Econs, M. J., Murer, H., Lemieux, N., & Tenenhouse, H. S. (1994). Localization of a renal sodium phosphate co-transporter gene to human chromosome 5q35. *Genomics*, **19**, 176–7.

Levi, M., Kempson, S. A., Lotscher, M., Biber, J., Murer, H., & Levi, M. (1997). Role of microtubules in the rapid regulation of renal phosphate transport in response to acute alterations in dietary phosphate content. *J. Clin. Invest.*, **99**, 1302–12.

McPherson, J. D., Krane, M. C., Wagner-McPherson, C. B., Kos, C. H., & Tenenhouse, H. S. (1997). High resolution mapping of the renal sodium-phosphate co-transporter gene (SLC17A2) confirms its localization to human chromosome 5q35. *Pediat. Res.*, **41**, 632–4.

Mizgala, C. L. & Quamme, G. A. (1985). Renal handling of phosphate. *Physiol. Rev.*, **65**, 431–66.

Murer, H. (1992). Cellular mechanisms in proximal tubular Pi reabsorption: some answers and more questions. *J. Am. Soc. Nephrol.*, **2**, 1649–65.

Murer, H. & Biber, J. (1996a). Renal sodium-phosphate co-transport. *Curr. Opin. Nephrol. Hypertens.*, **3**, 504–10.

Murer, H. & Biber, J. (1996b). Molecular mechanisms of renal apical Na phosphate co-transport. *Ann. Rev. Physiol.*, **58**, 607–18.

Murer, H. & Biber, J. (1997). A molecular view of proximal tubular inorganic phosphate (Pi) reabsorption and of its regulation *Pflüger's Arch.*, **433**, 379–89.

Murer, H., Forster, I., Hilfiker, H., Pfister, M., Kaissling, B., Lotscher, M., & Biber, J. (1998). Cellular/molecular control of renal Na/Pi-co-transport. *Kid. Int. Suppl.*, **65**, S2–10.

Murer, H., Werner, A., Reshkin, S., Waurin, R., & Biber, J. (1991). Cellular mechanisms in proximal tubular reabsorption of inorganic phosphate. *Am. J. Physiol.*, **260**, C885–99.

Norbis, F., Boll, M., Stange, G., Markovich, D., Verrey, F., Biber, J., & Murer, H. (1997). Identification of a cDNA/protein leading to an increased Pi-uptake in *Xenopus laevis* oocytes. *J. Membrane Biol.*, **156**, 19–24.

Palmer, G., Bonjour, J-P., & Caverzasio, J. (1997). Expression of a newly identified phosphate transporter/retrovirus receptor in human SaOS-2 osteoblast-like cells and its regulation by insulin-like growth factor I. *Endocrinology*, **138**, 5202–9.

Pfister, M. F., Hilfiker, H., Forgo, J., Lederer, E., Biber, J., & Murer, H. (1998a). Cellular mechanisms involved in the acute adaptation of OK cell Na/Pi-co-transport to high- or low-Pi medium. *Pflüger's Arch.*, **435**, 713–19.

Pfister, M. K., Ruf, I., Stange, G., Ziegler, U., Lederer, E., & Biber, J. (1998b). Parathyroid hormone leads to the lysomal degradation of the renal type II Na/Pi co-transporter. *Proc. Natl Acad. Sci., USA*, **95**, 1909–14.

Rasmussen, H. & Tenenhouse, H. S. (1995). Mendelian hypophosphatemias. In *The Metabolic and Molecular Basis of Inherited Disease*, ed. C. R. Scriver, A. L. Beaudet, W. S. Sly, & D. Valle, pp. 3717–45. New York: McGraw Hill Book Co.

Schroder, B., Hattenhauer, O., & Breves, G. (1998). Phosphate transport in pig proximal small intestines during postnatal development: lack of modulation by calcitriol. *Endocrinology*, **139**, 1500–7.

Strom, T. M., Francis, F., Lorenz, B., Boeddrich, A., Econs, M., Lehrach, H., & Meitinger, T. (1997). *Pex* gene deletions in Gy and Hyp mice provide mouse models for X-linked hypophosphatemia. *Hum. Molec. Genet.*, **6**, 165–71.

Tenenhouse, H. S. (1997). Cellular and molecular mechanisms of renal phosphate transport. *J. Bone Miner. Res.*, **12**, 159–64.

Tenenhouse, H. S. (1999). Recent advances in epithelial sodium coupled phosphate transport. *Curr. Opin. Nephrol. Hypertens.*, **8**, 407–19.

The HYP Consortium (1995). A gene (PEX) with homologies to endopeptidases is mutated in patients with X-linked hypophosphatemic rickets. *Nat. Genet.*, **11**, 130–6.

Veldman, C. M., Schlapfer, I., & Schmid, C. (1998). Prostaglandin E_2 stimulates sodium-dependent phosphate transport in osteoblastic cells via a protein kinase C-mediated pathway. *Endocrinology*, **139**, 89–94.

Wagner, G. F., Vozzolo, B. L., Jaworski, E., Haddad, M., Kline, R. L., Olsen, H. S., Rosen, C. A., Davison, M. B., & Renfro, J. L. (1997). Human stanniocalcin inhibits renal phosphate excretion in the rat. *J. Bone Miner. Res.*, **12**, 165–71.

Walker, J. J., Yan, T. S., & Quamme, G. A. (1987). Presence of multiple sodium-dependent phosphate transport processes in proximal brush-border membranes. *Am. J. Physiol.*, **252**, F226–31.

Wehrle, J. P. & Pedersen, P. L. (1989). Phosphate transport processes in eukaryotic cells. *J. Membrane Biol.*, **111**, 199–213.

Yagci, A., Werner, A., Murer, H., & Biber, J. (1992). Effect of rabbit duodenal mRNA on phosphate transport in *Xenopus laevis* oocytes: dependence on 1,25-dihydroxy-vitamin-D_3. *Pflüger's Arch.*, **422**, 211–16.

9

Molecular genetic analysis of growth factor signaling in bone

Janet E. Henderson and David Goltzman

Introduction

Disorders of bone and cartilage metabolism, including osteoporosis and osteoarthritis, are amongst the leading causes of morbidity and mortality in our aging population. These disorders account not only for a tremendous outlay in health care costs, but also compromise the quality of life of a large percentage of the world's population. Recent advances in human and murine molecular genetics have identified many of the phylogenetically conserved proteins that regulate the related processes of bone development, fracture repair and bone remodeling. They include multifunctional growth factors and morphogens, their high affinity receptors, transcription factors, and target genes including the bone morphogenetic proteins. In the mouse, these signaling components are expressed in a time-dependent manner, and in spatially restricted patterns, in developing bones, in fracture callus and in adult bone, where they co-ordinate the passage of skeletal cells through stages of replication, maturation and apoptotic cell death. Despite recent advances, little is known about the way in which individual components interact with one another to co-ordinate bone growth and bone remodeling. One particularly powerful approach to this problem is to analyze mice with a congenital deficiency of one or more of the regulatory genes, to determine if their protein products are redundant or complementary in their effect on cartilage and bone cells. The signaling pathways can be investigated at the molecular biochemical level in vivo, in the limbs of wild-type and mutant mice, and in vitro in skeletal cells released from the developing bones. In this manner, we can identify the abnormal patterns of cell growth and maturation associated with the absence of specific genes and determine if we can correct the abnormality by treating the cells with specific agents. This combined in vivo and in vitro approach to disorders of bone and mineral metabolism, including osteoporosis, will identify key components of the regulatory pathways that co-ordinate bone development, fracture repair and skeletal homeostasis. These components then represent potential targets for the development of genetic screening tools and to assist in the design of effective therapeutic interventions to prevent or treat age-related bone and cartilage degradation.

As described in the preceding chapters, many hormones, growth factors, enzymes and matrix proteins have been implicated in the signaling pathways that co-ordinate bone growth and bone remodeling. In some instances, growth factors appear to mediate similar effects on cell proliferation and maturation and in others they appear to be quite different. For example, parathyroid hormone-related protein (PTHrP) enhances proliferation of skeletal cells and impedes progression to a differentiated phenotype. Conversely, signaling through fibroblast growth factor receptor 3 (FGFR3), inhibits the replication of chondrocytes and enhances their terminal differentiation. This chapter will describe the way that a molecular genetic approach can be used to define the potential interactive roles of signaling by PTHrP and FGFs in bone, using largely developmental processes as a paradigm.

Overview of skeletal development and bone remodeling

Bone formation

This occurs via two distinct, yet related, processes. The flat bones of the skull and the outer surfaces of bones of the appendicular skeleton are formed by intramembranous ossification, whereby mesenchymal precursors differentiate directly into bone forming osteoblasts (Erlebacher et al., 1995). The remaining skeletal elements are produced by endochondral bone formation, during which mesenchymal cells differentiate into chondrocytes that build a cartilage anlage, which is subsequently replaced by bone (Chapter 1, this volume). It is becoming increasingly evident that these processes, as well as those involved in fracture repair and bone remodeling, are regulated through signaling pathways that include a few phylogenetically conserved molecules (Lanske et al., 1996; Naski & Ornitz, 1998; Vortkamp et al., 1998; Schmitt et al., 1999). These include morphogens like hedgehog (HH), multifunctional growth factors, like PTHrP and FGFs, the Gli family of transcription factors and their putative target genes, the bone morphogenetic proteins (BMPs). These interdependent signaling pathways co-ordinate the orderly progression of committed chondroprogenitor and osteoprogenitor cells through stages of proliferation, differentiation and programmed cell death during bone formation. All of these molecules are expressed in a time-dependent manner and in spatially restricted patterns in the growth plates of developing mouse bones and, by virtue of targeted disruption or targeted over-expression they have also been shown to play critical, and sometimes complementary, regulatory roles in cartilage and bone development. During skeletogenesis (Fig. 9.1(a)), FGFR3, Indian hedgehog (IHH), Gli-1 and BMP6 have been identified within areas of condensed mesenchyme, which are

(*a*)

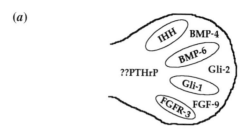

(*b*)   **Tibia**   **Growth plate**   **Zones**

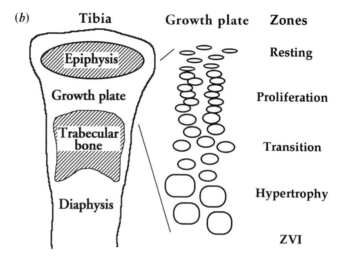

(*c*)

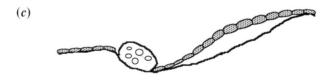

Fig 9.1   Skeletogenesis, endochondral bone formation and bone remodeling. The digits of the
hands and feet originate as condensations of mesenchymal cells that differentiate into
chondrocytes. Under the influence of different members of the HH/Gli/BMP families of
proteins, chondrocytes undergo further differentiation and build the cartilage template on
which bone is formed, whereas cells in the interdigital mesenchyme undergo apoptosis
(Fig 9.1(*a*)). After invasion of the cartilage anlage by blood vessels, longitudinal bone
growth is co-ordinated by conserved signaling pathways that regulate the progression of
growth plate chondrocytes through stages of differentiation during the process of
endochondral ossification (ZVI = zone of vascular invasion) (Fig 9.1(*b*)). In the adult
skeleton, similar signaling pathways regulate the co-ordinated activity of multinucleated
osteoclasts, which erode mineralized bone tissue, and of mononuclear osteoblasts, which
deposit and mineralize new bone (Fig 9.1(*c*)).

destined to become the bones. FGF-9, Gli-2 and BMP-9, on the other hand, are expressed in undifferentiated mesenchyme in the interdigital space destined for apoptosis. To date, PTHrP expression has not been evaluated at this early stage of development. During endochondral bone development (Fig. 9.1(*b*)), PTHrP enhances the proliferation and delays maturation of growth plate chondrocytes, whereas signaling through FGFR3 inhibits mitosis and enhances endochondral ossification. Furthermore, the biological activity of both PTHrP and FGFR has been linked to signaling through the conserved HH/Gli/BMP pathway during bone development.

Bone remodeling

Bone remodeling during adult life (Fig. 9.1(*c*)) takes place under the combined influence of local regulatory pathways, such as the one described above, and of many systemic factors, whose activity in bone is described in more detail elsewhere. In this context it is important to reiterate that the calciotropic hormone, PTH, and the locally derived growth factor, PTHrP, compete for binding to the same cell surface receptor on skeletal cells, as a consequence of 65% sequence homology at their amino termini. PTHrP is expressed at a much earlier stage than PTH, which makes it the predominant ligand in developing bone. PTH, on the other hand, regulates calcium homeostasis in the postnatal period. As such, it most probably has a greater influence on bone remodeling than does PTHrP, although both peptides have been shown to have anabolic effects in bone (Fraher et al., 1992, 1999). The major systemic factors that regulate bone metabolism are the calciotropic hormones, which include PTH (Chapters 6, 15 and 24, this volume) and vitamin D (Chapters 7 and 25, this volume), and steroid hormones like estrogen (Chapters 14 and 21, this volume) and testosterone (Chapter 16, this volume). At the local level, IGF-I and its binding proteins (Chapter 5) are important modulators of bone growth and remodeling, as are members of the transforming growth factor-ß (TGFß) superfamily, including the BMPs. More recently, PTHrP (Amizuka et al., 1994, 1995, 1996) and FGFs, through FGFR3 (Colvin et al., 1996; Naski & Ornitz, 1998) have been added to the list of agents that play a dual role in developmental and postnatal bone metabolism. Under physiologic circumstances, these hormones and growth factors regulate endochondral bone development during prenatal and early postnatal life (Chapter 1, this volume) and co-ordinate the coupled anabolic and catabolic activity of cells of the osteoblast (Chapter 2, this volume) and osteoclast (Chapter 3, this volume) lineages during bone remodeling. Thus, similar signaling pathways co-ordinate the development and maintenance of bones of the appendicular skeleton. The congenital absence, or acquired deficiency, of any one of the components of these pathways in bone can result in the loss of structural and functional integrity and the development of osteopenia and osteoporosis.

(a) Mechanisms of PTHrP action

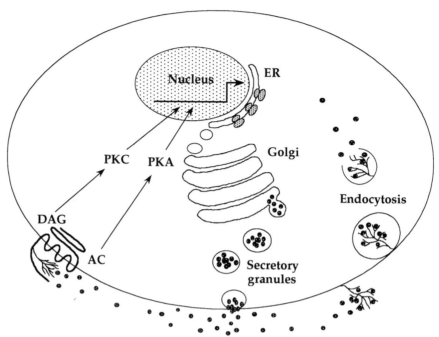

Fig 9.2(a)   Molecular mechanisms of PTHrP and FGFR3 action in bone. PTHrP is manufactured with a signal peptide that is co-translationally cleaved as the nascent protein enters the secretory pathway. Once PTHrP is released from the cell, it can bind to the G-protein-linked receptor that it shares with PTH, and activate signal transduction through protein kinase A (PKA) or C (PKC) pathways. Alternatively, PTHrP binds to an unidentified cell-surface protein and is endocytosed and released into the intracellular compartment to be translocated to the nuclear compartment.

Conserved signaling pathways in bone

PTHrP

PTHrP is a growth factor, which was discovered as a tumor-derived peptide that elicits a common paraneoplastic syndrome called humoral hypercalcemia of malignancy (Goltzman & Henderson, 1996, 1997). PTHrP and PTH activate the same G-protein-coupled cell surface receptor (PTH1R) through which they elicit a similar spectrum of biological activity (Henderson & Goltzman, 1998). PTHrP also influences cell function directly in the nucleus of chondrocytes and bone forming osteoblasts (Henderson et al., 1995, 1996; Aarts et al., 1999a, b) (Fig. 9.2(a)). PTHrP is expressed in a wide variety of embryonic, fetal and adult tissues (Broadus & Stewart, 1994) where it acts primarily at the local level to regulate cell prolifera-

(b)   Signaling through FGFR3

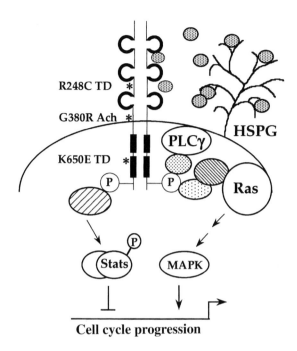

Fig 9.2(*b*)   FGFR3 is one of four high affinity receptors for the FGF ligands. Ligand binding, which is assisted by heparan sulfate proteoglycan (HSPG) causes dimerization and initiates signaling through phospholipase C γ, Ras or STAT to mediate changes in cell cycle progression. Point mutations in the extracellualr, transmembrane and intracellular kinase domain result in amino acid substitutions which render the receptor ligand independent. The mutations result in the human chondrodysplasias, thanatophoric dysplasia (TD) and achondroplasia (Ach).

tion and differentiation. In developing bone, PTHrP is expressed primarily by undifferentiated chondrocytes and osteoblasts, whereas PTH1R is expressed predominantly on more differentiated cells (Amizuka et al., 1994, 1995, 1996). Signaling by PTHrP in bone has been linked to the conserved HH/Gli/BMP pathway (Vortkamp et al., 1996).

FGFR3

FGFR3 is a receptor tyrosine kinase and is one of four high affinity receptors for the FGF family of ligands (Basilico and Moscatelli, 1992) (Fig. 9.2(*b*)). Alternative splicing generates variants of the IgG-like extracellular domain with different ligand-binding specificites (Ornitz et al., 1996). Ligand binding to FGFRs is facilitated by heparan sulfate proteoglycan and results in receptor dimerization, autophosphorylation and signal transduction through the ras-raf-MAPK, phospholipase-Cγ or STAT signal transduction pathways (Mohammadi et al., 1992; Su et al., 1997). FGFR-3 is expressed predominantly in resting and proliferating chondrocytes and has been linked to signaling through the same IHH/Gli/BMP pathway as PTHrP (Naski & Ornitz, 1998). Point mutations that result in amino acid substitutions throughout FGFR-3 result in lethal (thanatophoric) and non-lethal (achondroplasia) forms of chondrodysplasia and abnormal bone development. Although in vitro studies have identified FGF-1 and FGF-9 as preferred ligands for FGFR3, its endogenous ligand/s in developing bone remain unidentified.

Gli

Gli proteins are transcription factors that have been identified as components of the signaling pathways used by PTHrP and FGFR3 in skeletal cells. The Gli-1 gene was originally isolated from a glioblastoma, while Gli-2 and Gli-3 were cloned on the basis of homology with Gli-1 in the zinc finger domain (Kinzler et al., 1988). These DNA binding proteins have been associated with both neoplastic and developmental disorders and are believed to represent mammalian homologues of the *Drosophila* gene *cubitis interruptus,* which lies downstream of the HH morphogens (Fig. 9.3(*a*) and (*b*)). In developing bone, Gli-1 appears to be restricted to chondrogenic cells whereas Gli-2 and Gli-3 share overlapping fields of expression in regions of non-chondrogenic mesenchyme that is destined for apoptosis (Fig. 9.1(*a*)) (Buscher et al., 1997; Mo et al., 1997). Mice homozygous-null for targeted disruption of Gli-2 exhibit defects in bone formation associated with an apparent increase in chondrocyte proliferation and defective mineralization (unpublished observations). A spontaneous intragenic deletion in the Gli-3 gene is responsible for Greig cephalopolysyndactyly syndrome in humans and the *Xtra toes (Xt)* mutation in mice (Hui & Joyner, 1993; Johnson, 1967). Given that PTHrP, Gli-2 and Gli-3 are associated with apoptosis in developing bone, the presence of a Gli consensus sequence (Yoon et al., 1998) in the 5' regulatory region of PTHrP suggests that it may represent a downstream target for one or more of the Gli proteins.

BMPs

BMPs are growth factors that were discovered by virtue of their capacity to induce exogenous, *de novo,* bone formation at the site of implantation of demineralized bone fragments (Urist, 1965). Subsequently their potential use as anabolic agents in bone, both in fracture repair and in the treatment of osteopenic disorders, has been the subject of intensive investigation (Schmitt et al., 1999). Like PTHrP and FGFs, BMPs appear to influence both the replication and maturation of skeletal

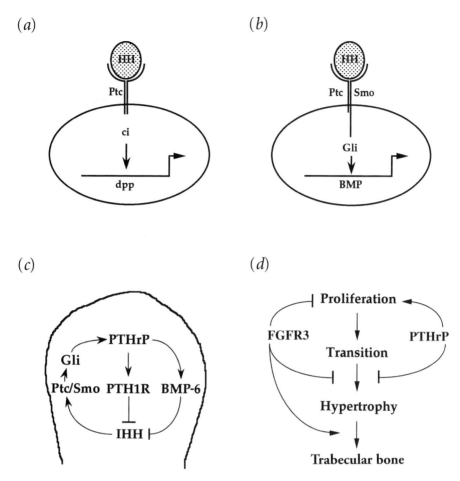

Fig 9.3   Conserved signaling pathways in bone development. The *HH/Gli/BMP* signaling pathway represents the mammalian homologue of the *hh/ci/dpp* pathway that regulates *Drosophila* development (Fig 9.3(*a*)). Binding of the morphogen HH to Ptc releases inhibition on Smo, which transduces the signal through Gli to BMP (Fig 9.3(*b*)). Signaling through FGFR3 and PTHrP have both been linked to the HH/Gli/BMP pathway to regulate the passage of growth plate chondrocytes through stages of replication and differentiation during endochondral bone formation (Fig 9.3(*c*)). In the tibial epiphysis, IHH expression is correlated with expression of type X collagen and chondrocyte maturation. PTHrP is believed to inhibit production of IHH through BMP-6 (Fig 9.3(*d*)). HH = hedgehog; Ptc = patched; Smo = smothen; ci = cubitis interruptis; dpp = decapentaplegic; gli = glioma; BMP = bone morphogenetic protein.

cells, perhaps in a ligand concentration-dependent manner. For instance, low concentrations might stimulate proliferation whereas higher concentrations could promote differentiation. These effects could also be dependent on expression of specific receptor subunits on target cells, or on the presence of BMP binding proteins in the bone microenvironment (Hogan, 1996). BMPs 4 and 6 have been implicated as downstream effectors of signaling through PTH1R and through FGFR-3. BMP-6 is thought to be involved in a long-range feedback loop that involves PTHrP, which inhibits cartilage maturation and endochondral bone formation (Fig. 9.3(c)). It has been proposed that binding of the morphogen, IHH, to its receptor patched (Ptc) allows signaling to proceed through the co-receptor smothen (Smo) to increase PTHrP production. PTHrP then inhibits IHH expression indirectly through BMP-6. Transgenic expression of a constitutively active FGFR-3 in cartilage also inhibits IHH as well as BMP-4 expression, which may co-ordinate endochondral (trabecular) and intramembranous (cortical) bone formation. It is therefore possible that although the signaling pathways downstream of PTHrP and FGFR-3 mediate complementary effects in bone development, they might share common components, such as IHH and BMPs (Fig. 9.3(d)).

Murine models of disorders of bone metabolism

History of gene targeting

Until 1985 murine models of human disease were restricted to those that arose from naturally occurring mutations, which were carried in the mouse germline. One of the first successful attempts at targeted disruption of the mouse genome was published by Smithies et al. who replaced the endogenous *β-globin* gene with the gene encoding a selectable marker (Smithies et al., 1985). Since that time, gene targeting technology has advanced to the extent that investigators can now target murine genes for removal (knockout), for replacement with an altered copy (knockin) and for conditional expression in restricted tissues, or at a specific developmental stage (cre-recombinase technology). The extensive training required to acquire such expertise, combined with the high cost of maintenance for the colonies required for generating mutant mice, has led many investigators to use commercial laboratories, or academic institutions, on a fee for service basis to generate mice with a mutation of interest.

The mouse knockout and mutation database

This comprehensive index of mutations in the murine germline is edited by Ian Jackson and published online at http://biomednet.com/db/mkmd. There are currently more than 2000 entries, which characterize targeted and spontaneous mutations in the mouse genome. Additional unlisted mutant phenotypes are available through collaboration with the individuals who generated the mutant strain. Mice hemizygous or homozygous null for many of these mutations exhibit a skeletal phenotype of largely unknown etiology. Given the restricted number of phylogenetically conserved proteins that regulate bone development and bone remodeling, these animals represent a rich source of potential models in which to study bone disease at the molecular genetic level. Two of the more striking skeletal phenotypes that have been documented recently are exhibited by mice with targeted disruption of the genes encoding PTHrP and FGFR-3.

Targeted disruption of PTHrP and FGFR-3 in mice

The congenital absence of PTHrP in mice results in a lethal phenotype (Amizuka et al., 1994; Karaplis et al., 1994; Tucci et al., 1996), which is characterized by decreased chondrocyte proliferation and premature bone formation, and resembles that of humans with Blomstrand dysplasia. Forced expression of PTHrP in cultured chondrocytes leads to increased proliferation of chondrocytes, inhibits their maturation and rescues serum-deprived cells from apoptosis (Henderson et al., 1995, 1996). Transgenic over-expression of PTHrP in cartilage in vivo has similar effects (Weir et al., 1996). Targeted disruption of FGFR-3 in mice results in continued elongation of the limbs in the postnatal period, as a result of increased proliferation of growth plate chondrocytes and delayed bone formation (Colvin et al., 1996). Conversely, transgenic expression of a constitutively active FGFR-3, carrying the achondroplasia mutation (FGFR-3^{Ach}), in the growth plates of mice (Naski & Ornitz, 1998) results in a short-limbed phenotype similar to that seen in humans with achondroplasia. Expression of the same mutant FGFR-3^{Ach} in cultured chondrocytes leads to profound inhibition of cell proliferation and differentiation, which is associated with altered cell matrix interactions (Henderson et al., 2000). In total, these observations suggest that PTHrP mediates a positive influence on bone growth, whereas FGFR-3 is a negative regulator of endochondral bone development.

Targeted disruption of the genes encoding PTHrP and FGFR-3 has, therefore, revealed critical and apparently complementary roles for the proteins during bone development. Further investigation of adult mice hemizygous for PTHrP (Amizuka et al., 1995) revealed osteopenic lesions in the proximal tibia and dysmorphic features, similar to those seen in newborn homozygous-null animals. Conversely, the epiphyseal growth plates of adult FGFR-3-null mice (Colvin et al., 1996) showed hypercellularity of the proliferative zone and an extended region of hypertrophic cells, compared with wild-type littermates, in whom the epiphyses had effectively fused. Furthermore, the tibia and femur became bowed and the mice developed severe kyphosis due to continued longitudinal growth of bones undergoing endochondral ossification. In the case of PTHrP, osteopenia may have been a consequence of developmental abnormalities in chondrogenic and osteogenic cells, or may have developed due to PTHrP haploinsufficiency in the postnatal period. Conversely, the congenital deficiency of FGFR-3 is manifested in the postnatal period by the continued presence of growth cartilage capable of undergoing endochondral ossification. Given their seemingly overlapping signaling pathways, it is reasonable to hypothesize that the congenital absence of FGFR-3 could compensate for PTHrP deficiency during bone development, and that reconstitution of the haploinsufficient neonate with PTHrP might prevent premature osteopenia. The first hypothesis is being addressed by generating compound PTHrP$^{+/-}$ FGFR-3$^{-/-}$ mutant mice, and the second by using gene therapy in neonatal PTHrP$^{+/-}$ mice.

Analysis of compound mutant mouse bones

Single and compound mutant mice, and their wild-type littermates can be identified at birth by analysis of genomic DNA harvested from an ear or tail clipping. Informative progeny are then sacrificed at monthly intervals after administration of agents to label proliferating cells and to identify regions of the bone that are undergoing active mineral deposition.

The skeletons of representative mice are differentially stained to identify cartilaginous and mineralized components, while the leg bones of other animals are embedded and sectioned for microscopic analysis. Many of the signaling molecules, such as PTHrP, FGFR-3, Gli, IHH and its putative co-receptors patched (Ptc) and smothen (Smo), are in low abundance and lack high affinity antibodies with which to identify their presence. In such cases, the mRNA encoding the protein, rather than the protein itself, is identified by *in situ* hybridization with an antisense riboprobe. In contrast, matrix proteins like collagens, osteopontin, osteocalcin and matrix Gla protein, are in relatively high abundance and easily identified by immunocytochemistry using monoclonal antibodies or polyclonal antisera (Chapter 4). The combined use of *in situ* hybridization and immunocytochemistry provides a comprehensive picture of functional and developmental alterations in the bones of compound mutant mice. These molecular analyses are then correlated with tetracycline labeling, to monitor the rate of bone apposition, enzyme histochemistry to identify anabolic (osteoblastic) and catabolic (osteoclastic) activity, and scanning electron microscopy, to reveal the overall trabecular architecture of the bone. If the increase in cellular proliferation and delayed maturation observed in the bones of FGFR$^{-/-}$ mice can compensate for the defects, which lead to osteopenia in PTHrP$^{+/-}$ mice, the bones of the compound mutant animals should closely resemble those of wild-type mice by 3 months of age.

Gene therapy in PTHrP$^{+/-}$ neonatal mice

An alternative approach to investigate the pathogenesis of premature osteopenia in PTHrP$^{+/-}$ mice is to reconstitute the haploinsufficient animal at birth with recombinant PTHrP, secreted into the bone microenvironment by transduced bone marrow stromal cells. Bone marrow transplantation is gaining popularity amongst investigators as a form of 'gene therapy' to deliver osteogenic compounds to correct congenital and acquired disorders of bone metabolism (Musgrave et al., 1999; Pereira et al., 1998; Vu et al., 1998). To achieve high levels of PTHrP expression, and to trace the PTHrP-producing cells in vivo, PTHrP can be expressed from a retroviral vector (Galipeau et al., 1999), as a fusion protein with green fluorescent protein (GFP), which is normally expressed in jellyfish. Retroviral-mediated gene transfer is preferred for its extremely high efficiency (virtually 100%) compared with more conventional methods, in which the foreign DNA is transferred in liposomes or attached to calcium phosphate precipitates, and enters only 25% to 50% of the target cells. Bone marrow stromal cells are harvested from donor mice by conventional methods and grown in tissue culture dishes where they are treated with virus carrying the DNA encoding the PTHrP-GFP fusion protein. The presence of recombinant protein in the transduced cells is verified by immunochemical means, using antisera directed against PTHrP, and by fluorescence microscopy in live cells, to identify GFP. Three to four weeks after transplantation of the stromal cells into the recipient PTHrP$^{+/-}$ mice, green fluorescent cells are identified in the long bones. Their concentration will indicate the seeding efficiency of the transplanted cells and their location will verify the identity of cells derived from the GFP-expressing progenitors. An alternative mechanism for determining transplantation and seeding efficiency is to use male donor mice and female recipient mice, and perform *in situ* hybridization with a male-specific probe like Sry, which is expressed exclusively in male germ cells. To improve the efficiency of exogenous gene expression the recipient mice are subjected to a sublethal dose of radiation prior to transplantation, which results in partial immunosuppression and improved survival of the transplanted stromal cells. As PTHrP has been shown to be an anabolic agent in adult bone, the haploinsufficient mice should demonstrate an increase in trabecular bone and an improvement in overall bone density.

Acknowledgements

The work was supported in part by grants from the Medical Research Council of Canada (JEH and DG), from the National Cancer Institute (DG) and from the Kidney Foundation of Canada (JEH). JEH is a Chercheur Boursier of the Fonds de la Recherche en Sante du Quebec.

REFERENCES

Aarts, M. M., Levy, D., He, B., Stregger, S., Chen, T., Richard, S., & Henderson, J. E. (1999a). Parathyroid hormone related protein (PTHrP) interacts with RNA. *J. Biol. Chem.*, 274, 4832–8.

Aarts, M., Rix, A., Guo, R., Bringhurst, R., & Henderson, J. E. (1999b). The nucleolar targeting signal (NTS) of parathyroid hormone related protein (PTHrP) mediates endocytosis and nuclear translocation. *J. Bone Miner. Res.*, In Press.

Amizuka, N., Henderson, J. E., Hoshi, K., Warshawsky, H., Ozawa, H., Goltzman, D., & Karaplis, A. C. (1996). Programmed cell death of chondrocytes and aberrant chondrogenesis in mice homozygous for parathyroid hormone-related peptide gene deletion. *Endocrinology*, 137, 5055–67.

Amizuka, N., Karaplis, A. C., Henderson, J. E., Warshawsky, H., Lipman, M. L., Matsuki, Y., Ejiri, S., Tanaka, M., Izumi, N., Ozawa, H., & Goltzman, D. (1995). Haploinsufficiency of parathyroid hormone-related peptide (PTHrP) results in abnormal post-natal bone development. *Dev Biol.*, 175, 166–76.

Amizuka, N., Warshawsky, H., Henderson, J. E., Goltzman, D., & Karaplis, A. C. (1994). Parathyroid hormone-related peptide (PTHrP)-depleted mice show abnormal epiphyseal cartilage development and altered endochondral bone formation. *J. Cell Biol.*, 126, 1611–23.

Basilico, C. & Moscatelli, D. (1992). The FGF family of growth factors and oncogenes. In *Advances in Cancer Research*, ed. G. F. V. Woude & G. Kleins, 115–65. San Diego, CA: Academic Press.

Broadus, A. E. & Stewart, A. F. (1994). Parathyroid hormone-related protein: structure, processing and physiological actions. In *The Parathyroids*, ed. J. P. Bilezekian, M. A. Levine, & R. Markuss, pp. 259–94. New York: Raven Press.

Buscher, D., Bosse, B., Heymer, J., & Ruther, U. (1997). Evidence for genetic control of Sonic hedgehog by Gli3 in mouse limb development. *Mechanisms of Development*, 62, 175–82.

Colvin, J. S., Bohne, B. A., Harding, G. W., McEwen, D. G., & Ornitz, D. M. (1996). Skeletal overgrowth and deafness in mice lacking fibroblast growth factor receptor 3. *Nature Genet.*, 12, 390–7.

Erlebacher, A., Filvaroff, E. H., Gitelman, S. E., & Derynck, R. (1995). Toward a molecular understanding of skeletal development. *Cell*, 80, 371–8.

Fraher, L. J., Avram, R., Watson, P. H., Hendy, G. N., Henderson, J. E., Chong, K. L., Goltzman, D., Morley, P., Willick, G. E., Whitfield, J. F., & Hodsman, A. B. (1999). Comparison of the biochemical responses to parathyroid hormone (hPTH)-(1–31)NH$_2$ and hPTH-(1–34) in healthy humans. *J. Clin. Endocrinol. Metab.*, 84, 2739–43.

Fraher, L. J., Hodsman, A. B., Jonas, K., Saunders, D., Rose, C. I., Henderson, J. E., Hendy, G. N., & Goltzman, D. (1992). A comparison of the in vivo biochemical responses to exogenous parathyroid hormone (1–34) and parathyroid hormone-related peptide (1–34) in man. *J. Clin. Endocrinol. Metab.*. 75, 417–23.

Galipeau, J., Li, H., Paquin, A., Sicilia, F., Karpati, G., & Nalbantoglu, J. (1999). Vesicular stomatitis virus G pseudotyped retrovector mediates effective in vivo suicide gene delivery in experimental brain cancer. *Can. Res.*, 59, 2384–94.

Goltzman, D. & Henderson, J. E. (1996). Expression of PTHrP in disease. In *Principles of Bone Biology*, ed. J. P. Bilezekian, L. G. Raisz, & G. A. Rodan, pp. 809–26. San Diego, CA: Academic Press.

Goltzman, D. & Henderson, J. E. (1997). Parathyroid hormone-related peptide and hypercalcemia of malignancy. In *Cancer Treatment and Research: Endocrine Neoplasms*, ed A. Arnold, pp. 193–216. Boston, MS: Academic Publishers.

Henderson, J. E. & Goltzman, D. (1998). Osteoblast receptors. In *Advances in Organ Biology: Molecular and Cellular Biology of Bone*, Series ed. E.E. Bittar, guest ed. M. Zaidi, pp. 499–512. Stamford, CT: JAI Press.

Henderson, J. E., Amizuka, N., Warshawsky, H., Biasotto, D., Lanske, B. M. K., Goltzman, D., & Karaplis, A. C. (1995). Nucleolar targeting of PTHrP enhances survival of chondrocytes under conditions that promote cell death by apoptosis. *Mol. Cell. Biol.*, **15**, 4064–75.

Henderson, J. E., He, B., Goltzman, D., & Karaplis, A. C. (1996). Constitutive expression of parathyroid hormone-related peptide (PTHrP) stimulates growth and inhibits differentiation of CFK2 chondrocytes. *J. Cell Physiol.*, **169**, 33–41.

Henderson, J. E., Naski, M. C., Aarts, M., Wang, D., Cheng, L., Goltzman, D., & Ornitz, D. M. (1999). Expression of FGFR3 with the G380R achondroplasia mutation inhibits proliferation and maturation of CFK2 chondrocytic cells. *J. Bone Miner. Res.*, In Press.

Hogan, B. L. M. (1996). Bone morphogenetic proteins: multifunctional regulators of vertebrate development. *Genes and Dev.*, **10**, 1580–94.

Hui, C. C. & Joyner, A. L. (1993). A mouse model of Greig cephalopolysyndactyly syndrome: the extra-toes mutation contains an intragenic deletion of the Gli3 gene. *Nat. Genet.*, **3**, 241–6.

Johnson, D. R. (1967). Extra toes: a new mutant gene causing multiple abnormalities in the mouse. *J. Embryol. Exp. Morph.*, **17**, 543–81.

Karaplis, A. C., Luz, A., Glowacki, J., Bronson, R. T., Tybulewicz, V. L. J., Kronenberg, H. M., & Mulligan, R. C. (1994). Lethal skeletal dysplasia from targeted disruption of the parathyroid hormone-related peptide (PTHrP) gene. *Genes Dev.*, **8**: 277–89.

Kinzler, K. W., Rupert, J. M., Bigner, S. H., & Vogelstein, B. (1988). The Gli gene is a member of the Kruppel family of zinc finger proteins. *Nature*, **332**, 371–4.

Lanske, B., Karaplis, A. C., Lee, K., Luz, A., Vortkamp, A., Pirro, A., Karperien, M., Defize, L. H. K., Ho, C., Mulligan, R. C., Abou-Samra, A. B., Juppner, H., Segre, G. V., & Kronenberg, H. M. (1996). PTH/PTHrP receptor in early development and Indian Hedgehog-regulated bone growth. *Science*, **273**, 663–6.

Mo, R., Freer, A. M., Zinyk, D. L., Crackowr, M. A., Michaud, J., Heng, H. H. Q., Chik, K. W., Shi, X. M., Tsui, L. C., Cheng, S. H., Joyner, A. L., & Hui, C. C. (1997). Specific and redundant functions of Gli2 and Gli3 zinc finger genes in skeletal patterning and development. *Development*, **124**, 113–23.

Mohammadi, M., Dionne, C. A., Li, W., Li, N., Spivak, T., Honegger, A. M., Jaye, M., & Schlessinger, J. (1992). Point mutation in FGF receptor eliminates phosphatidylinositol hydrolysis without affecting mitogenesis. *Nature*, **358**, 681–4.

Musgrave, D. S., Bosch, P., Ghivizzani, S., Robbins, P. D., Evans, C. H., & Huard, J. (1999). Adenovirus-mediated direct gene therapy with bone morphogenetic protein-2 produces bone. *Bone*, **24**, 541–8.

Naski, M. C. & Ornitz, D. M. (1998). Repression of hedgehog signalling and BMP4 expression by fibroblast growth factor receptor 3 in growth plate cartilage of transgenic mice. *Development*, 125, 4977–88.

Ornitz, D. M., Xu, J., Colvin, J. S., McEwen, D. G., MacArthur, C. A., Coulier, F., Gao, G., & Goldfarb, M. (1996). Receptor specificity of the fibroblast growth factor family. *J. Biol. Chem.*, 271, 15292–7.

Pereira, R. F., O'Hara, M. D., Leptev, A. V., Halfrd, K. W., Pollard, M. D., Class, R., Simon, D., Livezey, K., & Prockop, D. J. (1998). Marrow stromal cells as a source of progenitor cells for nonhematopoietic tissues in transgenic mice with a phenotype of osteogenesis imperfecta. *Proc. Natl Acad. Sci., USA*, 95, 1142–7.

Schmitt, J. M., Hwang, K., Winn, S. R., & Hollinger, J. O. (1999). Bone morphogenetic proteins: an update on basic biology and clinical relevance. *J. Orthop. Res.*, 17, 269–78.

Smithies, O., Gregg, R. G., Boggs, S. S., Koralewski, M. A., & Kucherlapati, R. S. (1985). Insertion of DNA sequences into the human chromosomal beta-globin locus by homologous recombination, *Nature*, 317, 230–4.

Su, W. C. S., Kitagawa, M., Xue, N., Xie, B., Garofalo, S., Cho, J., Deng, C., Horton, W. A., & Fu, X. Y. (1997). Activation of STAT-1 by mutant fibroblast growth factor receptor in thanatophoric dysplasia typeII dwarfism. *Nature*, 386, 288–92.

Tucci, J., Hammond, V., Senior, P. V., Gibson, A., & Beck, F. (1996). The role of fetal parathyroid hormone related protein in transplacental calcium transport. *J. Mol. Endo.*, 17, 159–64.

Urist, M. R. (1965). Bone: formation by autoinduction. *Science*, 150, 893–9.

Vortkamp, A., Lee, K., Lanske, B., Segre, G. V., Kronenberg, H. M., & Tabin, C. J. (1996). Regulation of rate of cartilage differentiation by Indian Hedgehog and PTH-related protein. *Science*, 273, 613–22.

Vortkamp, A., Pathi, S., Peretti, G. M., Caruso, E. M., Zaleske, D. J., & Tabin, C. J. (1998). Recapitulation of signals regulating embryonic bone formation during postnatal growth and in fracture repair. *Mech. Develop.*, 71, 65–76.

Vu, T. H., Shipley, J. M., Bergers, G., Berger, J. E., Helms, J. A., Hanahan, D., Shapiro, S. D., Senior, R. M., & Werb, Z. (1998). MMP-9/gelatinase B is a key regulator of growth plate angiogenesis and apoptosis of hypertrophic chondrocytes. *Cell*, 93, 411–22.

Weir, E., Philbrick, W., Amling, M., Neff, L., Baron, R., & Broadus, A. (1996). Targeted over-expression of parathyroid hormone-related peptide in chondrocytes causes chondrodysplasia and delayed endochondral bone formation. *Proc. Natl Acad. Sci., USA*, 93, 10240–5.

Yoon, J. W., Liu, C. Z., Yang, J. T., Swart, R., Iannaccone, P., & Waterhouse, D. (1998). Gli activates transcription through a herpes simplex viral protein 16-like activation domain. *J. Biol. Chem.*, 273, 3496–501.

Part II

Determinants of peak bone mass

10

Genetic determinants of osteoporosis

Millan S. Patel, Laurence A. Rubin and David E. C. Cole

Introduction

Osteoporosis may be defined as a reduction in bone mineral density (BMD) of at least 2.5 standard deviations (SD) accompanied by microarchitectural changes and increased bone fragility (Schapira & Schapira, 1992). Genetic studies of osteoporosis have principally focused on the first part of this definition, BMD heritability, due to the large patient populations required for genetic analyses and the relative ease with which BMD measurements can now be obtained. From a public health perspective, however, bone fragility is of critical importance and thus increasing attention is being devoted to the genetics of fracture risk. Integral to any discussion of BMD and bone strength is the issue of bone loss. It is the genetics of these key determinants of progression to osteoporosis, the genetics of bone mass, bone loss and bone fragility, that form the subject matter for this chapter (Fig. 10.1).

Genetics of BMD – a quantitative trait

Like serum sodium or arterial blood pressure, bone mineral density values lie along a continuum; thus BMD is termed a quantitative trait. Genetic studies of quantitative traits are difficult to perform since family members cannot be neatly divided into affected and unaffected categories, as can be done with Mendelian (single gene) disorders. As well, collection of large pedigrees of affecteds is much more difficult with late age-onset disorders such as osteoporosis. Finally, many quantitative traits are specified by more than one gene (polygenic inheritance) resulting in the failure of traditional linkage analysis to detect the effects of any single locus without prohibitively large sample collection.

Human geneticists use two other methods in addition to linkage analysis to detect genes or loci involved in the specification of quantitative traits (Lander & Schork, 1994). The first, sib pair mapping, is an approach to locating chromosome regions shared between affected sibs that is independent of the underlying method

- Up to 80% of the variance in Caucasian peak bone mass at the hip and spine may be genetically determined.

- There are no clinically applicable genetic tests for osteoporosis or fracture risk yet available.

- Genetic syndromes causing osteoporosis can be distinguished by focusing on key historical points - dental, skin and eye abnormalities and conducting a careful physical examination which includes dental examination.

- Genes involved in osteoporosis can be found or tested using association studies, allele-sharing studies and linkage analysis.

Fig. 10.1   Key points.

of inheritance. The power of this method is limited when the trait under study is controlled by a large number of genes. The second method, the genetic association study, occupies a central place in the genetic analysis of quantitative traits. Association studies test for whether a candidate allele has a higher frequency in the case vs. the control group. There are two types of genetic association studies, depending on the nature of the control group (Spielman & Ewens, 1996). The first uses population-based controls and has been the method of convenience for much of the work to date in osteoporosis genetics. A given allele of a gene is said to be associated with a trait if it occurs at higher frequency in a group of unrelated, affected individuals than in a race-matched control group of unrelated, unaffected individuals.

Such a study methodology can be compromised by several mechanisms (Econs & Speer, 1996), the most germane of which is called population stratification. For example, imagine studying the genetics of BMD in a case population of whites who have a background admixture of 30% non-white-derived alleles and comparing the allele frequency at a given locus to a control population of whites who have a background admixture of 15% non-white-derived alleles. The allele under study may show a higher frequency in the case population, not because it predisposes to low BMD, but because its frequency simply reflects stratification of the case and control groups by degree of non-white ancestry. The effects of population stratification are notoriously difficult to control for and have prompted the development of a second type of genetic association study which utilizes family-based controls instead. Since family members serve as the controls for a population of affected individuals in such studies, ethnicity is automatically controlled for (assuming paternity is unambiguously determined).

The transmission – disequilibrium test (TDT)

The most powerful family-based association study currently available is the transmission–disequilibrium test (TDT) (Allison, 1997; Schaid, 1998; Spielman & Ewens, 1996). The TDT relies on the random segregation of alleles: the prior probability of allele transmission from heterozygous parent to their offspring is 0.5 for each allele. This rule holds if the child is affected and the locus under study is not involved in trait determination. However, if the allele under study is involved in trait determination, it will more likely be transmitted to an affected child. Even small deviations from the expected 50:50 ratio of allele transmission can be detected in a robust manner. This study design has several strengths. Family collection is less arduous since only singleton affecteds and their parents need be ascertained and the clinical status of the parents need not be determined. The sample size required to detect a given allele effect is considerably lower than that required for other study designs (Risch & Merikangas, 1996). Most importantly, the TDT tests for linkage or association and can therefore be used to prove causation (linkage) when association has previously been shown (Spielman & Ewens, 1996). This latter feature will be crucial for the success of genome-wide high density scans in mapping novel loci involved in osteoporosis genetics (Risch & Merikangas, 1996).

The TDT is limited, especially in late-onset disorders, by the need to sample parental DNA. This limitation may be partly circumvented by sampling DNA from multiple sibs and inferring parental genotypes from those data (Schaid & Li, 1997). The power of the TDT also depends on the underlying model of inheritance. Weak, recessive alleles require exceedingly large sample sizes for an effect to be demonstrated. The statistical foundations of the TDT continue to be actively refined and, despite the limitations of this method, it holds great promise for the future.

BMD heritability

The broadest indicator of a genetic contribution to osteoporosis comes from observations of marked ethnic differences in BMD and fracture rates (Melton, 1993). Such differences were recognized as early as 430 BC by the Greek historian Herodotus when he surveyed the ground 40 years after the battle of Pelusium. He wrote that '. . . if you strike the Persian skulls, even with a pebble, they are so weak that you break a hole in them; but the Egyptian skulls are so strong that you may smite them with a stone and you will scarcely break them in' (Smith et al., 1973).

The genetic contribution to BMD is further supported by the finding that daughters (Seeman et al., 1989) and relatives (Evans et al., 1988) of women with osteoporosis have lower BMD, on average, than age- and gender-matched controls. An autosomal dominant high bone density phenotype (greater than 3 SD above the mean) has been mapped in one family to chromosome 11q12–13 (Johnson et al., 1997). The magnitude of the genetic contribution to BMD variance is termed heritability and has been quantitatively estimated in several twin and family studies.

Twin studies involve comparison of the intrapair differences in BMD of monozygotic (MZ) twins with the intrapair differences of dizygotic (DZ) twins. Since identical twins share 100% of their genetic material, all intrapair differences are assumed to arise as a result of environmental factors. In DZ twins, intrapair differences may arise from both genetic and environmental factors. Therefore, demonstration of less intrapair variation in MZ twins allows the inference that genetic factors are responsible for the observed differences.

Twin studies examining the heritability of BMD at the femoral neck and lumbar spine have indicated that 50–80% of the variance in Caucasian female BMD at these sites is due to shared genetic factors. When older twins are compared with younger twins, the heritability of BMD is modestly decreased, suggesting that an accumulation of environmental influences with aging dilutes the genetic effect (Slemenda et al., 1991; Smith et al., 1973). An elegant study on peak bone mass accumulation by Hopper et al. (1998) further illustrates the point that genetic effects on BMD vary with age. Studying 215 Australian Caucasian female twin pairs aged 10–26 years, they showed that genetic effects on spinal and femoral BMD predominated in the 10–13-year-old and 18–26-year-old age groups while environmental effects predominated in the 14–17-year-old age group. After age 17, as an increasing proportion of the twin pairs began to live apart, the evidence for shared environmental effects on BMD decreased to non-detectable levels while the strength of the genetic effects steadily increased (Hopper et al., 1998). These data are in broad agreement with a study involving 129 French Caucasian nuclear families (Gueguen et al., 1995). These authors showed that, while genetic effects on total body BMD were independent of age, an individual-specific residual factor varied with age in a non-linear fashion, reaching a minimum at age 26. This corresponded to a maximum value for heritability at this age of 84%.

Twin studies provide a powerful methodology for estimating the genetic contribution to a trait, but are limited by their assumptions. One assumption is that MZ twin pairs experience no less environmental diversity than DZ twin pairs. A second assumption is that there are no gene interactions (e.g., dominance or epistasis) involved in trait determination. These assumptions were tested for BMD at the lumbar spine and femoral neck by Slemenda et al. (1991) and found to be violated. These authors noted that MZ twins tended to be much more alike than DZ twins for confounding traits such as cigarette smoking, and calcium and caffeine intake. Evidence for gene interactions was also found. Their data suggest that current estimates of the genetic contribution to BMD may be artificially inflated. This is supported by data from family studies (Krall & Dawson-Hughes, 1993; Sowers et al., 1992) indicating that the variance in male and female Caucasian BMD at the lumbar spine and femoral neck due to genetic factors is closer to 45–67%. Furthermore, some studies show that BMD of the lumbar spine, a site with about 80% trabecular bone, has higher heritability than BMD of the femoral neck, a site with about 50% trabecular bone. In the end, the exact magnitude of the genetic effect may not be as important as the actual demonstration of an effect. One way or the other, the evidence from twin and family studies is overwhelmingly in favor of a significant genetic contribution to BMD. The challenge will be to dissect this genetic contribution into its constituent parts.

Bone turnover heritability

Biochemical markers of bone formation appear to be under significant genetic control. Bone-specific alkaline phosphatase (BSAP) and serum carboxyterminal propeptide of type I collagen (PICP) are two markers of bone formation which have been shown in several twin studies to have high levels of heritability. Intriguingly, an allele of the transforming growth factor beta 1 gene has been shown to be associated with levels of BSAP (Langdahl et al., 1997).

Markers of bone resorption have been found to be heritable in some studies but not in others. A study of 120 postmenopausal twin pairs showed that a clear genetic contribution to markers of bone turnover was only significant for those markers which did not change markedly at the menopause (Garnero et al., 1996). Several family studies have also indicated that BMD correlation coefficients in mother–daughter pairs are higher for premenopausal than postmenopausal mothers, suggesting that pre- and postmenopausal bone turnover characteristics are under separate control. In a 16-year longitudinal study on the rate of bone loss in aging male twins, the intrapair variance was the same for identical and non-identical twins, suggesting a lack of genetic effects on the rate of bone loss (Slemenda et al., 1996). In contradistinction to these findings, the Sp1 allele (see below) of the collagen IA1 gene was shown to have effects on BMD which increased with time since menopause. Since the allelic frequencies were the same in all age strata (arguing against allele-specific mortality effects), this observation suggests that the Sp1 allele may be a risk factor for increased postmenopausal bone loss.

Genetics of bone fragility

Fracture risk is an extremely broad topic with numerous epidemiological predictors but few genetic ones. On a mechanistic level, for instance, hip fracture is predicted by a number of parameters which have little to do with bone *per se*. These include propensity to fall, thickness of the greater trochanteric fat pad and visual acuity. Each of these factors likely has a genetic component specified by a number of genes. Within bone, femoral geometry – specifically hip axis length (HAL) – is an independent predictor of fracture risk (Kanis & McCloskey, 1996). A genetic component to HAL is suspected based on ethnic differences in HAL between black and white women (Theobald et al., 1998). Of the two twin studies which have examined HAL heritability, only one showed a strong genetic effect.

The candidate gene approach has demonstrated promise for the detection of alleles which predispose to fracture. The Sp1 allele of collagen IA1 confers a relative risk for fracture equivalent to that of a 1 SD decrease in BMD, an effect that is partly independent of BMD. Future work in the area of bone fragility genetics will be extremely broad-based and susceptibility alleles for each of the epidemiological predictors of fracture risk await discovery.

Candidate genes

Association studies have been used extensively in the field of BMD genetics to examine the role of candidate genes. Most of the studies to date have utilized population-based controls. Since association studies are susceptible to false positive results, it is essential that each gene tested have a physiologically relevant role to play in bone and mineral metabolism. It is even more convincing if a functional allele is tested; that is, the allele is shown to alter the level of gene expression or protein function qualitatively or quantitatively. Because linkage disequilibrium or population-specific genotype–environment interactions may be present, positive results may apply only to the population being studied.

Collagen IA1

Type I collagen comprises 90% of the organic component of bone. Collagen fibrils are assembled from three tropocollagen molecules supplied by the collagen IA1 (COLIA1) gene and the collagen IA2 (COLIA2) gene. Mutations in either of these genes cause osteogenesis imperfecta (OI), a disease characterized by low BMD and increased bone fragility, making them ideal candidates for genetic studies of osteoporosis. In 26 individuals with a history of fractures and a strong family history of osteoporosis, the coding regions of the COLIA1 and COLIA2 genes were sequenced (Spotila et al., 1994). Mutations of COLIA1 were found in three individuals, suggesting that OI is a minor cause of osteoporosis in such situations.

Subsequent studies have focused on more prevalent polymorphisms of the COLIA1 locus. The most promising allele examined to date is an Sp1 binding site polymorphism. Sp1 is an ubiquitous, nuclear matrix-associated transcription factor thought to play a role in the relaxation of higher-order chromatin structure to facilitate gene expression. An Sp1 binding site in the first intron of COLIA1 contains a polymorphism in about 22% of Caucasians which causes reduced binding affinity for the Sp1 protein (Grant et al., 1996). This allele has been shown to associate with postmenopausal BMD in Scottish (Grant et al., 1996), English (Grant et al., 1996), Dutch (Uitterlinden et al., 1998), Danish (Langdahl et al., 1998) and French (Roux et al., 1998) Caucasian populations. In the largest study to date, 1778 postmenopausal Dutch women were studied (Uitterlinden et al., 1998). The effects of the Sp1 allele on BMD were found to be dependent on age since menopause, suggesting that this allele may play a role in determining the rate of postmenopausal bone loss. The overall effect on BMD at the spine and femoral neck was small, however, with the Sp1 allele accounting for 2% of the variance in BMD in women aged 75 to 80 years. This is consistent with a polygenic model of inheritance for BMD with many genes playing a role, each with small effects.

More importantly, several studies have shown an effect of the Sp1 allele on fracture risk. Grant et al. (1996) reported a small case-control study documenting a relative risk of vertebral fracture of 3.2 (95% CI 2.0–14.6) while Uitterlinden et al. (1998) found a relative risk for any fracture type of 1.5 (95% CI 1.1–4.4). This finding is especially important since the Sp1 allele is the first genetic marker shown to be associated with significant fracture risk. A Danish case-control study (Langdahl et al., 1998) confirmed and extended these findings, showing that the Sp1 allele conferred an elevated risk for vertebral fracture (OR 11.8; 95% CI 2.6–53) in men and women, a risk that was only partly dependent on BMD. The fracture risk conferred by the Sp1 allele is comparable to the relative risks for vertebral and hip fracture conferred by a 1 SD decrease in vertebral and femoral neck BMD (pooled odds ratio 2.3 to 2.6; Marshall et al., 1996).

The effects of the COLIA1 Sp1 allele must be confirmed prospectively and in a wider range of populations before its clinical utility can be judged. With the preliminary data currently available, it appears to be a very promising factor for the future prediction of postmenopausal BMD and fracture risk.

Vitamin D receptor

Morrison and colleagues (1994) reported the first genetic marker to be associated with BMD, a *BsmI* restriction fragment length polymorphism (RFLP) of the vitamin D receptor (VDR) gene. Based on studies of a heterogeneous population of pre- and postmenopausal female twins as well as a population-based sample of unrelated individuals, they found that the VDR *BsmI* RFLP accounted for 75% of the variance in BMD. This claim was not substantiated (Eisman, 1996) when the study was revised and expanded. In the larger study groups, no VDR allele effect was seen for the twin sample, although a small effect remained in the population-based sample.

Numerous publications have since investigated the potential association of VDR

3′ polymorphisms with BMD. While some showed no association, others showed an effect only at the femur (Fleet et al., 1995; Houston et al., 1996; Riggs et al., 1995), only at the spine (Salamone et al., 1996; Yamagata et al., 1994), and some found an effect at both sites (Spector et al., 1995). A meta-analysis of many of these studies confirmed a small effect of the *B* allele (the allele without the *BsmI* restriction site) on lowering BMD (Cooper & Umbach, 1996). However, several large studies showed that the *B* allele was associated with higher BMD (Houston et al., 1996; Uitterlinden et al., 1996) and other large studies showed no effect whatsoever (Hustmyer et al., 1994; Jorgensen et al., 1996). Several explanations that have been proposed to reconcile these diverse and seemingly contradictory findings are discussed below.

Studies examining the physiological implications of VDR genotype have shown that the *BsmI* RFLP and two others (*ApaI, TaqI*) in the 3′ region of the VDR gene are associated with differences in intestinal absorption of calcium (Dawson-Hughes et al., 1995; Wishhart et al., 1997) and in differing BMD responses to calcium supplementation (Krall et al., 1995) or vitamin D supplementation (Graafmans et al., 1997).

It should be emphasized that the 3′ alleles of VDR have not been definitively shown to be associated with functional changes in gene expression or with changes in VDR protein function. Therefore, any import of the polymorphisms in a biological sense are likely to be mediated through their linkage to nearby polymorphism with functional effects. The putative linked polymorphism may be located within the VDR gene or possibly in a nearby gene on chromosome 12. This phenomenon, whereby some alleles in a population are found to be linked to other alleles at proportions in excess of what would be expected due to random chance, is termed linkage disequilibrium (not to be confused with the transmission disequilibrium tested for by the TDT).

Equilibrium arises in a population of randomly mating individuals through the progressive scrambling of neighboring alleles by DNA recombination, such that their association with one another is random (or in equilibrium) in the population. Linkage disequilibrium arises when two alleles are physically very close to one another on a chromosome and insufficient evolutionary time has passed to allow equilibrium to become established. Alternatively, when a new mutation occurs, linkage disequilibrium exists between this new allele and its neighboring alleles until a sufficient number of recombination events in the population have rendered their relationships random, thereby restoring equilibrium.

If the VDR 3′ polymorphisms are in linkage disequilibrium (LD) with a neighboring functional polymorphism(s), the strength and presence or absence of a significant LD will vary between populations. Since each population has a unique genetic history, this relationship would explain why some studies show positive effects of the *B* allele of VDR, some negative effects of the *B* allele, and others no effect. Several candidates exist for the putative functional allele, including a *FokI* RFLP which alters the translation start site of VDR, a variable-length 3′ poly-A tract and other RFLPs in the 3′ region of VDR.

Several alternative explanations exist to explain the variability seen in association studies as typified by the VDR story. First, some studies are too small to detect the modest effect on BMD variance conferred by the VDR locus. Secondly, if an environmental factor is interacting with the VDR/BMD association, the strength of the association will depend upon the magnitude of this interaction. In this regard, Kiel et al. (1997) found no effect of VDR 3′ alleles on BMD initially but went on to stratify the study population by calcium intake. Such stratification for calcium intake revealed environmentally dependent VDR effects. In another large study population, the association between VDR and BMD was strengthened by stratification for calcium intake (Rubin et al., 1999). Such gene–environment interactions will probably play a prominent role in future studies on the genetics of osteoporosis. A third cause of variability in association studies is genotype–genotype interaction whereby alleles at one locus interact with alleles at another locus to modify trait expression. This has been found in the context of VDR and estrogen receptor alpha alleles (Gennari et al., 1998; Willing et al., 1998).

While controversy remains, it is likely that 3′ VDR alleles are associated with BMD in an effect mediated through linkage disequilibrium. Their effect is strongest for female Caucasian BMD at the hip, where they account for less than 10% of the variance in peak BMD. Their effects at the spine are weaker and in perimenopausal individuals have generally been difficult to appreciate.

Estrogen receptor alpha

The role of estrogen in the accumulation and maintenance of bone mass is unequivocal (Civitelli et al., 1993). Allelic variation at the estrogen receptor alpha (ER1) locus as a determinant of BMD has been examined by several investigators. In two Japanese studies of postmenopausal women (Kobayashi et al., 1996; Sano et al., 1996), alleles at ER1 were shown to be associated with lumbar spine BMD. A study of peak BMD found significant association of two RFLPs in the first intron of ER1 with femoral neck BMD in a population of 501 Caucasian women (Willing et al., 1998). The RFLPs have no known functional consequences for gene expression and therefore any effects on BMD are likely mediated through other functional ER1 variants in linkage disequilibrium. Furthermore, when VDR genotypes were stratified by ER genotypes, a significant genotype–genotype interaction was detected – that is, VDR alleles were found to account for significant additional variance in peak BMD (Willing et al., 1998). A similar effect has been seen at the lumbar spine in a postmenopausal Caucasian population, the only other population to date in which this intriguing genotype–genotype interaction has been examined (Gennari et al., 1998).

Such an interaction is difficult to explain physiologically but is not without support. VDR-deficient mice display an estrogen insufficiency phenotype accompanied by failure of ovarian folliculogenesis (Yoshizawa et al., 1997). Furthermore, the enzyme responsible for the final, rate-limiting step in estrogen synthesis, P450 aromatase, is upregulated by 1,25 dihydroxyvitamin D_3 in a VDR-dependent manner (Tanaka et al., 1996). Early physiological evidence from in vitro and in vivo studies therefore supports interaction(s) between these pathways. Studies in other populations will be needed to establish the relevance of this connection to human bone density determination.

Transforming growth factor beta

The transforming growth factor beta (TGF-β) superfamily of growth factors comprises more than 30 members grouped in several subfamilies (for review, see Alevizopoulos & Mermod, 1997). The prototypic member of the TGF-β subfamily is TGF-β1, a multifunctional hormone which plays key roles in cell growth and differentiation, wound healing, inflammation and morphogenesis. In growing bone, TGF-β1–3 isoforms are expressed in defined regions of the growth plate, suggesting a role in control of bone growth. In mature bone, TGF-β1 may be one of the factors which regulates the central interaction of bone turnover – osteoblast–osteoclast coupling. In vitro studies have indicated that estrogen promotes TGF-β1 synthesis by osteoblasts and that both estrogen and TGF-β1 promote osteoclast apoptosis (Hughes et al., 1996).

Langdahl et al. (1997) discovered a rare allele of the TGF-β1 gene – a one-base pair deletion in intron 4 designated 713–8delC – which was associated with very low bone mass and increased bone specific alkaline phosphatase in osteoporotic women. Yamada et al. (1998) reported the association of a coding polymorphism (designated T29C) which results in the substitution of proline for leucine in the signal peptide of TGF-β1 with lumbar bone density and vertebral fracture frequency in two different Japanese populations of osteoporotics, as compared to normal controls. However, since the case and control groups had different allele frequencies, it is possible that these alleles are associated with survival rather than the osteoporotic phenotype (Yamada et al., 1998).

Other candidate genes

Alleles of other candidate genes have been shown to associate with BMD. These include interleukin-6, insulin-like growth factor-I, calcitonin receptor (Masi et al., 1998), osteopontin (Willing et al., 1998), HLA (Tsuji et al., 1998) and apolipoprotein E (Shiraki et al., 1997). Mapping studies in mice and humans will corroborate a role for some of these genes as determinants of BMD as well as identify novel loci involved in the genetic control of BMD, bone turnover and bone fragility.

Table 10.1. Syndromic causes of low bone density

Syndrome name	Select features	OMIM #
Turner (XO)	Short stature, primary amenorrhea	–
Klinefelter (XXY)	Tall stature, gynecoid features	–
Osteogenesis imperfecta	Blue sclerae, dental abn., hyperhidrosis	166200
Ehlers–Danlos	Joint hypermobility +/− dislocation	130060
Cutis laxa	Lax skin, premature aged appearance	219100
Geroderma osteodysplasticum	Short stature, lax skin, droopy face, dental abnormalities	231070
Marfan	Tall stature, lens dislocation, aortic root dilation	154700
Homocystinuria	Tall stature, lens dislocation, thrombosis	236270
Lysinuric protein intolerance	Dietary protein avoidance	222700
Cleidocranial dysplasia	Sloped shoulders, dental abnormalities	119600
Osteoporosis-pseudogliom	Poor vision, early fractures	259770
Werner	Short stature, premature aging	277700
Hereditary sensory neuropathies	Insensitivity to pain	162400
Hajdu–Cheney	Short stature, hirsutism, clubbing	102500
Singleton–Merten	Diffuse aortic calcification, psoriasis, dental abnormalities	182250

Notes:

Further information about the conditions listed may be obtained from the Online Mendelian Inheritance in Man (OMIM) website located at: www3.ncbi.nlm.nih.gov/omim/

Genetic syndromes featuring osteoporosis

Postmenopausal osteoporosis is not one but many diseases. Part of the heterogeneity of this condition may be due to the presence of osteoporosis in a number of genetic syndromes (Table 10.1). Patients with a syndromic cause of osteoporosis may present with a wide variety of manifestations, making targeted history taking and careful physical examination of critical importance in screening for this subgroup of patients. However, many will show an early onset of disease and will have specific syndromic features. Patients with syndromic osteoporosis may not respond to conventional therapy, may require alternate treatment modalities or may have associated abnormalities. Family members should be offered screening for the condition, and relatives making reproductive decisions may be offered counseling for their risks of having affected children.

Several features are common to a number of the syndromes listed in Table 10.1. During tooth eruption, osteoclasts degrade bone superiorly while osteoblasts synthesize bone inferiorly. Malfunction of either cell type results in failure of tooth eruption or abnormally timed eruption. Thus, too few teeth, persistent deciduous or abnormally shaped teeth are all potential signposts for a syndromic osteoporosis. Likewise, easy bruising, hyperextensible skin, bluish sclerae, joint hypermobility and deeply wrinkled skin are signs of collagen defects and the concurrence of two or more of these signs should prompt a search for a heritable disorder of connective tissue.

The proportion of postmenopausal osteoporosis accounted for by Mendelian disorders is unknown but likely to be small. However, a mutation causing an autosomal recessive disease which has an incidence of 1 in 40000 live births will be carried by 1% of the general population. It is possible that being a carrier for one or more such mutations predisposes to lower bone mass. For the dominant syndromes, it is possible that a range of milder alleles exist in the population which also predispose to low bone mass, as has been demonstrated in the case of osteogenesis imperfecta.

Conclusions

Bone mineral density is a highly heritable trait. Important strides have already been made towards identifying some potential genetic predictors of low bone mass and fracture risk. At the present time, however, there are no clinically applicable genetic markers for predicting bone mass or fracture risk. The current global effort to sequence the human genome and characterize human genetic diversity will provide crucial starting points for the future study of these traits and will allow mapping and association studies on a previously unattainable scale. The effects of most genes or loci will be mediated through interaction with the environment and dissection of such gene–environment interactions will likely prove to be a formidable challenge. A thorough understanding of the genetic basis for osteoporosis should allow therapy to be individualized for those affected and in the long term, will bring preventive therapy to those at greatest risk.

Acknowledgements

This work was supported in part by a grant-in-aid from the Dairy Farmers of Canada to DECC and LAR.

REFERENCES

Alevizopoulos, A. & Mermod, N. (1997). Transforming growth factor-beta: the breaking open of a black box. *Bioessays*, **19**(7), 581–91.

Allison, D. B. (1997). Transmission–disequilibrium tests for quantitative traits. *Am. J. Hum. Genet.*, **60**(3), 676–90.

Christian, J. C., Yu, P. L., Slemenda, C. W., & Johnston, C. C. Jr. (1989). Heritability of bone mass: a longitudinal study in aging male twins. *Am. J. Hum. Genet.*, 44(3), 429–43.

Civitelli, R., Villareal, D. T., & Armamento-Villareal, R. (1993). Estrogen status and bone mass in the premenopausal period: is osteoporosis a developmental disease? *J. Endocrinol. Invest.*, 16(10), 829–39.

Cooper, G. S. & Umbach, D. M. (1996). Are vitamin D receptor polymorphisms associated with bone mineral density? A meta-analysis. *J. Bone Miner. Res.*, 11, 1841–9.

Dawson-Hughes, B., Harris, S. S., Finneran, S., & Parry, P. (1995). Calcium absorption on high and low calcium intakes in relation to vitamin D receptor genotype. *J. Clin. Endocrinol. Metab.*, 80, 3657–61.

Econs, M. J. & Speer, M. C. (1996). Genetic studies of complex diseases: let the reader beware. *J. Bone Miner. Res.*, 11, 1835–40.

Eisman, J. A. (1996). Genetics of osteoporosis. In *Osteoporosis 1996*, ed. S. E. Papapoulos et al., pp. 131–5. Elsevier Science B.V.

Evans, R. A., Marel, G. M., Lancaster, E. K., Kos, S., Evans, M., & Wong, S. Y. (1988). Bone mass is low in relatives of osteoporotic patients. *Ann. Int. Med.*, 109(11), 870–3.

Fleet, J. C., Harris, S. S., Wood, R. J., & Dawson-Hughes, B. (1995). The BsmI vitamin D receptor restriction fragment length polymorphism (BB) predicts low bone density in premenopausal black and white women. *J. Bone Miner. Res.*, 10, 985–90.

Garnero, P., Arden, N. K., Griffiths, G., Delmas, P. D., & Spector, T. D. (1996). Genetic influence on bone turnover in postmenopausal twins. *J. Clin. Endocrinol. Metab.*, 81(1), 140–6.

Gennari, L., Becherini, L., Masi, L., Mansani, R., Gonnelli, S., Cepollaro, C., Martini, S., Montagnani, A., Lentini, G., Becorpi, A. M., & Brandi, M. L. (1998). Vitamin D and estrogen receptor allelic variants in Italian postmenopausal women: evidence of multiple gene contribution to bone mineral density. *J. Clin. Endocrinol. Metab.*, 83(3), 939–44.

Graafmans, W. C., Lips, P., Ooms, M. E., van Leeuwen, J. P., Pols, H. A., & Uitterlinden, A. G. (1997). The effect of vitamin D supplementation on the bone mineral density of the femoral neck is associated with vitamin D receptor genotype. *J. Bone Miner. Res.*, 12(8):1241–5.

Grant, S. F. A., Reid, D. M., Blake, G., Herd, R., Fogelman, I., & Ralston, S. H. (1996). Reduced bone density and osteoporosis associated with a polymorphic Sp1 binding site in the collagen type Ia1 gene. *Nat. Genet.*, 14, 203–5.

Gueguen, R., Jouanny, P., Guillemin, F., Kuntz, C., Pourel, J., & Siest, G. (1995). Segregation analysis and variance components analysis of bone mineral density in healthy families. *J. Bone Miner. Res.*, 10(12), 2017–22.

Herodotus (430 BC). *The Persian Wars*. Book III, Chapter 12.

Hopper, J. L., Green, R. M., Nowson, C. A., Young, D., Sherwin, A. J., Kaymakci, B., Larkins, R. G., & Wark, J. D. (1998). Genetic, common environment, and individual specific components of variance for bone mineral density in 10– to 26-year-old females: a twin study. *Am. J. Epidemiol.*, 147(1), 17–29.

Houston, L. A., Grant, S. F. A., Reid, D. M., & Ralston, S. H. (1996). Vitamin D receptor polymorphism, bone mineral density, and osteoporotic vertebral fracture: studies in a UK population. *Bone*, 18, 249–52.

Hughes, D. E., Dai, A., Tiffee, J. C., Li, H. H., Mundy, G. R., & Boyce, B. F. (1996). Estrogen promotes apoptosis of murine osteoclasts mediated by TGF-beta. *Nat. Med.*, 2(10), 1132–6.

Hustmyer, F. G., Peacock, M., Hui, S., Johnston, C. C., & Christian, J. (1994). Bone mineral density in relation to polymorphism at the vitamin D receptor gene locus. *J. Clin. Invest.*, **94**, 2130–4.

Johnson, M. L., Gong, G., Kimberling, W., Recker, S. M., Kimmel, D. B., & Recker, R. R. (1997). Linkage of a gene causing high bone mass to human chromosome 11 (11q12–13). *Am. J. Hum. Genet.*, **60**, 1326–32.

Jorgensen, H. L., Scholler, J., Sand, J. C., Bjuring, M., Hassager, C., & Christiansen, C. (1996). Relation of common allelic variation at vitamin D receptor locus to bone mineral density and postmenopausal bone loss: cross sectional and longitudinal population study. *Br. Med. J.*, **313**, 586–90.

Kanis J. A. & McCloskey, E. V. (1996). Evaluation of the risk of hip fracture. *Bone*, **18**(Suppl. 3), 127S–32S.

Kiel, D. P., Myers, R. H., Cupples, L. A. et al. (1997). The *BsmI* vitamin D receptor restriction fragment length polymorphism (bb) influences the effect of calcium intake on bone mineral density. *J. Bone Miner. Res.*, **12**, 1049–57.

Kobayashi, S., Inoue, S., Hosoi, T., Ouchi, Y., Shiraki, M., & Orimo, H. (1996). Association of bone mineral density with polymorphism of the estrogen receptor gene. *J. Bone Miner. Res.*, **11**, 306–11.

Krall, E.A. & Dawson-Hughes, B. (1993). Heritable and life-style determinants of bone mineral density. *J. Bone Miner. Res.*, **8**(1), 1–9.

Krall, E. A., Parry, P., Lichter, J. B., & Dawson-Hughes, B. (1995). Vitamin D receptor alleles and rates of bone loss: influences of years since menopause and calcium intake. *J. Bone Miner. Res.*, **10**, 978–84.

Lander, E. S. & Schork, N. J. (1994). Genetic dissection of complex traits. *Science*, **265**, 2037–48.

Langdahl, B. L., Knudsen, J. Y., Jensen, H. K., Gregersen, N., & Eriksen, E. F. (1997). A sequence variation: 713–8delC in the transforming growth factor-beta 1 gene has higher prevalence in osteoporotic women than in normal women and is associated with very low bone mass in osteoporotic women and increased bone turnover in both osteoporotic and normal women. *Bone*, **20**(3), 289–94.

Langdahl, B. L., Ralston, S. H., Grant, S. F., & Eriksen, E. F. (1998). An Sp1 binding site polymorphism in the COLIA1 gene predicts osteoporotic fractures in both men and women. *J. Bone Miner. Res.*, **13**(9), 1384–9.

Marshall, D., Johnell, O., & Wedel, H. (1996). Meta-analysis of how well measures of bone mineral density predict occurrence of osteoporotic fractures. *Br. Med. J.*, **312**, 1254–9.

Masi, L., Becherini, L., Colli, E., Gennari, L., Mansani, R., Falchetti, A., Becorpi, A. M., Cepollaro, C., Gonnelli, S., Tanini, A., & Brandi, M. L. (1998). Polymorphisms of the calcitonin receptor gene are associated with bone mineral density in postmenopausal Italian women. *Biochem. Biophys. Res. Commun.*, **248**(1), 190–5.

Melton, L. J. (1993). Hip fractures: a worldwide problem today and tomorrow. *Bone*, **14**(Suppl. 1), S1–S8.

Morrison, N. A., Cheng, Q. I., Tokita, A., Kelly, P. J., Crofts, L., Nguyen, T. V., Sambrook, P. N., & Eisman, J. A. (1994). Prediction of bone density from vitamin D receptor alleles. *Nature*, **367**, 284–7.

Riggs, B. L., Nguyen, T. V., Melton, III L. J., Morrison, N. A., OíFallon, W. M., Kelly, P. J., Egan,

K. S., Sambrook, P. N., Muhs, J. M., & Eisman, J. A. (1995). The contribution of vitamin D receptor gene alleles to the determination of bone mineral density in normal and osteoporotic women. *J. Bone Miner. Res.*, **10**, 991–6.

Risch, N. & Merikangas, K. (1996). The future of genetic studies of complex human diseases. *Science*, **273**, 1516–17.

Roux, C., Dougados, M., Abel, L., Mercier, G., & Lucotte, G. (1998). Association of a polymorphism in the collagen IA1 gene with osteoporosis in French women. *Arthritis Rheum.*, **41**(1), 187–8.

Rubin, L. A., Hawker, G. A., Peltekova, V.D., Fielding, L., Rideout, R., & Cole, D. E. (1999). Determinants of peak bone mass: clinical and genetic analyses in a young female Canadian cohort. *J. Bone Miner. Res.*, **14**, 633–43.

Salamone, L. M., Ferrell, R., Black, D. M., Palermo, L., Epstein, R. S., Petro, N., Steadman, N., Kuller, L. H., & Cauley, J. A. (1996). The association between vitamin D receptor gene polymorphisms and bone mineral density at the spine, hip and whole-body in premenopausal women. *Osteoporos. Int.*, **6**, 63–8.

Sano, M., Inoue, S., Hosoi, T., Ouchi, Y., Emi, M., Shiraki, M., & Orimo, H. (1996). Association of an estrogen receptor dinucleotide repeat polymorphism with osteoporosis. *Biochem. Biophys. Res. Commun.*, **217**, 378–83.

Schaid, D. J. (1998). Transmission disequilibrium, family controls, and great expectations. *Am. J. Hum. Genet.*, **63**(4), 935–41.

Schaid, D. J. & Li, H. (1997). Genotype relative-risks and association tests for nuclear families with missing parental data. *Genet. Epidemiol.*, **14**(6), 1113–18.

Schapira, D. & Schapira, C. (1992). Osteoporosis: the evolution of a scientific term. *Osteoporos. Int.*, 2(4), 164–7.

Seeman, E., Hopper, J. L., Bach, L. A., Cooper, M. E., Parkinson, E., McKay, J., & Jerums, G. (1989). Reduced bone mass in daughters of women with osteoporosis. *New Engl. J. Med.*, **320**, 554–8.

Shiraki, M., Shiraki, Y., Aoki, C., Hosoi, T., Inoue, S., Kaneki, M., & Ouchi, Y. (1997). Association of bone mineral density with apolipoprotein E phenotype. *J. Bone Miner. Res.*, **12**(9), 1438–45.

Slemenda, C. W., Christian, J. C., Williams, C. J., Norton, J. A., & Johnston, C. C. Jr. (1991). Genetic determinants of bone mass in adult women: a reevaluation of the twin model and the potential importance of gene interaction on heritability estimates. *J. Bone Miner. Res.*, **6**(6), 561–7.

Slemenda, C. W., Turner, C. H., Peacock, M., Christian, J. C., Sorbel, J., Hui, S. L., & Johnston, C. C. (1996). The genetics of proximal femur geometry, distribution of bone mass and bone mineral density. *Osteoporosis. Int.*, **6**(2), 178–82.

Smith, D. M., Nance, W. E., Kang, K. W., Christian, J. C., & Johnston, C. C. Jr. (1973). Genetic factors in determining bone mass. *J. Clin. Invest.*, **52**, 2800–8.

Sowers, M. R., Boehnke, M., Jannausch, M. L., Crutchfield, M., Corton, G., & Burns, T. L. (1992). Familiality and partitioning the variability of femoral bone mineral density in women of child-bearing age. *Calcif. Tissue Int.*, **50**(2), 110–14.

Spector, T. D., Keen, R. W., Arden, N. K., Morrison, N. A., Major, P. J., Nguyen, T. V., Kelly, P. J., Baker, J. R., Sambrook, P. N., Lanchbury, J. S., & Eisman, J. A. (1995). Influence of the vitamin

D receptor genotype on bone mineral density in postmenopausal women: a twin study in Britain. *Br. Med. J.*, **310**, 1357–60.

Spielman, R. S. & Ewens, W. J. (1996). The TDT and other family-based tests for linkage disequilibrium and association. *Am. J. Hum. Genet.*, **59**(5), 983–9.

Spotila, L. D., Colige, A., Sereda, L., Constantinou-Deltas, C. D., Whyte, M. P., Riggs, B. L., Shaker, J. L., Spector, T. D., Hume, E., & Olsen, N. (1994). Mutation analysis of coding sequences for type I procollagen in individuals with low bone density. *J. Bone Miner. Res.*, **9**(6), 923–32.

Tanaka, S., Haji, M., Takayanagi, R., Tanaka, S., Sugioka, Y., & Nawata, H. (1996). 1,25-Dihydroxyvitamin D3 enhances the enzymatic activity and expression of the messenger ribonucleic acid for aromatase cytochrome P450 synergistically with dexamethasone depending on the vitamin D receptor level in cultured human osteoblasts. *Endocrinology*, **137**(5), 1860–9.

Theobald, T. M., Cauley, J. A., Gluer, C. C., Bunker, C. H., Ukoli, F. A., & Genant, H. K. (1998). Black–white differences in hip geometry. Study of Osteoporotic Fractures Research Group. *Osteoporosis Int.*, **8**(1), 61–7.

Tsuji, S., Munkhbat, B., Hagihara, M., Tsuritani, I., Abe, H., & Tsuji, K. (1998). HLA-A*24–B*07–DRB1*01 haplotype implicated with genetic disposition of peak bone mass in healthy young Japanese women. *Hum. Immunol.*, **59**(4), 243–9.

Uitterlinden, A. G., Burger, H., Huang, Q., Yue, F., McGuigan, F. E., Grant, S. F. A., Hofman, A., van Leeuwen, J. P., Pols, H. A., & Ralston, S. H. (1998). Relation of alleles of the collagen type Ialpha1 gene to bone density and the risk of osteoporotic fractures in postmenopausal women. *N. Engl. J. Med.*, **338**(15), 1016–21.

Uitterlinden, A. G., Pols, H. A., Burger, H., Huang, Q., Van Daele, P. L., Van Duijn, C. M., Hofman, A., Birkenhager, J. C., & Van Leeuwen, J. P. (1996). A large-scale population-based study of the association of vitamin D receptor gene polymorphisms with bone mineral density. *J. Bone Miner. Res.*, **11**(9):1241–8.

Willing, M., Sowers, M. F., Aron, D., Clark, M. K., Burns, T., Bunten, C., Crutchfield, M., D'Agostino, D., & Jannausch, M. (1998). Bone mineral density and its change in white women: estrogen and vitamin D receptor genotypes and their interaction. *J. Bone Miner. Res.*, **13**(4), 695–705.

Wishart, J. M., Horowitz, M., Need, A. G., Scopacasa, F., Morris, H. A., Clifton, P. M., & Nordin, B. E. C. (1997). Relations between calcium intake, calcitriol, polymorphisms of the vitamin D receptor gene, and calcium absorption in premenopausal women. *Am. J. Clin. Nutr.*, **65**, 798–802.

Yamada, Y., Miyauchi, A., Goto, J., Takagi, Y., Okuizumi, H., Kanematsu, M., Hase, M., Takai, H., Harada, A., & Ikeda, K. (1998). Association of a polymorphism of the transforming growth factor-beta1 gene with genetic susceptibility to osteoporosis in postmenopausal Japanese women. *J. Bone Miner. Res.*, **13**(10), 1569–76.

Yamagata, Z., Miyamura, T., Iijima, S., Asaka, A., Sasaki, M., Kato, J., & Koizumi, K. (1994). Vitamin D receptor polymorphism and bone mineral density in healthy Japanese women. *Lancet*, **344**, 1027.

Yoshizawa, T., Handa, Y., Uematsu, Y. et al. (1997). Mice lacking the vitamin D receptor exhibit impaired bone formation, uterine hypoplasia and growth retardation after weaning. *Nat. Genet.*, **16**, 391–6.

11

Non-genetic determinants of peak bone mass

Velimir Matkovic and John D. Landoll

Introduction

Osteoporosis is becoming one of the most common chronic diseases affecting millions of people worldwide, primarily due to the aging of the world's population. Since bone fractures are closely related to diminished bone mass and reduced bone mineral density, we have to identify all underlying causes responsible for inadequate accumulation of bone tissue during skeletal growth and consolidation, and excessive losses thereafter. Maximizing bone mass during skeletal growth, therefore, has been the goal of the primary prevention of osteoporosis, while the reduction of bone loss during menopause and aging is the problem in secondary prevention programs. Until recently, the concern for patients with osteoporosis dictated a simple approach to preventive medicine, that is to reduce the number of women suffering from it. They were considered the minority, while the majority of the population without fractures was considered normal. This approach was primarily based on the X-ray diagnosis which assumed that women fall into just two categories, namely those who have the disease and those who do not (Matkovic et al., 1995b). That there is no clear distinction between the bone health and osteoporosis was originally proposed by Newton-John and Morgan (1970) and shown for the first time in a study of fracture rates among two populations with different peak bone mass (Matkovic et al., 1979). Those with high peak bone mass had lower incidence of hip fractures and vice versa (Fig. 11.1). Newton John and Morgan suggested that there is a continuum in the disease severity, that is, there is an increase in the number of bone fractures with a decline in bone mineral density in the population rather than a bimodal distribution of bone mass with a sharp distinction between bone health and osteoporosis. There is a continuum in bone mass and bone mineral density in any age segment of the female population (Fig. 11.2). This variability in bone mass, which is to a great extent genetically determined and modified by the environment, has major implications for bone health. Current thought is that those who have higher bone mass as young adults may be at lower risk of developing osteoporosis later in life. Starting bone mass, therefore, seems to be the main predictor of subsequent bone mass measurements over time. This applies to

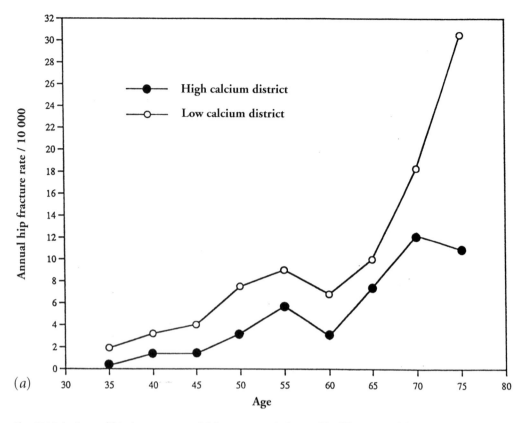

Fig. 11.1(*a*) Annual hip fracture rates (*a*) in two populations with different peak bone mass as indicated by the cortical area (CA) of the second metacarpal bone. Adapted from Matkovic et al., 1979.

growing individuals with the resultant net-positive increment in bone mass, and to the elderly in whom bone loss dominates. Hormonal factors, exercise and nutrition play very important roles in peak bone mass acquisition and maintenance.

Peak bone mass

Peak bone mass is defined as the highest level of bone mass achieved as a result of normal growth. Peak bone mass is important because it determines resistance or susceptibility to fracture (Heaney & Matkovic, 1995). The ecological study from Croatia suggested that peak bone mass may be modified by the environment (nutrition) and laid background for primary prevention programs (Matkovic et al., 1979, 1980). The study compared two farming communities accustomed to a heavy physical labor but with different dietary habits and found a difference in bone mass and hip fracture rates. It appeared that both populations were losing bone with age

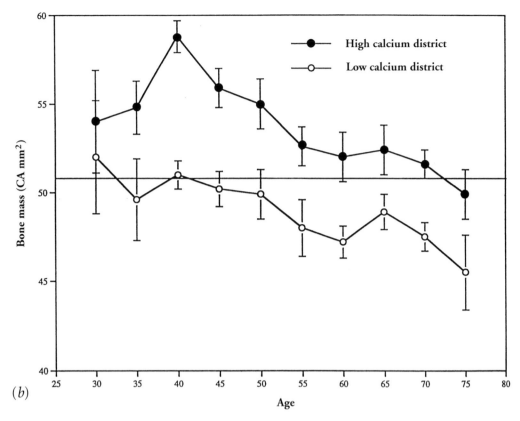

(b)

Fig. 11.1(b)   Results presented as a mean ± SE. The horizontal line marks the level at which one population started and the other finished. Adapted from Matkovic et al., 1979.

at about the same rate, but those who started with more bone, ended up having higher bone mass and lower incidence of hip fractures. It was concluded that, other things being equal, a high peak bone mass provided a larger reserve later in life. The difference in bone mass and fracture rates were attributed to nutritional factors, primarily calcium and/or protein intake. The differences in bone mass between the communities were established at an early age (30 y), implying that, if calcium intake is important, it may be during skeletal growth that it has its greatest impact. This was the first proposal of the hypothesis that increasing peak bone mass by calcium supplementation during skeletal formation may contribute to osteoporosis prevention (Matkovic et al., 1979). Results of a similar ecological study conducted in China on populations accustomed to different calcium intakes over their lifetime confirmed the above finding and reiterated the importance of adequate calcium intake for skeletal formation and peak bone mass (Hu et al., 1993). Positive relations between the bone mineral density of adult women and their milk consumption in childhood, adolescence, or throughout life, were also found in several

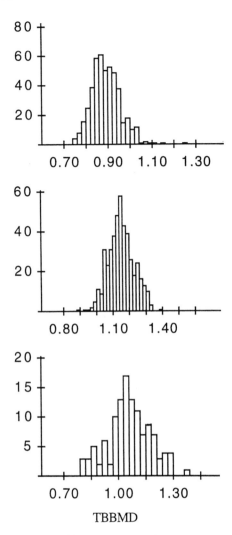

Fig. 11.2   Frequency histograms of total body bone mineral areal density (TBBMD) in girls ($n=464$, 10 ± 2 y) (top), young adult females ($n=454$, 37 ± 7) (middle), and postmenopausal elderly women ($n=131$, 64 ± 8) (bottom). Mean TBBMD for girls, young adult females, and the elderly women is as follows: 0.89 ± 0.07 g/cm², 1.15 ± 0.08 g/cm², and 1.07 ± 0.11 g/cm², respectively.

retrospective studies (Cauley et al., 1988; Halioua & Anderson, 1989; Murphy et al., 1994; Sandler et al., 1985; Soroko et al., 1994) which further strengthen the hypothesis. Overall, it is likely that variations in calcium nutrition early in life may account for as much as a 5–10% difference in peak adult bone mass. Such a difference, although small, probably contributes to more than 50% of the difference in the hip fracture rate later in life.

The same trend exists when comparing bone mass and hip fracture rates between

Table 11.1. Bone size, bone mass and bone density variables of daughters at ages 14 and 16 years as % of their mother's value

Variable	Daughters	
	Age 14	Age 16
Bone size		
Ht (cm)	99	100
L (mm)	99	100
TA (mm²)	90	93
MA (mm²)	130	113
Bone mass		
CA (mm²)	85	90
DPA (g)	87	97
Bone density		
CA/TA	95	98
SPAf1 (g/cm²)	80	91
SPAf2 (g/cm²)	87	94
DPA (g/cm)	95	101

Notes:
Ht = total height; L = length; TA = total area; MA = medullary area;
CA = cortical area;
SPAf1 = single photon absorptiometry of the distal forearm;
SPAf2 = single photon absorptiometry of the proximal forearm;
DPA = dual photon absorptiometry.
Source: From Matkovic et al., 1990.

men and women, and between Caucasians and African Americans. Both men and people of African descent have higher peak bone mass and lower hip fracture rates than their counterparts (Matkovic et al., 1995c). This again confirms the hypothesis that people with greater bone mass in early adulthood are able to resist the effects of age-related bone loss.

A knowledge of the timing of peak bone mass and bone mineral density is essential if preventive measures are to be adequately implemented. One study reports that, by the age of 14, values for bone size, mass, and density of adolescent girls are similar to the corresponding values of their mothers (Table 11.1) (Matkovic et al., 1990). Such an early attainment of peak bone mass is supported by the observation that, from age 14, longitudinal bone growth diminishes, although consolidation continues. By age 16, most epiphyses are closed, and endosteal bone apposition ceases as well. Subsequently, several other studies indicate an early attainment of peak bone mass, although the entire age range from childhood to menopause was

Table 11.2. Age of the inflection point at which most of the bone mass is being accumulated for various bone parameters with estimates of bone variable at the inflection point and R-squared of each model (Mean ± SE)

ROI	N	R^2	Inflection point age (years)	Estimate of bone variable
Height	234	0.692	16.25 ± 0.04	162.8 cm
TBBMC	231	0.624	18.33 ± 0.07	2432 g
TBBMD	231	0.587	18.70 ± 0.08	1.11 g/cm²
Skull	231	0.642	21.77 ± 0.12	2.29 g/cm²
Fem. neck	232	0.425	17.23 ± 0.07	1.04 g/cm²
Wards	232	0.328	18.49 ± 0.09	1.02 g/cm²
Trochanter	232	0.229	16.72 ± 0.12	0.86 g/cm²
L_{2-4} BMC	231	0.657	18.79 ± 0.07	48.05 g
L_{2-4} BMD	231	0.630	18.45 ± 0.07	1.18 g/cm²
L_3 body vol.	228	0.583	19.18 ± 0.10	16.46 cm³
L_3 body BMC	229	0.482	20.02 ± 0.10	4.20 g
L_3 body-lat.	229	0.274	23.97 ± 0.19	0.77 g/cm²
L_3 body-mid	229	0.237	23.15 ± 0.24	0.73 g/cm²
L_3 body dens.[a]	227	0.131	27.18 ± 0.06	0.257 g/cm³
Radius	223	0.673	17.82 ± 0.07	0.65 g/cm²
Wrist	222	0.407	22.32 ± 0.18	0.34 g/cm²

Notes:
The inflection point marks the transition between the rapid accumulation of bone mass during growth and skeletal maturity of young adulthood.
ROI, regions of interest; TBBMC, total body bone mineral content; TBBMD, total body bone mineral density; BMC, bone mineral content; BMD, bone mineral density.
[a] True bone mineral density (g/cm³). *Source:* From Matkovic et al., 1994.

not evaluated (Bonjour et al., 1991; Gilsanz et al., 1988; Glastre et al., 1990; Lu et al., 1994; Theintz et al., 1992). The results of our cross-sectional study (Matkovic et al., 1994) conducted in 265 premenopausal females, age 8–50 y show that most of the bone mass at multiple skeletal locations (forearm, AP and lateral spine, hip, total body) is accumulated by late adolescence (Table 11.2). This is particularly notable for bone mineral density of the proximal femur and the vertebral body, which begin to decline immediately following peak bone mass formation at the age of ∼18 y.

Based on this cross-sectional model, bone size, bone mass, and bone mineral density of the regional skeletal sites increased by an average of about 4% /y between preadolescence (age 8 y) and late adolescence when most of the bone mass has been accumulated. This ranged from 1.2% for the estimate of true density of the body of L_3 vertebra to 6.6% for the femoral neck. The relatively smaller increments in true density (mass/volume ratio in g/cm^3) are of interest, indicating that most of the changes we measure during growth using either single photon absorptiometry (SPA) or dual X-ray absorptiometry (DXA) are predominantly due to the change in bone volume, and to a much lesser extent to increases in bone mineral density. A similar observation was previously documented using ash weight/volume ratio of the human radii in vitro in a study by Trotter & Hixon (1974) and by calculating apparent bone mineral density in the study of Katzman et al. (1991). Trotter and Hixon also studied skeletal weights throughout the lifespan and found maximal skeletal weight to be at age 20, with relatively rapid decline thereafter. However, there were only a few subjects in the third and fourth decades in their study, making the assessment of precise timing difficult.

Bone mass of the other regions of interest is either no different in women between the age of 18 and menopause or is maximal in 50-year-old women (skull, forearm, AP spine, total body), indicating slow but permanent bone accumulation continuing at some sites up to the time of menopause (Fig. 11.3). This gain in bone mass in premenopausal adult women is probably the result of continuous periosteal expansion with age. Periosteal apposition has previously been described for the skull (Israel, 1968; Susanne, 1979) vertebrae (Ericksen, 1976; Mosekilde & Mosekilde, 1990) and tubular bones including ribs (Epker & Frost, 1966), shaft of the femur (Bohr & Schaadt, 1990; Smith & Walker, 1964) and metacarpal bones (Garn et al., 1967, 1992). In a study of human ribs, Epker & Frost (1966) used tetracycline labeling in vivo to reveal continued apposition of periosteal bone after age 20. All of the above studies indicate that the periosteal bone surface remains active throughout life and is probably responsible for the positive net bone tissue balance, resulting in the increase in bone mass with age seen at various skeletal sites measured in this study. This expansion of the periosteal envelope most likely plays a significant role with regard to the biomechanical integrity of bone mass at the specific skeletal region of interest.

Bone loss at some skeletal locations proceeds immediately after bone mass has been consolidated and reaches its peak by late adolescence. This is documented thus far for two skeletal regions of interest: trabecular bone of the body of the vertebra and proximal end of the femur. The significance of this phenomenon with regard to the subsequent development of crush fracture syndrome and hip fractures is not yet clear, although it is assumed that any reduction in bone mass or bone mineral density prior to the onset of menopause could proportionally increase the risk of subsequent fracture. This loss of trabecular bone was previously documented by different techniques: compressive strength and ash measurements of the vertebrae in vitro (Arnold, 1973), by iliac crest bone histomorphometric analysis

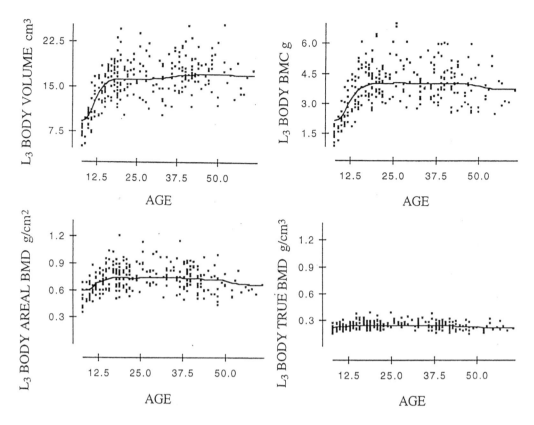

Fig. 11.3   Scatter plots with Trewess smooth of the volume, bone mineral content (BMC), bone mineral areal density, and the true density (mass per volume) of the body of the third lumbar vertebre in premenopausal women ages 8–55 years. (Adapted from Matkovic et al., 1994.)

(Marcus et al., 1983), as well as by computerized tomography of the vertebrae (Block et al., 1989).

Despite the fall in true density of the body of the L_3 vertebra, the bone mineral content of AP L_{2-4} steadily increased in the population under study, at a rate of about 0.23%/y (total of 7% between the age of 19 and 50) (Matkovic et al., 1994). This is presumably due to increase in the volume of the entire vertebrae including the spinal processes. It has been previously documented that the bodies of the lumbar vertebrae become significantly broader with age (Ericksen, 1976); this is most likely the explanation for third decade bone gain (0.6%/y) in the lumbar spine in women, as assessed by DXA (Recker et al.,1992). Trabecular bone loss in the body of the vertebra, however, does not necessarily mean a decrease in strength, since bony expansion and maintenance or even increase of bone mass at these sites may adequately compensate for trabecular density changes (Matkovic et al., 1994). If the relationship between bone mass and bone mineral density is driven by a feedback loop with a mechanostat (Frost, 1992), then the decrease in trabecular volume may reflect the increase in bone mass that results from periosteal expansion of the vertebrae (Matkovic et al., 1994). Only the lack of periosteal bone expansion in the vertebrae may weaken the biomechanical integrity of the vertebral body with significant predisposition to the development of crush fracture syndrome which is usually manifested at an early stage as anterior wedging. This requires confirmation through a longitudinal study.

While the loss and/or thinning of trabecular bone structure within the body of the vertebra may be compensated biomechanically by the expansion of the periosteal envelope, this may not be the case with the neck of the femur which lacks the periosteum. In a study by Matkovic et al. (1994) older premenopausal women had lower bone mineral density in the hip region (neck of the femur, Ward's triangle, and trochanter) than younger women; maximal values were found in ~18-year-old females. This suggests that the decline in the bone mineral density of the proximal end of the femur begins immediately following the acquisition of peak bone mass. The cross-sectional apparent decrease was about −0.3%/y for the trochanteric region, −0.4%/y for the femoral neck, and −0.6%/y for Ward's triangle. A disproportionately higher decline in the bone mineral density at Ward's triangle corresponds to the early disappearance of trabecular architecture in the region visible on standard skeletal radiographs of the hip. A difference of about 15.5% is found in the proximal femur between the ages of 17 and 50 (Matkovic et al., 1994). The same phenomenon has been very well documented previously in similar cross-sectional studies (Beck et al., 1992; Elliott et al., 1990; Hedlund & Gallagher, 1989). The significance of this premenopausal bone loss needs to be further clarified, probably through longitudinal studies, with particular focus on its contribution to the development of hip fractures later in life.

Hormonal status and peak bone mass

Human growth and skeletal maturation are dynamic processes which start in utero and end sometime during the third decade of life. This is the period when endogenous factors (heredity, hormones), in interaction with the environment (nutrition and physical exercise), modulate the skeleton and produce what will be an individual's peak bone mass. It has been speculated that genetics contributes about 75–80% of the variance in bone mass and the remaining 20–25% is affected by one's environment, although the exact contribution of each major determinant of bone mass is unknown. The emphasis here will be limited to the phase of bone mass acquisition and its maintenance up to the time of menopause.

The role of estrogens in the pathogenesis of postmenopausal bone loss is very well established; however, its role in bone mass acquisition is not completely understood or appreciated. Bone mass gain during the second decade of life is non-linear and is linked to sexual maturation more than chronological age. When relating bone mass to pubertal developmental stage, it becomes obvious that most of the bone mass (37%) is accumulated between pubertal stage 2 and 4 (Matkovic et al., 1994). This rapid accumulation of bone mass correlates with the rate of growth and probably also requires the concerted action of growth hormone, insulin-like growth factor-I (IGF-I) and sex steroids (including receptors). The increase in circulating IGF-I at early puberty correlates with sexual development and results from the interaction between sex steroids and growth hormone. Specifically, the surge in sex steroids in turn increases the secretion of growth hormone, which stimulates the production of insulin-like growth factor-I.

The amount of estrogen required to stimulate longitudinal bone growth is very small. Doses of 100 ng/kg/day produce maximal growth in agonadal individuals. This dose seems to be insufficient to cause either the development of secondary sexual characteristics or an increase in sex hormone binding globulin (Speroff et al., 1989). These low dose effects are consistent with the observation that girls attain peak height velocity early in puberty at serum estradiol levels of <30 pg/ml which is one-fifth the mean level found in young adult women. During this phase of rapid skeletal modeling (growth) bone mass is not yet consolidated and bone mass per bone volume ratio is relatively low (Garn, 1970). Presumably, this results in the high incidence of the bone fragility fractures (distal forearm) in children reaching the levels observed in women after menopause (Alffram & Bauer, 1962; Bailey et al., 1989; Matkovic et al., 1995a). A reduced bone mass was found in children with fractures (Goulding et al., 1998).

Bone consolidation proceeds by the cessation of longitudinal bone growth. This coincides with an increase in estradiol secretion by the beginning of menarche. Menarche marks the most powerful transition in skeletal development and bone physiology in young females. This suggests that it is more appropriate to express bone variables during adolescence in time since menarche than to chronological age. Estrogen driven endosteal apposition of bone is responsible for the increase in the relative amount of cortical bone (bone tissue within the bone volume) in premenopausal women as compared to men. This endosteal apposition of cortical bone starts at menarche and presumably ends at menopause (Garn, 1970).

Several studies document lower bone mineral density and higher fracture rate in adult women with a history of late menarche, as indicative of inadequate sex hormone levels during this critical period of skeletal development and/or a shorter time interval between menarche and menopause (Ilich et al., 1997a, b; Johnell et al., 1995; Rosenthal et al., 1989). Both young adult women and adolescents with hypothalamic amenorrhea have reduced bone mass at skeletal sites which should not be losing bone. This might lead to a reduction in bone mass at maturity and predispose this population to increased risk of osteoporosis later in life. The above-mentioned menstrual disturbances could be in part due to relative or absolute energy deficiency induced by weight loss or inadequate weight gain as seen in protein-calorie malnutrition, young athletic women, anorexics, and other clinical situations (Matkovic et al., 1997).

It is a well-known fact that, over the last century, there has been a trend in the western societies toward an earlier onset of menarche in young women, attributed to the improvement in nutritional status and body fatness. We were the first to show that the effects of nutrition on the reproductive function (age at menarche) in human females are being mediated by leptin (Matkovic et al., 1997). Leptin is a 167-amino acid peptide which is produced and released from adipose tissue (Zhang et al., 1994). It is considered a biochemical marker of obesity. Based on animal experimentation, leptin was considered a satiety factor which binds to specific receptors in the hypothalamus leading to reduced appetite and increased energy expenditure (Zhang et al., 1994). However, this has not yet been confirmed in humans. In homozygous mice the mutations of the obesity (*ob*) gene resulted in increased food intake, reduced energy expenditure, elevated insulin level, and subsequent obesity and the development of non-insulin dependent diabetes mellitus (Zhang et al., 1994). Administration of leptin to leptin-deficient homozygous *ob/ob* mice created the opposite effects.

To show the association between nutritional status and the age at menarche, Matkovic et al. (1997) measured body composition and serum leptin, and recorded timing of menarche in 343 young females over 4 years of follow-up. As delayed menarche and leanness are considered risk factors for osteoporosis, the relation between leptin and bone was examined as well. Body composition was measured by DXA and leptin by a new RIA. All participants were premenarcheal at baseline, ages 8–13 y. Leptin was strongly associated with body fat ($r=0.81$, $P<0.0001$) and its change ($r=0.58$, $P<0.0001$). An inverse relation between the age at menarche and leptin up to 12.2 ng/ml (95% CI 7.2–16.7) was found; an increase of 1 ng/ml in serum leptin lowered menarche by 1 month. Serum leptin of 12.2 ng/ml corresponded to a relative body fat of 29.7%, BMI of 22.3, and body fat of 16.0 kg. A gain in body fat of 1 kg lowered the timing of menarche by 13 days. The results of the study show that a critical blood leptin level is necessary to trigger reproductive ability in women suggesting that leptin is a mediator between fat cells and the gonads. In the above study leptin was positively related to bone area ($r=0.307$,

$P < 0.0001$) and its change ($r = 0.274$, $P < 0.0001$) (Matkovic et al., 1997). A direct effect of leptin on endocortical bone formation was described in *ob* mice receiving the peptide (Liu et al.,1997). The results of both studies suggest that leptin may mediate the effect of obesity on cortical bone.

Nutrition and peak bone mass

From infancy through young adulthood (about 30 years of age) the activity of bone formation predominates, resulting in a steady accumulation of bone mass. As the rate of growth changes with age, so skeletal modeling goes through phases of different intensity with time. These changes in skeletal modeling are paralleled by concomitant changes in calcium metabolism. Although calcium is the most obvious and persistent of the micronutrients and the fifth most abundant element in the body, it is more difficult to measure the adequacy of calcium intake during growth and consolidation of skeletal mass than other nutrients.

Calcium intake and skeletal modeling/turnover are the most important determinants of calcium balance during growth (Matkovic, 1991). When comparing the maximal calcium retention in the body, the highest requirements for calcium are during infancy and adolescence and then during childhood and young adulthood. This results from the high velocity of growth during infancy and puberty, as well as from skeletal consolidation that continues through late adolescence. These two determinants of bone volume and bone mineral density exert a major influence on calcium requirements. To meet these high calcium requirements, infants and adolescents have higher calcium absorption than children and young adults. Such a high calcium absorption during these developmental phases is mediated by calcitriol [$1,25(OH)_2D_3$] (Aksnes & Aarskog, 1982; Ilich et al., 1997a).

Another determinant of calcium balance in the body, and presumably bone mass, is urinary calcium. Urinary calcium increases with age and reaches its maximum by the end of puberty. It was shown that calcium intake has little influence on urinary calcium excretion during the period of most rapid skeletal formation. A stronger relationship between urinary and dietary calcium was previously documented only in adults. During their most intensive growth periods, young individuals retain most of the calcium they absorb rather than excrete it in the urine. That urinary calcium excretion is an important determinant of bone mass was shown recently in a study conducted in 381 Caucasian females in pubertal stage 2, aged 8–13 y. Urinary sodium was found to be one of the most important determinants of urinary calcium while calcium intake had relatively little impact. Urinary calcium was much higher at calcium intake of 37.5 mmol/d (1500 mg/d), supporting the notion that calcium is a threshold nutrient. Calcium intake had a significant positive influence on the bone mineral content and density of the

Table 11.3. Threshold intake and threshold balance by age group

Age group	R[a]	Threshold intake mg/day	Threshold balance mg/day
0–1 y	+0.825	1090	+503 ±91[b]
2–8 y	+0.555	1390	+246 ±126
9–17 y	+0.556	1480	+396 ±164
18–30 y	+0.601	957	+114 ±133

Notes: [a] Composite R. [b] x ± SD.
Source: From Matkovic & Heaney, 1992.

whole body and radius shaft while urinary calcium had a negative influence, presumably by reducing calcium accretion into the skeleton. The conclusion from this study is that low calcium intake and relatively high obligatory calcium loss in the urine, potentiated by sodium intake during rapid growth, may reduce calcium retention in the skeleton with a concomitant reduction in peak bone mass. Thus, higher sodium intake increases dietary requirement for calcium (Matkovic et al., 1995a).

Calcium is an essential threshold nutrient. An intake threshold is defined as the level below which skeletal accumulation is a function of intake, and above which skeletal accumulation is constant, irrespective of further increases in intake. This indicates that retained calcium below the threshold level cannot saturate the skeletal mass, while maximal saturation can be achieved at the threshold level and above. This type of threshold behavior is consistent with current models of bone growth, in which the bone modeling/remodeling process would tear down existing bone if calcium intake were insufficient to meet the demands of growth. However, at fully adequate intakes, the amount of bone deposited would depend not upon intake, but upon what was programmed into the growth process; hence additional increases in intake would not result in further skeletal retention. Below a certain threshold level of dietary calcium intake, young persons would not be able to reach their genetically predetermined peak bone mass, while adults would lose bone tissue at a faster rate than is necessary. Adequate calcium intake above a certain threshold level is therefore absolutely required for bone health during skeletal growth and consolidation, as well as for prevention of excessive bone loss with advancing age. Calcium intake thresholds with corresponding threshold balances were recently reported for growing individuals (Table 11.3) (Matkovic & Heaney, 1992).

The assumption is that dietary calcium intake at/or above the threshold level is necessary throughout the entire bone modeling and consolidation phase (from childhood to young adulthood) if genetically predetermined peak bone mass is expected to be reached. Several clinical trials indicated that children and teenagers particularly, may benefit from higher calcium intake with further gain in bone mass (Bonjour et al., 1997; Cadogan et al., 1997; Chan et al., 1995; Johnston et al., 1992; Lee et al., 1994; Lloyd et al., 1993; Matkovic et al., 1990). However, all of the intervention studies either with calcium supplements or dairy products in children and adolescents completed to date were relatively short in duration (1 to 3 y). The increase in bone mass observed in those studies could be explained to a large extent by the remodeling transient phenomenon emphasized recently by Heaney (1995a). According to Heaney (1995a), an intervention study should be long enough and of adequate sample size to allow for the assessment of the slope of the rate of change (gain) in the measured bone variable after the initial effect on the bone remodeling transient is expected to be completed (up to 40–60 weeks). In the continuation of the intervention study with calcium among identical twins during the fourth year (calcium withdrawn, codes released) the difference in bone mass between the groups has been diminishing, indicating that some of the relative gain has been lost (Slemenda at al., 1997), presumably as the result of the second transient. Similar findings were observed in the studies of Lee et al. (1996), and Lloyd et al. (1996). Another contributing factor for the lack of difference between the groups could be due to natural tendency of the placebo group to increase calcium intake to 'catch-up with skeletal mineralization.' It is, therefore, unclear from these short-term studies if a positive effect of a surplus intake of calcium on bone tissue can be maintained. Longitudinal bone growth and the periosteal bone expansion are the driving forces in bone mass acquisition during puberty and under the influence of strains imposed on the bone tissue from muscle action and loads. The endosteal apposition seems to be of a secondary importance early in puberty and it could be sacrificed to accomplish the expansion of the bone volume. If calcium intake is far below the calcium intake threshold required for optimal skeletal development, a permanent deficit in peak bone mass is expected. This could primarily be due to inadequate development of bone structures (thin cortex and/or reduced formation of trabecular network) within the expanding bone as an organ. Borderline calcium deficiency during growth may not result in a permanent deficit in bone mass at skeletal maturity (age 18 y) due to its effect on bone remodeling and the potential for recovery with the decline in calcium requirement proceeding after menarche and associated with the cessation of longitudinal bone growth. A long-term intervention study with calcium supplementation extending from childhood to young adulthood (age 18 y) at various calcium intake levels seems to be mandatory to answer these important questions.

During young adulthood (ages 18–30 years) bones are no longer growing along the longitudinal axis. The cycle of bone resorption and formation continues at a slower rate than during adolescence. There is small but continuous periosteal envelope expansion with age, which can contribute to the net positive bone tissue balance at most of the skeletal locations, including the spine, forearm, shaft of the femur, metacarpal bones, and the skull. In addition, there is also a minimal endo-steal apposition of bone mass by the beginning of young adulthood indicating consolidation of skeletal mass (Matkovic et al., 1994). The above events contribute to the bone mineral gain in young adult women during the third decade of life (Recker at al., 1992). This gain was in the range of 4.8% for the forearm, 6% for the lumbar spine, and 12.5% for the total body. In this 5-year longitudinal observational study, dietary calcium (calcium/protein ratio) and physical activity strongly influenced mineral apposition. When the gain in the total body bone mineral content is translated into calcium content, approximately 150 g of calcium is incorporated into the skeleton during this time interval. Net skeletal calcium accretion per day during this period could therefore be about +41 mg, a figure close to the one obtained from metabolic balance studies (Matkovic, 1991). This indicates that a window of opportunity for the restoration of skeletal mass in young adults under adequate nutrition is possible, but seems to close by the age of 30 years (Recker et al., 1992). The period of young adulthood is characterized by a decline in calcium absorption and calcium retention with a concomitant increase in calcium output (Matkovic, 1991; Matkovic & Heaney, 1992; Weaver et al., 1995). An analysis of calcium balances showed that, across all intake ranges from 500 mg/day to 1600 mg/day, calcium absorption and retention were substantially lower in young adults than in the younger groups. On the other hand, calcium output (urine and feces) was the highest. Young adults are in positive calcium balance of about 100 mg/day. When skin losses of about 60 mg/day (Charles et al., 1983) are subtracted from this amount, about 40 mg of calcium remains for bone accretion. To provide this small amount of extra calcium for bone building and to match higher urinary calcium output with the body's decreasing ability to absorb it, calcium intake among young adults should be above the recently established threshold of 960 mg/day. The current dietary reference intakes for calcium for young adults aged 19–30 years are set up at 1000 mg/day. Young athletes could lose a lot of calcium through sweat; this may be up to 60–80 mg/h of intensive training. Low calcium intake may lead to a negative calcium balance and bone loss, as reported for basketball players (Klesges et al., 1996).

Phosphorus is essential for normal bone and teeth formation and, therefore, plays a very important role during skeletal development. Out of about 700 g of phosphorus contained in the human body, approximately 85% is in the bone while the remaining part is in the soft tissues where it plays an important role in energy storage and release systems. Phosphorus is an ubiquitous element present in almost all of the foods we consume. Major dietary contributors of phosphorus are protein-rich foods and cereal grains; about half of the food phosphorus comes from milk and dairy products, as well as meat, poultry, and fish. Although phosphorus deficiency has been reported in adults taking large amounts of antacids, a widespread phosphorus deficiency syndrome in humans is practically unknown. This is to a large extent explained by the phosphorus homeostasis in the body. Most of the consumed phosphorus is excreted in the feces and urine. Phosphorus balance studies in adults showed that phosphorus output is equal to input at various intake levels from 700–1800 mg/day indicating excellent adaptation (Nordin, 1976). Due to the lack of balance studies at very low phosphorus intakes, Nordin (1976) concludes that it is almost impossible to calculate phosphorus requirements for adults. There is presumably an intake below which adult humans go into negative balance, however, this figure is unknown. As phosphorus is an essential component of the calcium hydroxyapatite crystal, growing individuals should be in a positive phosphorus balance. As in adults, phosphorus output (urinary and fecal excretion) is highly related to phosphorus input (dietary phosphorus), however, most adolescents are in a positive phosphorus balance of about 100 mg/day irrespective of their phosphorus intake. The analysis of phosphorus balances in adolescents show that the regression line of phosphorus output on phosphorus intake at range 800–2000 mg/day has a slope of 0.96 which is almost parallel to the line of equality and an intercept of -58. The difference between the lines is due to phosphorus retention in the body ($\sim$100 mg/day) required primarily for skeletal development (Landoll et al., 1998). As the girls in this study were postpubertal (2 years since menarche) they had a slower rate of growth and mineral accretion. A positive phosphorus balance of about 150–200 mg/d is expected during the pubertal growth spurt at age $\sim$12 y. Most of the recent concern of the nutrition community has centered around the excessive consumption of phosphorus relative to calcium, with consequent development of secondary hyperparathyroidism which could potentiate bone loss. High phosphate intake and abnormally low calcium to phosphate ratio (i.e., 1: 6) was implicated in the development of osteoporosis and secondary hyperparathyroidism in laboratory animals (Krook & Barrett, 1962; Krook et al., 1963; Krook & Lowe, 1964). Although this has not been rigorously studied in humans, it has been suggested that excessive consumption of phosphate through soft drinks could be a risk factor for periodontal disease and osteoporosis (Krook et al., 1972). In one study, an increase in the consumption of carbonated beverages has been shown to produce an increased incidence of fractures in adolescents, but this requires further confirmation (Wyshak & Frisch, 1994). While this theory had several supporters among bone researchers (Calvo et al., 1990; Jowsey et al., 1974), it was never accepted by specialists in the field: periodontists and clinicians dealing with metabolic bone disease. The average Ca/P ratio in the diets of typical American teenagers is in the range of 0.3–1.3. Within this range, calcium intake rather than phophorus is the main determinant of fecal calcium. A person needs to consume

25–80 cans (44 mg of phosphorus per can) of cola daily depending on the calcium intake, to drastically disturb the Ca/P ratio. In addition, subsequent balance studies with varying amounts of phosphorus in the diet did not find abnormalities in calcium metabolism in the form of decreased absorption and increased fecal excretion of calcium (Heaney & Recker, 1982; Spencer et al., 1965, 1978). In a more recent study, phosphate supplementation (up to 2000 mg/day) in a group of young men did not show any effect on calcium homeostasis or bone turnover markers (Whybro et al., 1998). Just as milk and dairy products are the main source of calcium in the diet, they are also a good source of phosphorus with a ratio of 1.3. The consumption of milk should, therefore, be encouraged among adolescents because it contains both minerals in a favorable ratio and is equally important for skeletal mineralization.

Vitamin D deficiency causes rickets in children and osteomalacia in adults, and also is related to calcium malabsorption and secondary hyperparathyroidism in the very elderly. Vitamin D deficiency is usually the result of inadequate exposure to sunlight and/or low dietary intake of vitamin D. Vitamin D facilitates calcium absorption from the diet. It stimulates active transport by inducing the synthesis of calcium-binding protein in intestinal mucosal cells. This function is particularly important for adaptation to low intakes. Most of the absorbed calcium, however, comes from the passive transport mechanism, which is not completely understood, and is not dependent on vitamin D. The proportion of absorption by the two mechanisms varies with intake; at high calcium intakes it is likely that active transport contributes relatively little to the total absorbed load. Nevertheless, vitamin D status can influence absorptive performance and influence calcium requirement (Heaney, 1995b). Seasonal deficiency of vitamin D has been recently described in children from Spain with corresponding increase in serum parathyroid hormone (PTH) (Docio et al., 1998). Out of 51 normal children studied in winter, 31% had levels of 25-hydroxyvitamin D [25(OH)D] below 12 ng/ml, and 80% had levels lower than 20 ng/ml. To what extent this may have implications with regard to skeletal mineralization and peak bone mass acquisition is unknown. To meet these high calcium requirements adolescents have higher calcium absorption than children and young adults. The high calcium absorption during puberty is mediated by calcitriol [$1,25(OH)_2D_3$] and is related to bone mass accrual (Ilich et al., 1997a).

Protein-calorie malnutrition during childhood can cause growth retardation and decreased formation of cortical bone (Garn et al., 1964), and therefore can interfere with the attainment of peak bone mass. This is probably mediated by IGF-I and leptin through its effect on the reproductive function. High protein intake may increase calcium excretion in the urine; however, this has not been confirmed in children who are in positive nitrogen balance which is required for protein synthesis during growth (Matkovic et al., 1995a).

The adolescent population may be susceptible to a mild to moderate zinc deficiency as a result of poor eating habits and increased requirements for growth. Although severe zinc deficiency is rarely seen in the US, mild zinc deficiency has been reported in children and adolescents, leading to the low growth percentiles, diminished taste acuity, and low hair levels. The effect on skeletal growth may be mediated through IGF-I; a direct link between zinc nutritional status and IGF-I was described in postmenopausal women (Devine et al., 1998). The implications of mild to moderate zinc deficiency with regard to peak bone mass are unknown, and warrants further investigation.

The Food and Nutrition Board National Academy of Sciences (1997), as well as the National Institutes of Health Consensus Panel on Optimal Calcium Intake (1994), increased calcium intake standards for teenagers to 1300 and 1500 mg/day, respectively. There is a concern that a high calcium intake may lead to a decreased absorption of other important minerals. However, recent clinical studies conducted among adolescents do not show any influence of high calcium intake ($\sim$1500 mg/day) on nutritional status of some of the major minerals and trace elements including magnesium (Andon et al., 1996), zinc (McKenna et al., 1997), iron (Ilich-Ernst et al., 1998), and selenium (Holben et al., 1996). This proves that the current recommendation for calcium intake is safe and should not trigger a concern among nutritionists that such a level may cause deficiency of other minerals or trace elements.

Acknowledgements

This work was supported in part by grants from NIH Ro1 AR40736-O1A1, CRC-NIH MO1-RR00034, and NRICGP/USDA-37200-7586.

REFERENCES

Aksnes, L. & Aarskog, D. (1982). Plasma concentrations of vitamin D metabolites in puberty: Effect of sexual maturation and implications for growth. *J. Clin. Endocrinol. Metab.*, **55**, 94–101.

Alffram, P. A. & Bauer, G. C. H. (1962). Epidemiology of fractures of the forearm. *J. Bone Joint Surg.*, **44A**, 105–14.

Andon, M. B., Ilich. J. Z., Tzagournis, M. A., & Matkovic, V. (1996) Magnesium balance in adolescent females consuming a low or high calcium diet. *Am. J. Clin. Nutr.*, **63**, 950–3.

Arnold, J. S. (1973). Amount and quality of trabecular bone in osteoporotic vertebral fractures. *Clin. Endocrinol. Metab.*, **2**, 221–38.

Bailey, D. A., Wedge, J. H., McCulloch, R. G., Martin, A. D., & Bernhardson, S. C. (1989) Epidemiology of fractures of the distal end of the radius in children associated with growth. *J. Bone and Jt. Surg.*, **71**-A(8), 1225–31.

Beck, T. J., Ruff, C. B., Scott, W. W., Plato, C. C., Tobin, J. D., & Quan, C. A. (1992). Sex differences in geometry of the femoral neck with aging: a structural analysis of bone mineral data. *Calcif. Tissue Int.*, **50**, 24–9.

Block, J. E., Smith, R., Glueer, C. C., Steiger, P., Ettinger, B., & Genant, H. K. (1989). Models of spinal trabecular bone loss as determined by quantitative computed tomography. *J. Bone Miner. Res.*, **2**, 249–57.

Bohr, H. & Schaadt, O. P. (1990). Structural changes of the femoral shaft with age measured by dual photon absorptiometry. *Bone Min.*, **11**, 357–62.

Bonjour, J. P., Carrie, A. L., Ferrarri, S., Clavien, H., Slosman, D., Theintz, G., & Rizzoli, R. (1997). Calcium-enriched foods and bone mass growth in prepubertal girls: a randomized, double-blind, placebo-controlled, trial. *J. Clin. Invest.*, **99**, 1287–94.

Bonjour, J. P., Theintz, G., Buchs, B., Slosman, D., & Rizzoli, R. (1991). Critical years and stages of puberty for spinal and femoral bone mass accumulation during adolescence. *J. Clin. Endocrinol. Metab.*, **73**, 555–63.

Cadogan, J., Eastell, R., Jones, N., & Barker, M. E. (1997). Milk intake and bone mineral acquisition in adolescent girls: randomised, controlled intervention trial. *Br. Med. J.*, **315**, 1255–60.

Calvo, M. S., Kumar, R., & Heath, H. III. (1990). Persistently elevated parathyroid hormone secretion and action in young women after four weeks of ingesting high phosphorus, low calcium diets. *J. Clin. Endocrinol. Metab.*, **70**, 1334–40.

Cauley, J. A., Gutai, J. P., Kuller, L. H., LeDonne, D., Sandler, R. B., Sashin, D., & Powell, J. G. (1988). Endogenous estrogen levels and calcium intakes in postmenopausal women. Relationships with cortical bone measures. *JAMA*, **260**, 3150–5.

Chan, G. M., Hoffman, K., & McMurray, M. (1995). Effect of dairy products on bone and body composition in pubertal girls. *J. Pediat.*, **126**, 551–6.

Charles, P., Taagehoj Jensen, F., Mosekilde, L., & Hvid Hansen, H. (1983). Calcium metabolism evaluated by 47Ca kinetics: estimation of dermal calcium loss. *Clin. Sci.*, **65**, 415–22.

Devine, A., Rosen, C., Mohan, S., Baylink, D., & Prince, R. L. (1998). Effects of zinc and other nutritional factors on insulin-like growth factor 1 and insulin-like growth factor binding proteins in postmenopausal women. *Am. J. Clin. Nutr.*, **68**, 200–6.

Docio, S., Riancho, J. A., Perez, A., Olmos, J. M., Amado, J. A., & Gonzales-Macias, J. (1998). Seasonal deficiency of vitamin D in children: a potential target for osteoporosis-preventing strategies. *J. Bone Miner. Res.*, **13**, 544–8.

Elliott, J. R., Gilchrist, N. L., Wells, J. E., Turner, J. G., Ayling, E., Gillespie, W. J., Sainsbury, R., Hornblow, A., & Donald, R. A. (1990). Effect of age and sex on bone density at the hip and spine in a normal caucasian New Zealand population. *NZ Med. J.*, **103**, 33–6.

Epker, B. N. & Frost, H. M. (1966). Periosteal appositional bone growth from age two to age seventy in man. *Anat. Rec.*, **154**, 573–8.

Ericksen, M. F. (1976). Some aspects of aging in the lumbar spine. *Am. J. Phys. Anthrop.*, **45**, 575–80.

Food and Nutrition Board (1997). Dietary Reference Intakes. Institute of Medicine, National Academy Press, Washington, DC.

Frost, H. M. (1992). The role of changes in mechanical usage set points in the pathogenesis of osteoporosis. *J. Bone Miner. Res.*, **7**, 253–61.

Garn, S. M. (1970). *The Earlier Gain and the Later Loss of Cortical Bone.* Springfield, IL: Charles C. Thomas Publ.

Garn, S. M., Pao, E. M., & Rihl, M. E. (1964). Compact bone in Chinese and Japanese. *Science,* 143, 1439–40.

Garn, S. M., Rohmann, C. G., Wagner, B., & Ascoli, W. (1967). Continuing bone growth throughout life: A general phenomenon. *Am. J. Phys. Anthrop.,* 26, 313–18.

Garn, S. M., Sullivan, T. V., Decker, S. A., Larkin, F. A., & Hawthorne, V. M. (1992). Continuing bone expansion and increasing bone loss over a two-decade period in men and women from a total community sample. *Am. J. Hum. Biol.,* 4, 57–67.

Gilsanz, V., Gibbens, D.T ., Roe, T. F., Carlson, M., Senac, M. O., Boechat, M. I., Huang, H. K., Schulz, E. E., Libanati, C. R., & Cann, C. C. (1988). Vertebral bone density in children: effect of puberty. *Radiology,* 166, 847–50.

Glastre, C., Braillon, P., David, L., Cochat, P., Meunier, P. J., & Delmas, P. D. (1990). Measurement of bone mineral content of the lumbar spine by dual energy X-ray absorptiometry in normal children: correlations with growth parameters. *J. Clin. Endocrinol. Metab.,* 70, 1330–3.

Goulding, A., Cannan, R., Williams, S. M., Gold, E. J., Taylor, R. W., & Lewis-Barned, N. J. (1998). Bone mineral density in girls with forearm fractures. *J. Bone Miner. Res.,* 13, 143–8.

Halioua, L. & Anderson, J. J. B. (1989). Lifetime calcium intake and physical activity habits: independent and combined effects on the radial bone of healthy premenopausal Caucasian women. *Am. J. Clin. Nutr.,* 49, 534–41.

Heaney, R. P. (1995a). Interpreting trials of bone-active agents. *Am. J. Med.,* 98, 329–30.

Heaney, R. P. (1995b). Nutrition and bone mass. *Phys. Med. Rehab. Clin. North. Am.,* 6(3), 551–6.

Heaney, R. P. & Recker, R. R. (1982). Effects of nitrogen, phosphorus, and caffeine on calcium balance in women. *J. Lab. Clin. Med.,* 99, 46–55.

Heaney, R. P. & Matkovic, V. (1995). Inadequate peak bone mass. In *Osteoporosis: Etiology, Diagnosis and Management,* ed. B. L. Riggs & L. J. Melton, 2nd edn, pp. 115–21. New York: Raven Press.

Hedlund, L. R. & Gallagher, J. C. (1989). The effect of age and menopause on bone mineral density of the proximal femur. *J. Bone Miner. Res.,* 4, 639–42.

Holben, D., Smith, A. M., Ha, E. J., Ilich, J. Z., & Matkovic, V. (1996). Selenium (Se) absorption, balance, and status in adolescent females throughout puberty. *Faseb J.,* 10, A532.

Hu, J. F., Zhao, X. H., Jia, J. B., Parpia, B., & Campbell, T. C. (1993). Dietary calcium and bone density among middle-aged and elderly women in China. *Am. J. Clin. Nutr.,* 58, 219–27.

Ilich, J. Z., Badenhop, N. E., Jelic, T., Clairmont, A. C., Nagode, L. A., & Matkovic, V. (1997a). Calcitriol and bone mass accumulation in females during puberty. *Calcif. Tissue Int.,* 61, 104–9.

Ilich, J. Z., Skugor, M., Badenhop, N. E., Landoll, J. D., & Matkovic, V. (1997b). Time since menarche is positively related to bone mass of total body and radius in premenopausal women. *J. Bone Miner. Res.,* 12, S252.

Ilich-Ernst, J. Z., McKenna, A. A., Badenhop, N. E., Clairmont, A. C., Andon, M. B., Nahhas, R. W., Goel, P., & Matkovic, V. (1998). Iron status, menarche, and calcium supplementation in adolescent girls. *Am. J.Clin. Nutr.,* 68, 880–7.

Israel, H. (1968). Continuing growth in the human cranial skeleton. *Arch. Oral Biol.,* 13, 133–7.

Johnell, O., Gullberg, B., Kanis, J. A., Allander, E., Elffors, L., Dequeker, J., Dilsen, G., Gennari,

C., Vaz, A. L., Lyritis, G., Mazzuoli, G., Miravet, L., Passeri, M., Cano, R. P., Rapado, A., & Ribot, C. (1995). Risk factors for hip fracture in European women: the MEDOS study. *J. Bone Miner. Res.*, **10**, 1802–15.

Johnston, C. C. Jr., Miller, J. Z., Slemenda, C. W., Reister, T. K., Hui, S., Christian, J. C., & Peacock, M. (1992). Calcium supplementation and increases in bone mineral density in children. *N. Engl. J. Med.*, **327**, 82–7.

Jowsey, J., Reiss, E., & Canterbury, J. M. (1974). Long term effects of high phosphate intake on parathyroid hormone levels and bone metabolism. *Acta Othop. Scand.*, **45**, 801–8.

Katzman, D. K., Bachrach, L. K., Carter, D. R., & Marcus, R. (1991). Clinical and anthropometric correlates of bone mineral acquisition in healthy adolescent girls. *J. Clin. Endocrinol. Metab.*, **73**, 1332–9.

Klesges, R. C., Ward, K. D., Shelton, M. L., Applegate, W. B., Cantler, E. D., Palmieri, G. M. A., Harmon, K., & Davis, J. (1996). Changes in bone mineral content in male athletes. Mechanisms of action and intervention effects. *JAMA*, **276**, 226–30.

Krook, L. & Barrett, R. B. (1962). Simian bone disease – a secondary hyperparathyroidism. *Cornell Vet.*, **52**, 459–92.

Krook, L. & Lowe, J. E. (1964). Nutritional secondary hyperparathyroidism in horse. *Path. Vet.*, **1**, S1–S98.

Krook, L., Barrett, R. B., Usui, K., & Wolke, R. E. (1963). Nutritional secondary hyperparathyroidism in the cat. *Cornell Vet.*, **53**, 224–40.

Krook, L., Whalen, J. P., Lesser, G. V., & Lutwak, L. (1972). Human periodontal disease and osteoporosis. *Cornell Vet.*, **62**, 371–91.

Landoll, J. D., Mobley, L. S., & Matkovic, V. (1998). The relationship between phosphorus intake and output during growth. *Bone*, **23**, S607.

Lee, W. T. K., Leung, S. S. F., Leung, D. M. Y., & Cheng, J. C. Y. (1996). A follow-up study on the effect of calcium-supplement withdrawal and puberty on bone acquisition of children. *Am. J. Clin. Nutr.*, **64**, 71–7.

Lee, W. T. K., Leung, S. S. F., Wang, S. F., Xu, Y. C., Zeng, W. P., Lau, J., Oppenheimer, S. J., & Cheng, J. C. Y. (1994). Double-blind, controlled calcium supplementation and bone mineral accretion in children accustomed to a low-calcium diet. *Am. J. Clin. Nutr.*, **60**, 744–50.

Liu, C., Grossmann, A., Bain, S., Strachan, M., Puerner, D., Bailey, C., Humes, J., Lenox, J., Yamamoto, G., Sprugel, K., Kuijper, J., Weigle, S., Durnam, D., & Moore, E. (1997). Leptin stimulates cortical bone formation in obese (ob/ob) mice. *J. Bone Miner. Res.*, **12**, S115.

Lloyd, T., Andon, M. B., Rollings, N., Martel, J. K., Landis, R. J., Demers, L. M., Eggli, D. F., Kieselhorst, K., & Kulin, H. E. (1993). Calcium supplementation and bone mineral density in adolescent girls. *JAMA*, **270**, 841–8.

Lloyd, T., Rollings, N., Andon, M. B., Eggli, D. F., Mauger, E., & Chinchilli, V. (1996). Enhanced bone gain in early adolescence due to calcium supplementation does not persist in late adolescence. *J. Bone Miner. Res.*, **11**, S154.

Lu, P. W., Briody, J. N., Ogle, G. D., Morley, K., Humphries, I. R. J., Allen, J., Howman-Giles, R., Sillence, D., & Cowell, C. T. (1994). Bone mineral density of total body, spine, and femoral neck in children and young adults: a cross-sectional and longitudinal study. *J. Bone Miner. Res.*, **9**, 1451–8.

McKenna, A. A., Ilich, J. Z., Andon, M. B., Wang, C., & Matkovic, V. (1997). Zinc balance in adolescent females consuming a low- or high-calcium diet. *Am. J. Clin. Nutr.*, **65**, 1460–4.

Marcus, R., Kosek, J., Pfefferbaum, A., & Horning, S. (1983). Age-related loss of trabecular bone in premenopausal women: A biopsy study. *Calcif. Tissue Int.*, **35**, 406–9.

Matkovic, V. (1991). Calcium metabolism and calcium requirements during skeletal modeling and consolidation of bone mass. *Am. J. Clin. Nutr.*, **54**, 245S–60S.

Matkovic, V. (1999). Can osteoporosis be prevented? Bone mineralization during growth and development. In *Human Growth in Context*, ed. F. E. Johnston, B. Eveleth, B. Zemel, vol. 17, pp. 1–17. London, UK: Smith-Gordon.

Matkovic, V. & Heaney, R. P. (1992). Calcium balance during human growth: evidence for threshold behavior. *Am. J. Clin. Nutr.*, **55**, 992–6.

Matkovic, V., Badenhop, N. E., Landoll, J. D., Ilich, J. Z., Rosen, C. J., & Buell, J. L. (1998). Skeletal growth in a nutrition perspective: genetic and endocrine interaction. In *Paediatric Osteology. Prevention of Osteoporosis – A Paediatric Task?*, ed. E. Shonau & V. Matkovic, pp. 53–71. New York: Elsevier Science.

Matkovic, V., Ciganovic, M., Tominac, C., & Kostial, K. (1980). Osteoporosis and epidemiology of fractures in Croatia. An international comparison. *Henry Ford Hosp. Med. J.*, **28**, 116–26.

Matkovic, V., Fontana, D., Tominac, C., Goel, P., & Chesnut, C. H. (1990). Factors which influence peak bone mass formation: A study of calcium balance and the inheritance of bone mass in adolescent females. *Am. J. Clin. Nutr.*, **52**, 878–88.

Matkovic, V., Ilich, J. Z., Andon, M. B., Hsieh, L. C., Tzagournis, M. A., Lagger, B. J., & Goel, P. K. (1995a). Urinary calcium, sodium, and bone mass of young females. *Am. J. Clin. Nutr.*, **62**, 417–25.

Matkovic, V., Ilich, J. Z., Skugor, M., Badenhop, N. E., Clairmont, A., Goel, P., Klisovic, D., Nasseh, R. W., & Landoll, J. D. (1997). Leptin is inversely related to age at menarche in human females. *J. Clin. Endo. Metab.*, **82**, 3239–45.

Matkovic, V., Ilich, J. Z., Skugor, M., & Saracoglu, M. (1995b). Primary prevention of osteoporosis. *Phys. Med. Rehab. Clin. North Am.*, **6**(3), 595–627.

Matkovic, V., Jelic, T., Wardlaw, G. M., Ilich, J. Z., Goel, P. K., Wright, J. K., Andon, M. B., Smith, K. T., & Heaney, R. P. (1994). Timing of peak bone mass in caucasian females and its implication for the prevention of osteoporosis. Inference from a cross-sectional model. *J. Clin. Invest.*, **93**, 799–808.

Matkovic, V., Klisovic, D., & Ilich, J. Z. (1995c). Epidemiology of fractures during growth and aging. *Phys. Med. Rehab. Clin. North Am.*, **6**(3), 415–39.

Matkovic, V., Kostial, K., Simonovic, I., Buzina, R., Brodarec, A., & Nordin, B. E. C. (1979). Bone status and fracture rates in two regions of Yugoslavia. *Am. J. Clin. Nutr.*, **32**, 540–9.

Mosekilde, L. & Mosekilde, L. (1990). Sex differences in age-related changes in vertebral body size, density and biomechanical competence in normal individuals. *Bone*, **11**, 67–73.

Murphy, S., Khaw, K. T., May, H., & Compston, J. E. (1994). Milk consumption and bone mineral density in middle aged and elderly women. *Br. Med. J.*, **308**, 939–41.

Newton-John, H. F. & Morgan, B. D. (1970). The loss of bone with age: osteoporosis and fractures. *Clin. Orthop.*, **71**, 229–32.

NIH Consensus Conference. (1994). Optimal calcium intake, *JAMA*, **272**, 1942–8.

Nordin, B. E. C. (1976). Nutritional consideration. In *Calcium, Phosphate and Magnesium Metabolism*, ed. B. E. C. Nordin, pp. 1–35. Edinburgh: Churchill Livingstone.

Recker, R. R., Davies, K. M., Hinders, S. M., Heaney, R. P., Stegman, M. R., & Kimmel, D. B. (1992). Bone gain in young adult women. *JAMA*, **268**, 2403–8.

Rosenthal, D. I., Mayo-Smith, W., Hayes, C. W., Khurana, J. S., Biller, B. M. K., Neer, R. M., & Klibanski, A. (1989). Age and bone mass in premenopausal women. *J. Bone Miner. Res.*, **4**, 533–8.

Sandler, R. B., Slemenda, C., LaPorte, R. E., Cauley, J. A., Schramm, M. M., Baresi, M., & Kriska, A. M. (1985). Postmenopausal bone density and milk consumption in childhood and adolescence. *Am. J. Clin. Nutr.*, **42**, 270–4.

Slemenda, C., Peacock, M., Hui, S., Zhou, L., & Johnston, C. C. Jr. (1997). Reduced rates of skeletal remodeling are associated with increased bone mineral density during the development of peak skeletal mass. *J. Bone Miner. Res.*, **12**, 676–82.

Smith, R. W. & Walker, R. R. (1964). Femoral expansion in aging women: Implications for osteoporosis and fractures. *Science*, **145**, 156–7.

Soroko, S., Holbrook, T. L., Edelstein, S., & Barrett-Connor, E. (1994). Lifetime milk consumption and bone mineral density in older women. *Am. J. Public Health*, **84**, 1319–22.

Spencer, H., Kramer, L., Osais, D., & Norris, C. (1978). Effect of phosphorus on the absorption of calcium and on calcium balance in men. *J. Nutr.*, **108**, 447–57.

Spencer, H., Menczel, J., Lewin, I., & Samachson, J. (1965). Effect of high phosphorus intake on calcium and phosphorus metabolism in men. *J. Nutr.*, **86**, 125–32.

Speroff, L., Glass, R. H., & Kase, N. G. (1989). *Clinical Gynecologic Endocrinology and Infertility*, 4th edn, pp. 379–437. Baltimore: Williams & Wilkins.

Susanne, C. (1979). Aging, continuous changes of adulthood. In *Human Physical Growth and Maturation. Methodologies and Factors*, ed. F. E. Johnston, A. F. Roche, & C. Susanne, pp. 161–175. New York: Plenum Press.

Theintz, G., Buchs, B., Rizzoli, R., Slosman, D., Clavien, H., Sizonenko, P. C., & Bonjour J. P. (1992). Longitudinal monitoring of bone mass accumulation in healthy adolescents: Evidence for a marked reduction after 16 years of age at the levels of lumbar spine and femoral neck in female subjects. *J. Clin. Endocrinol. Metab.*, **75**, 1060–5.

Trotter, M. & Hixon, B. (1974). Sequential changes in weight, density, and percentage ash weight of human skeletons from an early fetal period through old age. *Anat. Rec.*, **179**, 1–18.

Weaver, C. M., Martin, B. R., & Plawecki, K. L. (1995). Differences in calcium metabolism between adolescent and adult females. *Am. J. Clin. Nutr.*, **61**, 577–81.

Whybro, A., Jagger, H., Barker, M., & Eastell, R. (1998). Phosphate supplementation in young men: lack of effect on calcium homeostatis and bone turnover. *Eur. J. Clin.Nutr.*, **52**, 29–33.

Wyshak, G. & Frisch, R. E. (1994). Carbonated beverages, dietary calcium, the dietary calcium/phosphorus ratio, and bone fractures in girls and boys. *J. Adolesc. Health*, **15**, 210–15.

Zhang, Y., Proenca, R., Maffei, M., Barone, M., Leopold, L., & Friedman, J. M. (1994). Positional cloning of the mouse obese gene and its human homologue. *Nature*, **372**, 425–32.

12

Bone mineral acquisition during childhood and adolescence: physical exercise as a preventative measure

Heather A. McKay and Karim M. Khan

Introduction

The history of the human species has always included a lifestyle demanding heavy and prolonged physical work that was necessary for survival (Bortz, 1985). It has been estimated that the skeletal mass of humans living in the Late Paleolithic era exceeded that of humans in subsequent civilizations (Larsen, 1987; Wolpoff, 1980). This is attributed, in part, to the heavy physical exertion required for subsistence at that time (Eaton et al., 1988). Times, however, have changed and conditions of disuse have become firmly entrenched in our medical vocabulary.

It has been suggested that the ability of bone to adapt to mechanical loading is much greater in the immature, as compared to the mature, skeleton (Parfitt, 1994). Osteoporosis prevention, therefore, may begin early in life when optimal bone mineral accretion is critical to the attainment of a healthy adult skeleton (Bailey & McCulloch, 1992; Fassler & Bonjour, 1996; Parfitt, 1994). Peak bone mass is a major determinant of adult bone mass which is, in turn, related to fracture risk (Matkovic et al., 1979). Upwards of 90% of adult bone mass is achieved by the end of adolescence and subsequent gains are relatively small (Bonjour et al., 1991; Glastre et al., 1990; Slemenda et al., 1994; Theintz et al., 1992). Although peak bone mass is largely determined by genetics, which accounts for over half of the variance (Krall & Dawson-Hughes, 1993), other modifiable lifestyle factors, including physical activity, also play a role.

The aim of this chapter is to familiarize the reader with the association between physical activity, peak bone mass and adult skeletal health. To allow the reader to interpret existing evidence as well as recognize the limitations in current research, we will introduce the pattern of bone mineral accrual through childhood and adolescence. We will also discuss some of the methodological considerations when bone densitometry techniques are used to evaluate the pediatric skeleton. From that foundation we summarize the literature that evaluates childhood physical activity and peak bone mass.

Normal bone accrual and maintenance

In children and adolescents, the shape, architecture, and strength of bones are modulated by three key processes: growth, modeling and remodeling (Bailey et al., 1996). Growth of the skeleton occurs in two ways giving rise to the two primary structural types of bone: cancellous bone and cortical bone. Growth in length is achieved in cancellous bone by endochondral ossification whereas cortical bone is responsible for growth in width, primarily by periosteal apposition. Modeling is responsible for altering the shape and mass and for 'turning over' bone during growth. Unlike remodeling, absorption does not immediately precede formation and the outcome is a net gain of bone over time. Modeling is of particular interest as it appears that bone is much more capable of responding to external loads during growth than at any other time (Forwood & Burr, 1993; Haapasalo et al., 1998; Parfitt, 1994). Remodeling is a replacement process defined by the biological coupling of osteoblasts and osteoclasts. An activation phase is followed in sequence by a resorption and a formation phase (ARF sequence). Although remodeling is the dominant process affecting bone shape and mass in adults, it also occurs during growth. The net result of remodeling is to lose or maintain, but not to gain, bone (Frost, 1992).

Bone mineral accrual during growth

Adult bone mass is, at any time, a function of the bone accrued during the growing years and the amount of bone lost with advancing age. As low adult bone mineral density is associated with fracture risk (Melton et al., 1993) it is clear that bone mass accrual during the growing years should be optimized. While it is now generally accepted that bone mass continues to accrue after the cessation of linear growth, the debate as to when peak bone mass is achieved continues.

The pattern of normal bone mineral accrual during childhood and adolescence is only now coming to light. Most of what we know about normal bone mineral accrual comes from a large number of cross-sectional, and a few longitudinal, studies which generally report that bone mineral is accrued steadily throughout the growing years, accelerates rapidly at all skeletal sites with the onset of puberty, and plateaus as sexual maturity is reached (Bonjour et al., 1991; Faulkner et al., 1993a, b; Theintz et al., 1992). Cortical thickness is greater in boys than in girls at all ages, although this is not reflected in bone mineral density which is similar between boys and girls of the same age, until puberty. Although cross-sectional studies have added important information to our knowledge of bone mineral accrual the nature of these studies may misrepresent the timing and the intensity of peak events (Martin et al., 1997).

The general timing of peak bone mineral accrual appears to be specific to the type of bone (cortical or cancellous) (Bonjour et al., 1991; Faulkner et al., 1993a, b; Garn, 1970; Gilsanz et al., 1988; Mora et al., 1991; Theintz et al., 1992) and varies between boys and girls (Faulkner et al., 1993a, b; Gilsanz et al., 1994). When monitoring skeletal change, it is important to consider that girls have an approximately 2-year maturity advantage as compared with boys and that there is tremendous variability in maturity between same sex children of the same chronological age. Thus, biologically, maturity, is a more significant determinant of bone mineral than chronological age and is a major confound in research if it is not properly controlled for.

Important new information on the pattern of bone mineral accrual comes from a longitudinal study of boys and girls at the University of Saskatchewan where, approximately 200 boys and girls have been measured by DXA (Hologic 2000) yearly for 7 years (Bailey, 1997, 1999). Fig. 12.1 illustrates the normal pattern of bone mineral accrual from a longitudinal analysis for boys and girls at the 25th, 50th and 75th percentile from age 9 to 18 years. This is a 'distance' curve and is a plot of total body bone mineral content at any given age along the pathway to maturity. Distance curves for height are a more familiar clinical tool and are used to monitor a child's linear growth from birth to maturity. Fig. 12.2 is a 'velocity' curve which demonstrates the rate at which bone mineral is accrued in units of grams/year. Again, a velocity curve for height would measure a child's rate of growth in centimeters per year if height were measured annually. The velocity curves provide an excellent illustration of the sex difference in the timing of peak bone mineral accrual which occurs about 1.5 years earlier in girls than in boys, and is of a lesser magnitude (325 g/y for girls vs. 409 g/y for boys). The Saskatchewan group have also shown that the timing of peak bone mineral accrual velocity coincides with menarche (the first menstrual period) in girls and lags behind peak height velocity by approximately 1 year (McKay et al., 1998). This is of clinical interest as the dissociation between accelerated linear growth and peak bone mineral accrual may constitute a period of relative bone fragility that may explain the increased fracture rate observed during adolescence (Bailey et al., 1989; Parfitt, 1994).

During the pubertal years there is a 3- to 4-year window, sometimes referred to as the 'critical years', when a great proportion of bone mineral accrual occurs. In a study of healthy adolescents, maximal gain in lumbar spine and femoral neck BMC was observed at age 11–14 years with marked diminution of bone gain 2 years after (Theintz et al., 1992). A cross-sectional report from the University of Saskatchewan, which utilized 3020 DXA scans, determined the area under the curve (BMC accrued) between developmental ages 2 years on either side of peak height velocity (PHV) (Bailey, 1997). About 35% of total body, and lumbar spine BMC and over 27% of femoral neck BMC was laid down during the 4 years around

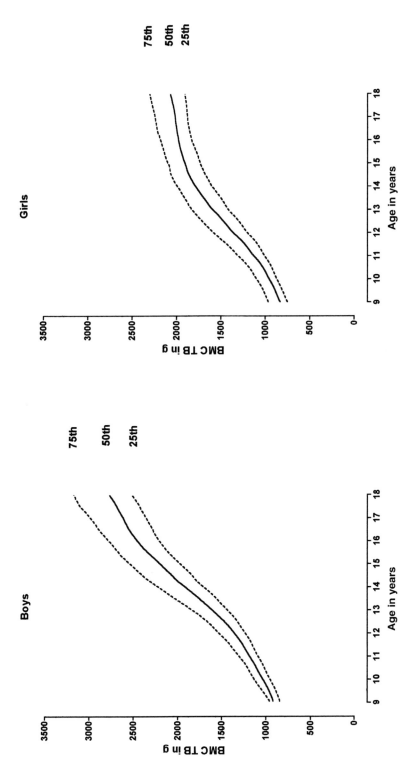

Fig. 12.1   Distance curves for total body bone mineral content (grams) for boys and girls derived longitudinal data. Curves representing the 25th, 50th and 75th percentile are provided.

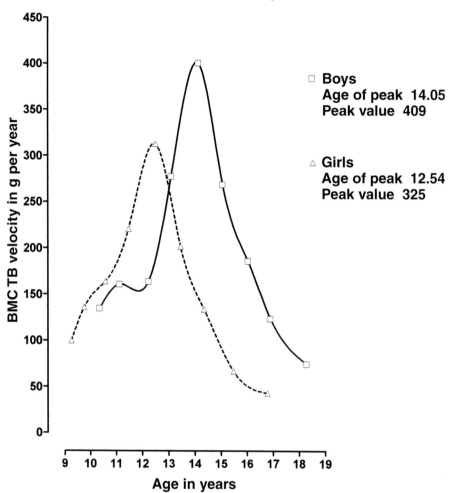

BMC TB velocity
General curve – cubic spline

□ **Boys**
Age of peak 14.05
Peak value 409

△ **Girls**
Age of peak 12.54
Peak value 325

Fig. 12.2   Velocity curves for total body bone mineral content (grams) for boys and girls, using a
cubic spline curve-fitting model derived from longitudinal data from the University of
Saskatchewan (Bailey et al., 1999). The sex difference in timing and magnitude of peak
bone mineral accrual is depicted. The girls reached peak bone mineral accrual velocity
approximately 1.5 years in advance of the boys and bone mineral accrual at peak was
325 g/yr as compared with 409 g/yr for boys.

PHV (Bailey, 1997). In a subsequent analysis of their 6-year longitudinal data these investigators found that, on average, 26% of adult total body bone mineral was accrued during the 2 years around peak bone mineral content velocity, at age 12.5 (0.9) y for girls and age 14.1 (1.0) y for boys. This amount was much greater than previous estimates, and demonstrates the limitations of cross-sectional designs for the study of growth (Bailey et al., 1999). In another cross-sectional study of girls, the growth spurt reportedly contributed 51% of peak bone mass (Gordon et al., 1991). As previously suggested, these gains in BMC appear to be more a function of pubertal stage than chronological age (Grimston & Hanley, 1992; Kröger et al., 1993).

On the other hand, true bone density does not appear to increase with size or age and reported increases in areal bone mineral density (BMD) or, as discussed previously, are a reflection of growth and an increase in size rather than an increase in bone mineral per unit volume (Kroger et al., 1992; Schonau et al., 1993).

Measurement of bone mineral

All branches of science and medicine depend on accurate and precise measurement of biological variables. Galileo said 'measure what can be measured and make measurable what cannot.' Various bone absorptiometry systems and techniques have been used extensively to measure bone mineral. These techniques are discussed in detail elsewhere in this volume. Of these techniques dual energy X-ray absorptiometry (DXA) is a readily available, relatively inexpensive and precise method. The low levels of radiation exposure make DXA the measurement system in popular use for studies involving children. DXA provides an assessment of bone area (cm), bone mineral content (BMC, g) and BMD of g/cm^2 for the total body, proximal femur and lumbar spine.

There is some confusion in the literature regarding the use of the term 'bone mass' which is often used interchangeably with BMC or BMD. The problem with the familiar use of this terminology is that current measurement systems do not measure bone mass *per se* but assesses the amount of bone mineral in bone. Bone density at maturity is a function of both the size of the bone and bone mass. It is important to make the distinction between the measurement of BMC and BMD and to understand what it is they represent.

Bone mineral content is the absolute amount of mineral present in the region of bone being measured. BMD is the relative amount of bone mineral per measured area of bone (BMC/bone area). Individuals familiar with the terminology will note immediately that BMD does not reflect true density (expressed as g/cm^3), but is a two-dimensional (length and width) representation of a three-dimensional (length, width and depth) bone. Therefore, BMD only partially controls for size differences, between boys and girls for example or between individuals of different ages or levels of maturity. 'True' bone mineral density (i.e., the amount of bone mineral per measured volume of bone) can only be assessed using quantitative computed tomography (QCT).

This presents a problem when BMD is used in longitudinal assessments of bone growth. An increase in overall size, if insufficiently accounted for, leaves the false impression of an increase in bone density where none exists. Thus, growth itself will lead to an increase in BMD, even if true, volumetric BMD remains constant (Carter et al., 1992). This has led to considerable confusion regarding the magnitude of change in BMD during growth.

In an attempt to address these concerns various mathematical equations based on geometric assumptions have been utilized to estimate bone volume and to derive what has been termed 'bone mineral apparent density (BMAD)' (Carter et al., 1992; Katzman et al., 1991) or corrected BMD (corr BMD) (Kröger et al., 1992). Using this approach, Kröger et al. found that much of the change in BMC with growth was due to bone expansion rather than to an increase in bone mineral per unit volume (Kröger et al., 1992). It has been suggested, however, that these formulae overcorrect, resulting in higher than expected values (Hillman, 1996). Clearly, a three-dimensional representation of bone as with QCT is the preferred bone density measure in developmental studies of growing children where bone size is changing. However, QCT is associated with substantial exposure to ionizing radiation.

Physical activity and bone

In the nineteenth century it was proposed that bone had the capacity to respond to mechanical loading (Wolff, 1892). More recently, it has been suggested that this response is controlled by a 'mechanostat' (Currey, 1984; Frost, 1987; Lanyon et al., 1982) that endeavors to keep strain in bone within an optimal level and adjusts the structure of bone in order to do so (Frost, 1987). Fig. 12.3 illustrates the four mechanical usage zones where bone undergoes gain or loss depending on the extent of loading.

In the trivial loading zone there is virtually no mechanical stimulus to bone and remodeling occurs. Studies conducted during bed rest (Bloomfield, 1997) or space flight (Oganov et al., 1992) reveal that this results in a net loss of bone over time. Thus, periods of bed rest (e.g., in pediatric illness) should be minimized. Strains in the physiologic loading zone maintain remodeling at a steady state which, in turn, maintains bone strength. In the overload zone modeling is stimulated and new bone is added in response to the mechanical demand. The result is an increase in

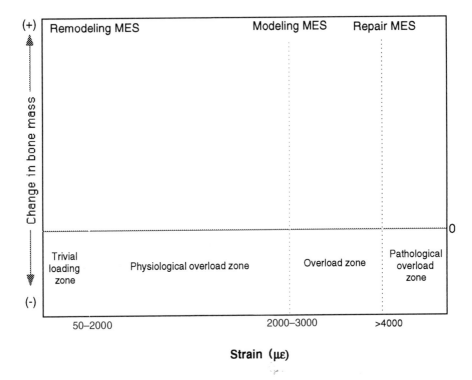

Strain (με)

1000 microstrain (με) = 0.1% change in length

4000 microstrain = 1/6 fracture strain

Fig. 12.3 A schematic representation of Frost's mechanostat theory (Frost, 1987). In the trivial loading zone there is virtually no mechanical stimulus to bone and remodeling occurs. Strains in the physiologic loading zone maintain remodeling at a steady state which, in turn, maintains bone strength. In the overload zone modeling is stimulated and new bone is added in response to the mechanical demand. Finally, in the pathological overload zone, bone suffers microdamage and woven (unorganized) bone is added as part of the repair process. (Adapted from Frost, 1987.)

bone strength. Finally, in the pathological overload zone, bone suffers microdamage and woven (unorganized) bone is added as part of the repair process.

It should be noted that a change in the set point thresholds would elicit a similar adaptive response (Frost, 1995). Also, the response to mechanical strain is site specific, therefore, one region of the skeleton may experience a net loss of bone while, simultaneously, another region experiences a net gain.

A prolific group of researchers well known for their animal work on the adaptive response of bone to mechanical loading introduced the error strain distribution hypothesis (Lanyon, 1996). This hypothesis suggested that bone cells respond to unfamiliar patterns of loading. That is, unusual strains of uneven distribution are more likely to elicit an osteogenic response than repetitive strains that are a function of everyday activity. The more unusual the strain distribution at a particular bone site, the greater its potential to increase bone density at that site (Lanyon, 1996).

Observational and experimental studies provide a degree of insight into several aspects of bone's response to physical activity but may also raise many questions. In this subsection we review studies that have addressed the following questions. First, does increased activity lead to increased bone mineral accretion? If so, what is the best type of exercise to promote bone mineral accretion? Secondly, is there a 'window of opportunity' during childhood or adolescence during which bone mineral accretion is optimized? Thirdly, are the benefits of a childhood or adolescent exercise program maintained during adulthood? And, finally, what happens to the skeleton in the absence of physical activity or during mechanical 'unloading'?

Does increased activity lead to increased bone mineral accretion?

Two recent reviews provide a detailed discussion of childhood and adolescent physical activity in relation to bone mineral (Bailey et al., 1996; Barr & McKay, 1998). Bailey et al. systematically reviewed 38 major studies and concluded that physical activity was positively associated with bone mineral accretion. There was, however, some degree of inconsistency in the results which could be attributed, at least in part, to limitations of study design. These include small numbers of subjects, short duration of prospective observations, the difficulty of accurately assessing usual physical activity in children and adolescents, and the tremendous variability in the tempo and timing of growth (Bailey et al., 1996). Unilateral control studies, in which the effect of genetics is controlled for within the study design, provided some of the most convincing evidence (Faulkner et al., 1993a, b; Kannus et al., 1995).

One such study from Kannus et al. at the UKK Institute for Health Promotion Research (Finland) provides an excellent illustration of the effect of childhood physical activity on bone. Bone mineral content of playing and non-playing arms was measured in 105 nationally ranked female racquet-sports players and 50 healthy women of similar age, height and weight who served as controls (Kannus et al., 1995). Although controls had approximately 4% higher bone mineral content in the dominant than the non-dominant humerus (attributed to activities of daily living), racquet sport players had on average ~13% side–side difference in humeral BMC, reflecting the strains experienced during tennis and squash.

Recent studies have provided further evidence to indicate that physical activity during youth is associated with higher bone mineral content or density (Boot et al., 1992; Cassell et al., 1996; Dyson et al., 1997; Gunnes & Lehmann, 1996; Morris et al., 1997; Ruiz et al., 1995). The University of Saskatchewan 6-year longitudinal study investigated the relationship between everyday physical activity and peak bone mineral accrual in a group of healthy Canadian children passing through adolescence (Bailey et al., 1999). These researchers compared children by quartiles of physical activity and, with height and weight at peak height velocity controlled for, demonstrated a 9% and 17% greater total body BMC for active boys and girls, respectively, over their inactive peers one year after the age of PBMCV. Similarly, the most active group accrued more bone than the least active group at peak velocity and in the 2 years around the bone mineral spurt for the total body and the femoral neck (but not the lumbar spine) ($P < 0.05$).

A 10-month study of normal 9- and 10-year-old schoolgirls appears particularly important as it utilized a prospective (but non-randomized) intervention design (Morris et al., 1997). The intervention schools added three weight bearing, physical education classes per week to their program. Gains in bone mineral content or density for girls in the intervention group averaged 5.5% greater for the whole body, 3.6% greater at the lumbar spine, and 10.3% greater at the femoral neck (Morris et al., 1997). The magnitude of these changes, if maintained into the later adult years, would substantially reduce the subjects' risk of osteoporosis.

What is the best type of exercise to promote bone mineral accretion? Both the mechanostat theory (Frost, 1987) and the error strain distribution hypothesis (Lanyon, 1996) give rise to this question. These theories predict that bone responds to activity with increased modeling only when the activity is associated with strain levels greater than those provided in the physiological loading zone (Frost, 1987) and that responses are greater when the strains are distributed in unusual patterns hypothesis (Lanyon, 1996). Studies that measured athletes in high intensity sports such as gymnastics and Olympic weightlifting provide partial answers.

It has been estimated that gymnastics activities produce forces as great as 18 times body weight during landings (Panzer et al., 1988) compared with only 1–2 times body weight for walking and running (Capozzo, 1983). In a 12-month prospective study of prepubertal elite female gymnasts ($n = 45$) and controls ($n = 48$) the gymnasts had a 30–85% greater increase in BMD than controls at the total body, spine and legs (Bass et al., 1998). The standard (z) scores increased with increasing duration of training. Similar results were reported in a smaller cross-sectional study of 7–11-year-old gymnasts and controls (Dyson et al., 1997).

In a cross-sectional study of 15–20-year-old male Olympic weightlifters, the mean distal and proximal forearm BMC of subjects was 51% and 41% above the age-matched controls, respectively (Virvidakis et al., 1990). These boys started training on average at age 14 years and had trained for an average of 4 years at the time of the study (personal communication from the author reported by Parfitt) (Parfitt, 1994).

Swimming, on the other hand, which serves to 'unload' the skeleton during periods of buoyancy during training, does not increase bone mass as measured by DXX. Although elite swimmers undertake intense training programs, their bone mineral density is similar to that of control subjects (Dyson et al., 1997; Taafe et al., 1995).

Is there a 'window of opportunity' during childhood or adolescence during which bone mineral accretion is optimized?

Are the benefits of a childhood or adolescent exercise program maintained during adulthood?

It has been suggested that childhood and adolescence represent a critical period where bone responds more favorably to mechanical loading than at other ages (Bailey & McCulloch, 1992; Bailey et al., 1996; Haapasalo et al., 1998; Kannus et al., 1995; Khan et al., 1998; Parfitt, 1994). A cross-sectional study of 7–17-year-old tennis players was conducted to see at what maturity level the side to side differences previously noted in older players, became evident (Haapasalo et al., 1998). The authors identified side-to-side BMD differences once girls reached the adolescent growth spurt (Tanner stage III). These data suggest a specific exercise effect which is dependent on, and closely linked to, maturational status. In the Kannus et al. study of female racquet-sports players referenced previously, when training was begun before menarche, difference in humeral bone mineral content ranged from 17% to 24% compared to 8% to 14% when training began after menarche (Kannus et al., 1995).

In a 3-year prospective observational study bone mineral accrual at the lumbar spine, the proximal femur and the distal radius was related to weight-bearing physical activity in prepubertal, but not in peripubertal children (Slemenda et al., 1994). A study of retired ballet dancers suggested that for BMD of the hip, the age range 10–12 years may represent a time when the proximal femur is particularly responsive to weight-bearing exercise (Khan et al., 1998). Among the former dancers, femoral neck bone mineral density was positively related to weekly hours of ballet undertaken between 10 and 12 years of age, but was not related to current physical activity or to years of full-time ballet training and performance.

In adults, it seems quite clear that beneficial effects on bone observed when an exercise program is initiated are lost during detraining (Dalsky et al., 1988) but whether this also occurs in response to exercise undertaken during growth is not clearly established. As bone can substantially change its shape during growth via the process of modeling, it is not inconceivable that long-term benefits from childhood activity are realized (Haapasalo et al., 1996, 1998). There is some evidence to suggest that higher levels of bone attained in childhood are maintained in gymnasts

(Kirchner et al., 1996). Whether childhood physical activity influences the rate or timing of adult bone loss is also not known. Studies specifically designed to answer these questions are needed.

What happens to the skeleton in the absence of physical activity or during mechanical 'unloading'?

An extreme example of unloading is provided by weightlessness experienced during space flight, but any time a patient is confined to bed we see a very real example of absence of regular loading. To return to the mechanostat hypothesis, bed-bound bones are in the trivial loading zone and thus rapidly lose bone mineral. A bed-rest study showed that trabecular bone was lost at the rate of about 1% per week (Krolner & Toft, 1983). Cortical bone is lost at about 1% per month (Whedon, 1984). It has been suggested that trabecular bone returns at about 1% per month, so that restoration of bone mineral is much slower than bone loss. However, as bone does not return to its previous level in all cases, patients should be encouraged to weight bear during periods of rehabilitation or recovery whenever possible.

Conclusions

Although prospective, randomized, intervention studies are needed to provide definitive answers, there is mounting evidence to suggest that physical activity undertaken in childhood has repercussions for the adult skeleton. Parfitt summed it up perfectly in stating 'in wild animals, by the time growth has ceased, the bones must be as strong as they will ever need to be, and attainment of further strength after cessation of growth would serve no useful purpose' (Parfitt, 1994). We need look no further than present-day studies reporting increases in television viewing and childhood obesity to see where our children are spending their time (Gortmaker et al., 1996, 1997). It seems plausible, that industrialization and convenience is won at the cost of our skeletons and that we play a dangerous game in ignoring the increasing trends towards physical inactivity in our children.

RECOMMENDED READING

Bailey, D. A., Faulkner, R. A., & McKay, H. A. (1996). Growth, physical activity, and bone mineral acquisition. In *Exercise and Sport Sciences Reviews*, ed. J. O. Holloszy, vol. 24, pp. 233–66. Baltimore: Williams & Wilkins.

Barr, S. & McKay, H. (1998). Nutrition, exercise and bone status in youth. *Int. J. Sports Nutr.*, 8(2), 124–42.

Forwood, M.R. & Burr, D. B. (1993). Physical activity and bone mass: exercises in futility? *Bone Miner.*, **21**, 89–112.

Parfitt, A. M. (1994). The two faces of growth: benefits and risks to bone integrity. *Osteoporos. Int.*, **4**, 382–98.

REFERENCES

Bailey, D. A. (1997). The Saskatchewan Pediatric Bone Mineral Accrual Study: bone mineral acquisition during the growing years. *Int. J. Sports Med.*, **18**(Suppl3), S191–4.

Bailey, D. A. & McCulloch, R. (1992). Are there childhood antecedents for an adult health problem? *Can. J. Pediat.*, **5**, 130–4.

Bailey, D. A., Faulkner, R. A., & McKay, H. A. (1996). Growth, physical activity, and bone mineral acquisition. *Exerc. Sport Sci. Rev.*, **24**, 233–66.

Bailey, D. A., Mirwald, R., McKay, H., Crocker, P., & Faulkner, R. (1999). The University of Saskatchewan Bone Mineral Accrual Study: a seven year longitudinal study of the relationship of physical activity to bone mineral accrual in growing children. *J. Bone Miner. Res.*, **14**(10), 1672–9.

Bailey, D. A., Wedge, J. H., McCulloch, R. G., Martin, A. D., & Bernhardson, S. C. (1989). Epidemiology of fractures of the distal end of the radius in children as associated with growth. *J. Bone Joint Surg. Am.*, **71**, 1225–31.

Barr, S. & McKay, H. (1998). Nutrition, exercise and bone status in youth. *Int. J. Sport Nutr.*, **8**, 124–42.

Bass, S., Pearce, G., Bradney, M., Hendrick, E., Delmas, P. D., Harding, A., & Seeman, E. (1998). Exercise before puberty may confer residual benefits in bone density in adulthood: studies in active prepubertal and retired female gymnasts. *J. Bone Miner. Res.*, **13**, 500–7.

Bloomfield, S. (1997). Changes in musculoskeletal structure and function with prolonged bed rest. *Med. Sci. Sports Exerc.*, **29**, 197–206.

Bonjour, J. P., Theintz, G., Buchs, B., Slosman, D., & Rizzoli, R. (1991). Critical years and stages of puberty for spinal and femoral bone mass accumulation during adolescence. *J. Clin. Endocrinol. Metab.*, **73**, 555–63.

Boot, A., de Ridder, M., Pols, H., Krenning, E., & de Muinck Keizer-Schrama, S. (1992). Bone mineral density in children and adolescents: relation to puberty, calcium intake and physical activity. *J. Clin. Endocrinol. Metab.*, **82**, 57–62.

Bortz, W. (1985). Physical exercise as an evolutionary force. *J. Hum. Evol.*, **14**, 145–55.

Capozzo, A. (1983). Force actions in the human trunk during walking. *J. Sports Med.*, **23**, 14–22.

Carter, D., Bouxsein, M., & Marcus, R. (1992). New approaches for interpreting projected bone densitometry data. *J. Bone Miner. Res.*, **7**, 137–45.

Cassell, C., Benedict, M., & Specker, B. (1996). Bone mineral density in elite 7- to 9-year-old female gymnasts and swimmers. *Med. Sci. Sports Exerc.*, **28**, 1243–6.

Currey J. D. (1984). *The Mechanical Adaptations of Bones.* Princeton University Press.

Dalsky, G. P., Stocke, K. S., Ehsani, A. A., Slatopolsky, E., Lee, W. C., & Birge Jr, S. J. (1988).

Weight-bearing exercise training and lumbar bone mineral content in postmenopausal women. *Ann. Int. Med.*, **108**, 824–8.

Dyson, K., Blimkie, C. J. R., Davison, K. S., Webber, C. E., & Adachi, J. E. (1997). Gymnastic training and bone density in pre-adolescent females. *Med. Sci. Sports Exerc.*, **29**, 443–50.

Eaton, S., Konner, M., & Shostak, M. (1988). Stone Agers in the fast lane: chronic degenerative diseases in evolutionary perspective. *Am. J. Med.*, **84**, 739–49.

Fassler, A. L. C. & Bonjour, J. P. (1996). Osteoporosis as a pediatric problem. *Ped. Nutr.*, **42**, 811–23.

Faulkner, R. A., Bailey, D. A., Drinkwater, D. T., Wilkinson, A. A., Houston, C. S., & McKay, H. A. (1993a). Regional and total body bone mineral content, bone mineral density and total body tissue composition in children 8–16 years of age. *Calcif. Tissue Int.*, **53**, 7–12.

Faulkner, R. A., Houston, C., Bailey, D., Drinkwater, D., McKay, H. A., & Wilkinson, A. (1993b). Comparison of bone mineral content and bone mineral density between dominant and non-dominant limbs in children 8–16 years of age. *Am. J. Hum. Biol.*, **5**, 491–9.

Forwood, M. & Burr, D. (1993). Physical activity and bone mass: exercises in futility? *Bone Miner.*, **21**, 89–112.

Frost, H. M. (1987). Bone 'mass' and the 'mechanostat': a proposal. *Anat. Rec.*, **219**, 1–9.

Frost, H. M. (1992). The role of changes in mechanical usage set points in the pathogenesis of osteoporosis. *J. Bone Miner. Res.*, **7**, 253–61.

Frost, H. M. (1995). Perspectives on a 'paradigm shift' developing in skeletal science. *Calcif. Tissue Int.*, **56**, 1–4.

Garn, S. M. (1970). *The Earlier Gain and Later Loss of Cortical Bone.* Springfield, IL: Charles C. Thomas Co.

Gilsanz, V., Boechat, M. I., Roe, T .F., Gilsanz, R., Loro, M. L., Sayre, J., & Goodman, W. G. (1994). Gender differences in vertebral body sizes in children and adolescents. *Radiology*, **190**, 673–7.

Gilsanz, V., Gibbens, D. T., Carlson, M., Boechat, M. I., Cann, C. E., & Schulz, E. E. (1988). Peak trabecular vertebral density in children: a comparison of adolescent and adult females. *Calcif. Tissue Int.*, **43**, 260–2.

Glastre, C., Braillon, P., David, L., Cochat, P., Meunier, P. J., & Delmas, P. D. (1990). Measurement of bone mineral content of the lumbar spine by dual energy X-ray absorptiometry in normal children: correlations with growth parameters. *J. Clin. Endocrinol. Metab.*, **70**, 1330–3.

Gordon, C. I., Halton, J. M., & Atkinson, S. A. (1991). The contribution of growth and puberty to peak bone mass. *Growth Dev. Aging*, **55**, 257–62.

Gortmaker, S. L., Dietz, W. H., Sobol, A. M., & Wehler, C. A. (1997). Increasing pediatric obesity in the United States. *Am. J. Dis. Child*, **141**, 535–40.

Gortmaker, S. L., Must, A., Sobol, A. M., Peterson, K., Colditz, G., & Dietz, W. H. (1996). Television viewing as a cause of increasing obesity among children in the United States, 1986–1990. *Arch. Pediatr. Adolesc. Med.*, **150**, 356–62.

Grimston, S. K. & Hanley, D. A. (1992). Bone mineral density in children is related to mechanical loading regime. *Med. Sci. Sports Exerc.*, **24**, S45.

Gunnes, M. & Lehmann, E. (1996). Physical activity and dietary constituents as predictors of forearm cortical and trabecular bone gain in healthy children and adolescents: a prospective study. *Acta Paediatr.*, **85**, 19–25.

Haapasalo, H., Kannus, P., Sievänen, H., Pasanen, M., Uusi-Rasi, K., Heinonen, A., Oja, P., & Vuori, I. (1996). Development of mass, density and estimated mechanical characteristics of bones in Caucasian females. *J. Bone Miner. Res.*, **11**, 1751–60.

Haapasalo, H., Kannus, P., Sievänen, H., Pasanen, M., Uusi-Rasi, K., Heinonen, A., Oja, P., & Vuori, I. (1998). Effect of long-term unilateral activity on bone mineral density of female junior tennis players. *J. Bone Miner. Res.*, **13**, 310–19.

Hillman L. (1996), Bone mineral acquisition in utero and during infancy and childhood. In *Osteoporosis*, ed. R. Marcus, D. Feldman & J. Kelsey, pp. 449–64. San Diego, CA: Academic Press.

Kannus, P., Haaspasalo, H., Sankelo, M., Sievänen, H., Pasanen, M., Heinonen, A., Oja, P., & Vuori, I. (1995). Effect of starting age of physical activity on bone mass in the dominant arm of tennis and squash players. *Ann. Int. Med.*, **123**, 27–31.

Katzman, D. K., Bachrach, L. K., Carter, D. R., & Marcus, R. (1991). Clinical and anthropometric correlates of bone mineral acquisition in healthy adolescent girls. *J. Clin. Endocrinol. Metab.*, **73**, 1332–9.

Khan, K., Bennell, K., Hopper, J., Flicker, L., Nowson, C., Sherwin, A., Crichton, K., Harcourt, P., & Wark, J. (1998). Self-reported ballet classes undertaken at age 10–12 years and hip bone mineral density in later life. *Osteoporos. Int.*, **8**, 165–73.

Kirchner, E., Lewis, R., & O'Connor, P. (1996). Effects of past gymnastics participation on adult bone mass. *J. App. Physiol.*, **80**, 226–32.

Krall, A. & Dawson-Hughes, B. (1993). Heritable and life-style determinants of bone mineral density. *J. Bone Miner. Res.*, **8**, 1–9.

Kröger, H., Kotaniemi, A., Kröger, L., & Alhava, E. (1993). Development of bone mass and bone density of the spine and femoral neck – a prospective study of 65 children and adolescents. *Bone Miner.*, **23**, 171–82.

Kröger, H., Kotaniemi, A., Vainio, P., & Alhava, E. (1992). Bone densitometry of the spine and femur in children by dual-energy x-ray absorptiometry. *Bone Miner.*, **17**, 75–85.

Krolner, B. & Toft, B. (1983). Vertebral bone loss: an unheeded side effect of therapeutic bed rest. *Clin. Sci.*, **64**, 537–40.

Lanyon, L. (1996). Using functional loading to influence bone mass and architecture. *Bone*, **18**, 37S-43S.

Lanyon, L. E., Goodship, A. E., Pye, C. J., & MacFie, J. H. (1982). Mechanically adaptive bone remodelling. *J. Biomech.*, **15**, 141–54.

Larsen, C. S. (1987). Bioarchaelogical interpretations of subsistence economy and behavior from human skeletal remains. *Adv. Archaeol. Meth. Theory*, **10**, 339–445.

McKay, H., Bailey, D., Mirwald, R., Davison, K., & Faulkner, R. (1998). Peak bone mineral accrual and age of menarche in adolescent girls – a six year longitudinal study. *J. Pediatr.*, **133**, 682–7.

Martin, A. D., Bailey, D. A., McKay, H. A., & Whiting, S. J. (1997). Bone mineral and calcium accretion during puberty. *Am. J. Clin. Nutr.*, **66**, 611–15.

Matkovic, V., Kostial, K., Simonovic, I., Buzina, R., Bordarec, A., & Nordin, B. E. C. (1979). Bone status and fracture rates in two regions of Yugoslavia. *Am. J. Clin. Nutr.*, **32**, 540–9.

Melton, L. J., Atkinson, E., O'Fallon, W., Wahner, H., & Riggs, B. (1993). Long-term fracture prediction by bone mineral assessed at different skeletal sites. *J. Bone Miner. Res.*, **8**, 1227–33.

Mora, S., Shulz, E., Roe, T., Sith, B. , & Gilsanz, V. (1991). Gains in cancellous and cortical bone during growth are determined by different factors. *J. Bone Miner. Res.*, **6**, S307.

Morris, F. L., Naughton, G. A., Gibbs, J. L., Carlson, J. S., & Wark, J. D. (1997). Prospective 10-month exercise intervention in premenarcheal girls: positive effects on bone and lean mass. *J. Bone Miner. Res.*, **12**, 1453–62.

Oganov, V., Grigor'ev, A., Voronin, L., Rakhmanov, A., Bakulin, A., Schneider, V., & LeBlanc, A. (1992). Bone mineral density in cosmonauts after 4.5–6 month long flights aboard orbital station MIR. *Aviak. Ekolog. Med.*, **26**, 20–4.

Panzer, V., Wood, G., Bates, B., & Mason, B. (1988). Lower extremity loads in landings of elite gymnasts. In *Biomechanics XI*, ed. G. de Groot, A. Hollander, P. Huijing & G. van Ingen Schenau, pp. 727–35. Amsterdam: Free University Press.

Parfitt, A. M. (1994). The two faces of growth: benefits and risks to bone integrity. *Osteoporos. Int.*, **4**, 382–98.

Ruiz, J., Mandel, J., & Garabedian, M. (1995). Influence of spontaneous calcium intake and physical exercise on the vertebral and femoral bone mineral density of children and adolescents. *J. Bone Miner. Res.*, **10**, 675–82.

Schonau, E., Wentzlik, U., Dietrich, M., Scheidhauer, K., & Klein, K. (1993). Is there an increase in bone density in children? *Lancet*, **342**, 689–90.

Slemenda, C., Reister, T., Hui, S., Miller, J., Christian, J., & Johnston, C. C. (1994). Influences on skeletal mineralization in children and adolescents: evidence for varying effects of sexual maturation and physical activity. *J. Pediatr.*, **125**, 201–7.

Taafe, T., Snow-Harter, C., Connolly, D., Robinson, T., Brown, M. D., & Marcus, R. (1995). Differential effects of swimming versus weight-bearing activity on bone mineral status of eumenorrheic athletes. *J. Bone Miner. Res.*, **10**, 675–82.

Theintz, G., Buchs, B., Rizzoli, R., Slosman, D., Clavien, H., Sizonenko, P. C., & Bonjour, J. P. (1992). Longitudinal monitoring of bone mass accumulation in healthy adolescents: evidence for a marked reduction after 16 years of age at the levels of lumbar spine and femoral neck in female subjects. *J. Clin. Endocrinol. Metab.*, **75**, 1060–5.

Virvidakis, K., Georgiou, E., Korkotsidis, A., Ntalles, K., & Proukakis, C. (1990). Bone mineral content of junior competitive weightlifters. *Int. J. Sports Med.*, **11**, 244–6.

Whedon, G. D. (1984). Disuse osteoporosis: physiological aspects. *Calcif. Tissue Int.*, **36**, S146–50.

Wolff J. (1892). *The Law of Bone Transformation*. Berlin: Hirschwald.

Wolpoff, M. H. (1980). *Paleoanthropology*. New York: Alfred A. Knopf.

13

Osteoporosis in children

Frank Rauch and Francis H. Glorieux

Introduction

This chapter deals with pediatric disorders which are characterized by increased bone fragility and decreased bone mass. Compared with adults, such diseases are relatively rare in children, but may have devastating consequences. Osteoporosis can occur as a primary bone disorder or may be secondary to other diseases and/or their treatment (Table 13.1). The primary forms of childhood osteoporosis comprise osteogenesis imperfecta and idiopathic juvenile osteoporosis. Secondary pediatric osteoporosis is most frequently seen as a consequence of immobilization and of long-term steroid treatment in a variety of chronic diseases.

Osteogenesis imperfecta

Osteogenesis imperfecta (OI), also called brittle bone disease, is a hereditary form of osteoporosis. In many patients the disease is due to abnormalities in collagen type I. Therefore, the disease manifests itself not only in bone, but also in other tissues that contain collagen type I, such as skin, teeth and sclerae. OI is thought to affect between 1/10000 and 1/15000 individuals of all racial and ethnic origins (Byers & Steiner, 1992).

Clinical presentation
Family history

In most familial cases of OI, heredity follows an autosomal dominant pattern. However, new mutations are frequent, especially in the more severe forms. There may also be germline mosaicism for OI mutations, so that unaffected parents can have more than one affected child (Rowe & Shapiro, 1998). In rare kindreds an autosomal recessive inheritance has been demonstrated.

Signs and symptoms

The severity of clinical expression of OI is extremely variable and ranges from stillbirth to perhaps lifelong absence of symptoms. Most patients have recurrent fractures. In the more severe cases chronic bone pain and skeletal deformities are

Table 13.1. Forms of osteoporosis in children, according to current literature

---

I. *Primary*
  Osteogenesis imperfecta
  Idiopathic juvenile osteoporosis

II. *Secondary*
  Endocrine disorders
    Cushing syndrome
    Glucocorticoid therapy
    Diabetes mellitus
    Thyrotoxicosis
    Gonadal dysgenesis
  Gastrointestinal disorders
    Biliary atresia
    Glycogen storage disease type 1
    Chronic hepatitis
    Malabsorption syndromes
  Inborn errors of metabolism
    Homocystinuria
    Lysinuric protein intolerance
  Other disorders
    Immobilization
    Anticonvulsant therapy
    Cyanotic congenital heart disease
    Acute lymphoblastic leukemia
    Anorexia nervosa
    Thalassemia

---

present. The most frequent extraskeletal findings are blue sclerae, ligamentous laxity with joint hypermobility, skin hyperlaxity with susceptibility to bruises, as well as fragile and discolored teeth (dentinogenesis imperfecta). Excessive sweating is a frequent but ill-explained finding in young children. Hearing loss can develop due to abnormalities in auditory ossicles, but is rarely evident in children.

Clinical classification

The most popular classification in present use was devised by Sillence (Sillence et al., 1979). Four forms of OI are distinguished according to clinical features. Type I OI comprises patients with a mild presentation and normal height, whereas type II OI is lethal in the perinatal period. Type III OI is the most severe form in children surviving the neonatal period. These patients have a well-defined phenotype including extremely short stature, growth plate abnormalities and progressive limb and spine deformities. Patients with a moderate to severe phenotype who do not fit into one of the above categories are classified as type IV OI. This classification has been useful in providing a framework for prognosis. However, the management of a given patient currently does not depend on whether one or another type is attributed, but rather is dictated by symptoms and disease severity.

Radiological features

The variability in clinical expression of OI is reflected in the radiological features. In most patients generalized osteopenia with thin cortices of long bones is apparent (Fig. 13.1). Wormian bones of significant number and size in the skull are a common but not pathognomonic feature of OI. Moderate to severe cases are characterized by modeling defects of long bones, such as decreased diameter of diaphyses and increased diameter of epiphyses and metaphyses. Deformities may result from recurrent fractures or simply from the lack of resistance to muscle pull. Such patients often also have deformities in the vertebrae, which can take a wedge-shaped, biconcave or even completely flattened appearance (Fig. 13.2). Platybasia, which can progress to basilar impression, and excessive pneumatization of the frontal and mastoid sinuses are common in severely affected patients. The pelvis can have a triradiate-shaped appearance. Prenatal diagnosis of severe OI is possible by ultrasound examination at 14 to 18 weeks of gestation. When the collagen mutation is known in a family, prenatal diagnosis can also be made by testing for the mutation in amniotic cells.

Radiological abnormalities may increase markedly during growth. 'Popcorn' calcifications are developmental defects in the regions of the epiphyses and metaphyses of major long bones (predominantly near the knees) that occur most often in type III OI patients. This finding is believed to result from traumatic fragmentation of the growth plate cartilage, which may severely limit long bone growth. When fractures occur in OI, they heal at normal rates. In a specific subtype, there is exuberant callus formation that in some cases has been mistaken for skeletal malignancy.

Laboratory findings

Routine biochemical studies of bone and mineral metabolism are typically unremarkable. Elevations in serum alkaline phosphatase and markers of bone resorption occur in patients with exuberant callus formation. Hypercalciuria is a common finding in severely affected children. Bone histology is characterized by increased turnover (Baron et al., 1983; unpublished observations), which may, in part, be due to periods of prolonged immobilization.

Differential diagnosis

The differential diagnosis for OI in infants and children includes idiopathic juvenile osteoporosis, Cushing's disease, homocystinuria, congenital indifference

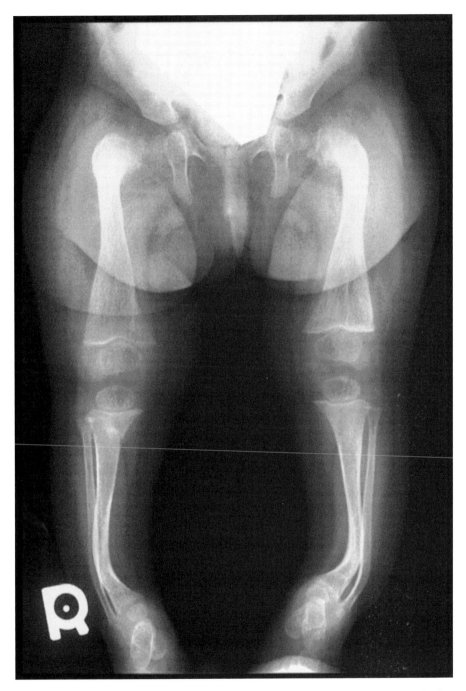

Fig. 13.1   Osteogenesis imperfecta. Severe deformities of the lower extremities in a 1-year-old girl
with OI type IV. Bilateral coxa vara and typical bowing of the lower leg are present. Note
the apparent absence of cortices in the distal half of the femora, flaring of the metaphyses
and thin diaphyses.

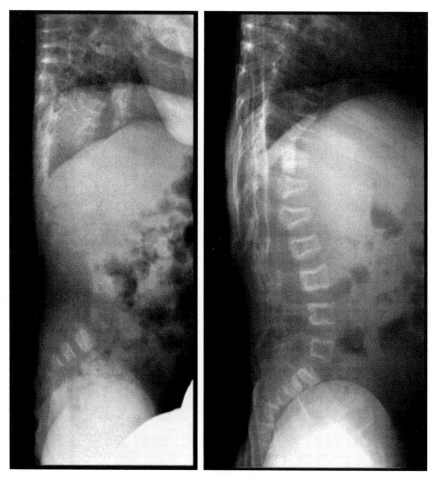

Fig. 13.2   Osteogenesis imperfecta. Left panel: Lateral view of the lumbar spine in a 20-month-old girl with OI type III. Some of the vertebrae are hardly discernible due to severe osteopenia. Almost all vertebral bodies are compressed. At the time this X-ray was taken, the areal bone density of L_1 to L_4 was −9.0 standard deviations below the age-specific mean value. Right panel: The same patient after 13 months of treatment with pamidronate. Vertebral bodies now show a markedly enhanced contrast due to thickened cortices. Also note the increased size and reshaping of vertebral bodies. The areal bone density has increased to −4.8 standard deviations below the mean.

to pain, child abuse, severe polyostotic fibrous dysplasia and some forms of Ehlers–Danlos syndrome. The correct diagnosis can usually be made from the patient's medical history, physical findings, and radiographic features. A positive family history is especially helpful, but many patients represent new mutations. The finding of a collagen type I abnormality strongly suggests the diagnosis of OI. However, OI cannot be ruled out in the absence of detectable collagen abnormalities.

Pathophysiology

OI is commonly assumed to be caused by mutations in one of the two genes that encode the alpha chains of collagen type I (Byers & Steiner, 1992). However, the actual prevalence of collagen mutations among patients who present the clinical picture of OI is currently unknown, as sufficiently sensitive sequencing strategies have only recently been developed (Korkko et al., 1998). The mechanisms by which genetic mutations lead to the clinical manifestations of the disease have not yet been elucidated.

Treatment

Medical treatment of OI has long been largely ineffective in altering the course of the disease. Recently, treatment with bisphosphonates has been shown to benefit children with severe forms of OI (Glorieux et al., 1998). Bone mineral density and physical activity increased markedly in these patients and fracture rate decreased by 65% (Fig. 13.2).

Supportive treatment requires a multidisciplinary approach including orthopedic surgeons, physiotherapists, occupational therapists, dentists and psychologists to care for recurrent fractures, limb deformities, kyphoscoliosis and dentinogenesis imperfecta (Engelbert et al., 1998). To stabilize the lower limbs the use of braces and rodding of femurs and tibiae are often necessary in severely affected patients. Support groups (e.g., Osteogenesis Imperfecta Foundation) are important sources of comfort and lay-language information for patients and their families.

Prognosis

Fracture rates decrease markedly after puberty, but may again increase in women after menopause (Paterson et al., 1984). Patients with mild forms of OI most commonly are not functionally impaired as adults. However, severely affected patients may remain wheelchair-bound for life. Life expectancy is close to normal in types I and IV, but is decreased in type III OI (Paterson et al., 1996). Respiratory infections are the main cause of death in such patients (McAllion & Paterson, 1996).

Idiopathic juvenile osteoporosis (IJO)

IJO is a transient, non-hereditary form of childhood osteoporosis without extraskeletal involvement. This is a very rare disease. About 100 cases have been reported in the literature.

Clinical features

Signs and symptoms

IJO typically develops in a prepubertal (mostly between 8 and 12 years of age), previously healthy child of either sex (Teotia et al., 1979). Symptoms begin with an insidious onset of pain in the lower back, hips and feet, and difficulty walking (Dent & Friedman, 1965). Knee and ankle pain and fractures of the lower extremities may be present. Vertebral compression fractures are frequent and cause the upper: lower segment ratio to decrease below unity. Long bone fractures, mostly at metaphyseal sites, may occur. Physical examination may be entirely normal or reveal thoracolumbar kyphosis or kyphoscoliosis, pigeon chest deformity, crown–pubis to pubis–heel ratio of less than 1.0, loss of height, deformities of the long bones, and limp.

Radiological features

On X-rays, the new bone formed in metaphyseal areas appears as a radiolucent band ('neo-osseous osteoporosis', Fig. 13.3) (Dent, 1977). Several vertebrae can have a wedge-shaped or biconcave appearance. Long bones usually have normal length and cortical width.

Laboratory findings

There are no known biochemical characteristics. Alterations of the markers of bone and mineral metabolism are non-specific and inconsistently noted. In some cases a negative calcium balance has been reported (Dent, 1977). Bone biopsy reveals markedly decreased activity of the osteoblast population on trabecular bone (unpublished observations).

Differential diagnosis

The diagnosis of IJO is made by the exclusion of OI and of diseases causing secondary osteoporosis (see below). The exclusion of most of these disorders usually is not difficult. However, it may be hard to distinguish between IJO and OI type I caused by a new mutation. Table 13.2 presents the typical distinguishing features between the two entities.

Pathophysiology

The cause of IJO is unknown. Whatever triggers the decrease in osteoblast performance, the effect obviously is that the skeleton no longer adequately adapts to the rapidly increasing mechanical loads during growth. Thus, the strain keeps increasing until the threshold is reached where fractures occur.

Treatment

There is no treatment with proven benefit to the patient. The effect of any kind of medical intervention is difficult to judge, because the disease is rare, has a variable course and usually resolves without treatment. Fluoride has been used with success in isolated cases (Glorieux et al., 1993). Bisphosphonates appear to yield promising results, but reliable data are still lacking (Brumsen et al., 1997).

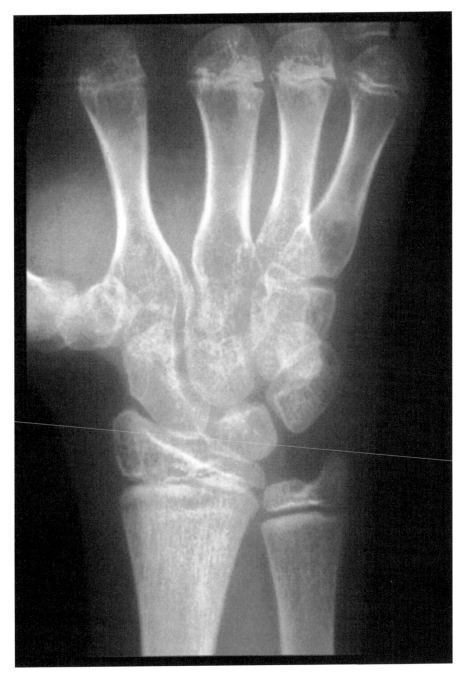

Fig. 13.3   Idiopathic juvenile osteoporosis. A radiolucent band in the radial metaphysis indicates the presence of 'neo-osseous osteoporosis'.

Table 13.2. Differential diagnosis between idiopathic juvenile osteoporosis (IJO) and osteogenesis imperfecta type I (OI)

	IJO	OI
Family history	Negative	May be positive
Onset	Late prepubertal	Birth or soon after
Duration	1–5 years	Lifelong
Clinical findings	Upper:lower segment ratio <1.0 Abnormal gait Metaphyseal fractures	Blue sclerae Frequently abnormal dentition Joint hyperlaxity Long bone fractures
Growth rate	Normal	Normal or decreased
Radiologic findings	Wedge compression in spine 'Neo-osseous osteoporosis'	Thin cortex of long bones Wormian bones in skull Thin ribs
Bone biopsy	Decreased bone turnover	Increased bone turnover
Connective tissue defect	No	Often collagen abnormalities

Prognosis

The disease process is only active in growing children and spontaneous recovery is the rule after 3–5 years of evolution. However, spine deformities and severe functional impairment may persist in severe cases (Smith, 1995).

Secondary osteoporosis

A variety of primary diseases and/or their therapies have been incriminated as causing osteoporosis in children (Table 13.1). It is important to note that not all of these disorders have been demonstrated to cause increased bone fragility. Often 'osteoporosis' has been diagnosed on the basis of decreased bone mass only. However, this criterion alone is not sufficient to establish that a disorder causes 'osteoporosis' in children, because decreased bone mass is the inevitable consequence of slower than normal bone growth. Slow growth rates are a common finding in many chronic pediatric disorders and do not necessarily indicate increased propensity for fractures. Therefore, we focus on two relatively common causes of increased bone fragility in children, corticosteroid excess and immobilization.

Corticosteroid-induced osteoporosis

This form of osteoporosis can result from excessive endogenous production of corticosteroids (Cushing syndrome). More frequently, it is a consequence of exogenously applied glucocorticoids, which are used to treat a variety of chronic inflammatory and immunologic disorders. An excess of corticosteroids in children affects longitudinal growth rate. In addition, glucocorticoids decrease osteoblast activity, while bone resorption is normal or even increased. This negative balance of bone remodeling leads to a loss of bone mass (Dempster, 1989). These effects are more pronounced in trabecular than in cortical bone. Therefore, corticosteroid-induced osteoporosis predominantly affects the spine, where vertebral compression fractures may occur.

Treatment of Cushing syndrome consists of surgical or medical suppression of endogenous corticoid secretion. Iatrogenic corticosteroid-induced osteoporosis in adults can be prevented and treated with bisphosphonates (Adachi et al., 1997; Saag et al., 1998). It is not yet known whether the same effects can be achieved in children.

Immobilization-induced osteoporosis

Acute immobilization decreases bone formation and increases bone resorption. Additionally, bone development is severely impaired in chronically immobilized children, due to lack of mechanical stimulation. Both factors combine to cause low bone mass. This typically results in vertebral compression fractures, but long bone fractures may also occur. Physiotherapy may help to stimulate bone and muscle development. Medical treatment with bisphosphonates has shown promising results in a small number of patients (Shaw et al., 1994), but this approach needs to be further evaluated.

REFERENCES

Adachi, J. D., Bensen, W. G., Brown, J., Hanley, D., Hodsman, A., Josse, R., Kendler, D. L., Lentle, B., Olszynski, W., Ste-Marie, L. G., Tenenhouse, A., & Chines, A. A. (1997). Intermittent etidronate therapy to prevent corticosteroid-induced osteoporosis. *N. Engl. J. Med.*, **337**, 382–7.

Baron, R., Gertner, J. M., Lang, R., & Vignery, A. (1983). Increased bone turnover with decreased bone formation by osteoblasts in children with osteogenesis imperfecta tarda. *Pediatr Res.*, **17**, 204–7.

Brumsen, C., Hamdy, N. A., & Papapoulos, S. E. (1997). Long-term effects of bisphosphonates on the growing skeleton. Studies of young patients with severe osteoporosis. *Medicine (Baltimore)*, **76**, 266–83.

Byers, P. H. & Steiner, R. D. (1992). Osteogenesis imperfecta. *Annu. Rev. Med.*, **43**, 269–82.

Dempster, D. W. (1989). Bone histomorphometry in glucocorticoid-induced osteoporosis. *J. Bone Miner. Res.*, **4**, 137–41.

Dent, C. E. (1977). Osteoporosis in childhood. *Postgrad. Med. J.*, **53**, 450–7.

Dent, C. E. & Friedman, M. (1965). Idiopathic juvenile osteoporosis. *Q. J. Med.*, **34**, 177–210.

Engelbert, R. H., Pruijs, H. E., Beemer, F. A., & Helders, P. J. (1998). Osteogenesis imperfecta in childhood: treatment strategies. *Arch. Phys. Med. Rehabil.*, **79**, 1590–4.

Glorieux, F. H., Bishop, N. J., Plotkin, H., Chabot, G., Lanoue, G., & Travers, R. (1998). Cyclic administration of pamidronate in children with severe osteogenesis imperfecta. *N. Engl. J. Med.*, **339**, 947–52.

Glorieux, F. H., Norman, M. E., Travers, R., & Taylor, A. (1993). Idiopathic juvenile osteoporosis. In *Proceedings. Fourth International Symposium on Osteoporosis and Consensus Development Conference*, ed. C. Christiansen & B. Rijs, pp. 200–2.

Korkko, J., Ala-Kokko, L., De Paepe, A., Nuytinck, L., Earley, J., & Prockop, D. J. (1998). Analysis of the COL1A1 and COL1A2 genes by PCR amplification and scanning by conformation-sensitive gel electrophoresis identifies only COL1A1 mutations in 15 patients with osteogenesis imperfecta type I: identification of common sequences of null-allele mutations. *Am. J. Hum. Genet.*, **62**, 98–110.

McAllion, S. J. & Paterson, C. R. (1996). Causes of death in osteogenesis imperfecta. *J. Clin. Pathol.*, **49**, 627–30.

Paterson, C. R., McAllion, S., & Stellman, J. L. (1984). Osteogenesis imperfecta after the menopause. *N. Engl. J. Med.*, **310**, 1694–6.

Paterson, C. R., Ogston, S. A., & Henry, R. M. (1996). Life expectancy in osteogenesis imperfecta. *Br. Med. J.*, **312**, 351.

Rouch, F., Travers, R., Norman, M. E., Taylor, A., Parfitt, A. M., & Glorieux, F. H. (2000). Deficient bone formation in idiopathic juvenile osteoporosis – a histomorphometric study of canellous iliac bone. *J. Bone Miner. Res.*, In press.

Rowe, D. W. & Shapiro, J. R. (1998). Osteogenesis imperfecta. In *Metabolic Bone Disease and Clinically Related Disorders*, ed. L. V. Avioli & S. M. Krane, pp. 651–95. San Diego, CA: Academic Press.

Saag, K. G., Emkey, R., Schnitzer, T. J., Brown, J. P., Hawkins, F., Goemaere, S., Thamsborg, G., Liberman, U. A., Delmas, P. D., Malice, M. P., Czachur, M., & Daifotis, A. G. (1998). Alendronate for the prevention and treatment of glucocorticoid-induced osteoporosis. Glucocorticoid-Induced Osteoporosis Intervention Study Group. *N. Engl. J. Med.*, **339**, 292–9.

Shaw, N. J., White, C. P., Fraser, W. D., & Rosenbloom, L. (1994). Osteopenia in cerebral palsy. *Arch. Dis. Child*, **71**, 235–8.

Sillence, D. O., Senn, A., & Danks, D. M. (1979). Genetic heterogeneity in osteogenesis imperfecta. *J. Med. Genet.*, **16**, 101–16.

Smith, R. (1995). Idiopathic juvenile osteoporosis: experience of twenty-one patients. *Br. J. Rheumatol.*, 34, 68–77.

Teotia, M., Teotia, S. P., & Singh, R. K. (1979). Idiopathic juvenile osteoporosis. *Am. J. Dis. Child*, **133**, 894–900.

Part III

Pathophysiology of the aging skeleton

14

Consequences of alterations in bone remodeling

Karen M. Prestwood and Lawrence G. Raisz

The key to understanding the pathogenesis of osteoporosis is an analysis of the bone remodeling process and of the mechanisms by which alterations in this process can lead to loss of bone mass and strength. Our knowledge of bone remodeling at the cellular and molecular level has increased greatly, but we still lack critical information on the factors which regulate bone remodeling in humans and which are likely to be responsible for bone loss. While the initial formation of the skeleton depends on direct apposition of new bone, or modeling, remodeling of the skeleton begins in early fetal life and becomes the dominant metabolic activity of the skeleton by the end of puberty.

During childhood and adolescence, rapid rates of bone remodeling are associated with a gain in bone mass. Once peak bone mass has been achieved, there is a period when skeletal remodeling remains in balance; that is, the rates of resorption and formation are relatively equal, or tightly 'coupled.' Bone loss probably begins before the menopause in women, but then accelerates at the menopause. Bone loss in men has not been clearly defined, but probably occurs at a slow rate beginning in the 50s and 60s and at an accelerated rate thereafter. Bone loss in postmenopausal women and older men represents an imbalance between the rates of resorption and formation, or 'uncoupled' bone remodeling. However, evidence suggests that, once bone loss begins, it is not constant or uniform throughout the skeleton, but can vary both in rate and site of loss. In this chapter we will describe the bone remodeling cycle, the basic multicellular units (BMU) of trabecular and cortical bone, and indicate some of the factors which can influence the remodeling cycle. Many hormones and local factors have been identified which influence bone remodeling, but their relative importance in physiologic and pathologic regulation is not well understood. Mechanical forces play a major role in the regulation of bone remodeling. Frost and others have described this regulation as being a 'mechanostat,' and further proposed that there is a 'set point' for the mechanostat which may vary with age and hormonal status (Frost, 1997). While this is a conceptually useful approach, we know little about the physical and biochemical signals which regulate the response to mechanical forces, and even less about how these signals are transduced with and between bone cells.

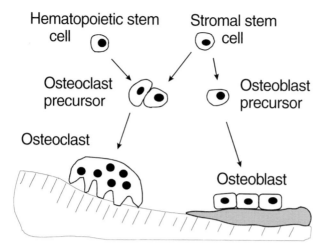

Fig. 14.1   The bone remodeling cycle. Osteoclast precursors are activated by interacting with osteoblast precursors and the mature osteoclasts resorb bone. After resorption is completed, the reversal phase begins and then osteoblasts appear on the surface of bone to lay down osteoid and to calcify new bone. Osteoclasts are derived from hematopoietic stem cells and osteoblast from stromal stem cells.

The bone remodeling cycle

As indicated in Fig. 14.1, the bone remodeling cycle begins with 'activation.' This process may be initiated by either local changes, such as mechanical force and microfractures, or by systemic hormones or local factors which influence overall bone turnover (Frost, 1997). The activation step is initiated by effects on cells of the osteoblast lineage, although it is likely that these responsor cells are not fully differentiated osteoblasts, but rather are either precursor cells in the marrow stroma or lining cells on the bone surface. These cells have receptors for factors which have been shown to influence bone resorption. The concept of osteoblast–osteoclast interaction as the first step in activation was proposed many years ago, but we have just begun to define the molecular mechanisms of this interaction. The factors which stimulate bone resorption can alter the expression of a surface molecule, variably called osteoclast differentiation factor (ODF), osteoprotegerin ligand (OPGL), TRANCE or RANK ligand (Matsuzaki et al., 1998; Yasuda et al., 1998). The latter two names come from other cell systems, specifically the activation of lymphocytes, in which these molecules are involved. The osteoblast not only makes this ligand, but also makes osteoprotegerin (OPG), which can bind to OPGL and block the interaction between the responser cells and osteoclast precursors (Simonet et al., 1997). The receptor molecule on osteoclast precursors with which the reponser cells interact is presumably a form of RANK (Fig. 14.2). In

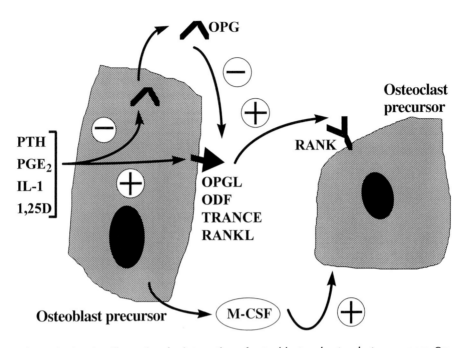

Fig. 14.2   Schematic drawing illustrating the interaction of osteoblast and osteoclast precursors. On
the surface of osteoblast precursors are molecules called by various names:
osteoprotegerin ligand (OPGL), osteoclast differentiating factor (ODF), TRANCE or RANKL.
These molecules interact with RANK on the surface of osteoclast precursors resulting on
activation of osteoclasts. PTH, PGE$_2$, IL-1 and 1,25D have a positive effect on OPGL
resulting in increased activation of osteoclasts and thus bone resorption. Osteoblasts also
make osteoprotegerin (OPG) which can bind to OPGL and block the interaction of
osteoblast and osteoclast precursors. PTH, PGE$_2$, IL-1, and 1,25D have a negative effect on
OPG production resulting in increased bone resorption. Osteoblast precursors also
produce M-CSF which acts by another pathway to activate osteoclasts. It appears that
both types of osteoblast–osteoclast interaction are necessary for activation of the bone
remodeling cycle.

this system, the usual terms of 'receptor' and 'ligand' may represent an over-
simplification, since it is likely that when these molecules bind to each other, signals
are transmitted to both interacting cells. Moreover, there may be other cell–cell
interactions between osteoblast and osteoclast which are important in the initial
steps of activation and osteoclastogenesis. Hormones and local factors which activate remodeling can increase the expression of OPGL and decrease the expression
of OPG (Tsukii et al., 1998). Regulation of the RANK receptor on osteoclast precursors probably also occurs, although it has not yet been demonstrated. The interaction between RANK and OPGL is necessary but not sufficient for the information
of active functional osteoclasts. At least one other factor, macrophage stimulating

factor (M-CSF or (CSF1), which can be produced by osteoblasts, is also important in osteoclastogenesis. M-CSF appears to play a role in the initial replication and activation of the osteoclast precursors, as well as in the subsequent steps of differentiation and fusion which lead to the fully activated osteoclast (Biskobing et al., 1995; Amano et al., 1998; Yao et al., 1998).

The function of the fully differentiated osteoclast has been described earlier in this volume. One important question in control of bone remodeling is how the depth and breadth of osteoclastic resorption are regulated. The limited extent of osteoclast resorption may be due to the finite lifespan of osteoclasts, whose nuclei undergo apoptosis. The lifespan and mortality of osteoclasts can be regulated by hormones, but the details of this regulation are not fully understood (Dempster, 1992).

Following osteoclastic resorption, the phase of remodeling called 'reversal' occurs, during which mononuclear cells present on the bone surface. The function of these cells is not understood; however, the mononuclear cells may be involved in further degradation of matrix, in the formation of the so-called 'cement line,' which is present between old and new bone, or in signaling of osteoblasts to migrate and differentiate to begin new bone formation at the resorption site (Baron et al., 1980). The initiation of the formation phase is probably not dependent on cell–cell interactions, but rather on local release of growth factors either from the matrix or from the various cells involved in the resorption and reversal process. These growth factors stimulate the subsequent replication, migration and differentiation of new osteoblasts in successive waves, which may also depend on signals from the differentiated osteoblasts themselves (Canalis et al., 1988). In younger individuals, the amount of new bone formed during the coupled phase of bone remodeling is approximately equal to that resorbed; however, the capacity of the osteoblast population to multiply and to lay down new bone decreases with aging. Therefore, the size of a BMU, or new packet of bone on a trabecular surface, as measured by 'mean wall thickness,' is decreased. In cortical bone, where the BMU is an osteon, the consequence of impaired osteoblast renewal is incomplete filling in of the Haversian canal, resulting in a porotic cortex (Parfitt et al., 1983).

Mechanisms of 'uncoupling'

The uncoupling of bone resorption and formation can result in loss of bone mass and strength in a number of different ways. Perhaps the simplest way is by an increase in the number of active BMUs, or 'activation frequency.' As a result of the increase in activation frequency, the amount of bone at each remodeling site decreases and this decrease results in lower bone mass. Moreover, multiple resorption sites both on trabecular surfaces and in the cortex may result in structural weakening of the bone. Further, there may also be an increase in the depth of resorption by more active osteoclasts or, more importantly, resorption that results in complete loss of trabecular architecture may occur. If the template on which the osteoblast initiates formation is lost, the resorbed bone cannot be replaced. Loss of connectivity in trabecular structures also results in an impairment of osteoblast formation by reducing the ability of osteoblasts to 'detect' mechanical forces, a requirement for initiating osteoblastic bone formation (Frost, 1997; Dempster, 1992). While the above changes result in uncoupling which could be independent of any defect in osteoblast function, the magnitude of the decrease in mean wall thickness with age suggests that osteoblast renewal remains a major factor in age-related bone loss (Jilka et al, 1996).

The pathogenesis of osteoporosis

Reduction of bone mass and strength sufficient to cause fractures that occur with minimal trauma can develop either because the skeleton never forms adequately (optimal peak bone mass is not achieved), or because bone is removed too rapidly (accelerated bone resorption), or because formation fails to keep pace with accelerated resorption. Probably all three processes are involved in the clinical expression of osteoporosis. The categorization of osteoporosis into type I (postmenopausal) or type II (senile) forms has been proposed on the basis of differences in the relative frequency of vertebral and hip fractures and on the relative importance of estrogen deficiency and secondary hyperparathyroidism. In fact, these two phenomena are interrelated, and there is considerable overlap between so-called type I and type II (Riggs et al., 1998). Changes in sex hormones and other systemic hormones, as well as local factors, probably all contribute to pathogenesis. In this chapter, we will summarize the most important actions and interactions of these factors and indicate the changes in the production or action of these factors that may occur with aging

Sex hormones

The accelerated rate of bone loss that occurs at menopause is largely due to estrogen deficiency. Decreased estrogen levels result in increased bone resorption and may also contribute to impaired formation, although we are still not sure how estrogen works. In rodent models, estrogen deficiency is associated with an increase in the activity of local cytokines, possibly in marrow as well as in bone cells.

Interleukin 1 (IL-1), tumor necrosis factor alpha 2 (TNFα 2), and interleukin 6 (IL-6) have all been implicated (Kimble et al., 1995, 1997; Manolagas & Jilka, 1995). Cytokine activity may be increased not only by greater production of cytokines, but also by changes in receptors or antagonists (Lorenzo et al., 1998). In rodents, the increased cytokine production associated with estrogen deficiency may stimulate bone resorption both directly and indirectly by increasing the local production of prostaglandins (Kawaguchi et al., 1995). Estrogen deficiency may result in decreased production of transforming growth factor beta (TGF-β), which can both inhibit bone resorption and stimulate bone formation. Estrogen treatment can shorten the lifespan of osteoclasts in vitro by increasing apoptosis, an event that may be mediated by an increase in TGF-β (Hughes et al., 1996). Finally, estrogen may affect other growth factors, including the growth hormone/insulin-like growth factor I (GH/IGF-I) system (Canalis, 1996), and may also impair calcium absorption in the intestine, resulting in increased levels of PTH, a potent stimulator of bone resorption (Prestwood & Kenny, 1998).

While estrogen deficiency plays a central role in postmenopausal osteoporosis, it may also be important in bone loss in men (Khosla et al., 1998). Men with aromatase deficiency who are unable to form estrogen from testosterone, as well as a single reported case of a man with a deficient estrogen receptor, showed increased bone turnover and low bone mass (Carani et al., 1997; Smith et al., 1995). Men with aromatase deficiency have been successfully treated with estrogen therapy (Bilezikian et al., 1998). Moreover, men with osteoporosis show lower estrogen levels than age-matched controls; and the increase in bone mass in response to testosterone administration correlates better with the change in estrogen levels than with changes in testosterone levels (Anderson et al., 1997; Vega et al., 1998). Testosterone may also have a direct effect on the skeleton, since receptors are present on osteoblasts (Abu et al., 1997). In postmenopausal women, testosterone has been shown to have an anabolic effect on bone (Raisz et al., 1996). Moreover, women with vertebral fractures were found to have lower testosterone and androstenedione levels than age-matched controls, but similar estradiol and estrone levels (Longcope et al., 1984).

Other hormones regulating bone turnover

There is an age-related decrease in the pulsatile excretion of growth hormone and in the circulating levels of IGF-I and IGF binding protein 3 (IGFBP3). Excessive thyroid hormone can cause bone loss, resulting from increased turnover. Glucocorticoid excess can result in both impaired bone formation and increased bone resorption. The latter probably occurs largely by indirect mechanisms (Prestwood & Kenny, 1998).

Local factors in osteoporosis

Examining the potential role of local factors in the pathogenesis of menopausal and age-related bone loss is important for several reasons. The predominance of trabecular over cortical bone loss in patients with vertebral osteoporosis suggests an influence of local factors. Further, many studies have been unable to detect a difference in the levels of systemic hormones between osteoporotic patients and age- and sex-matched controls, suggesting that other factors are involved. However, the analysis of local factors in humans is extremely difficult because: (i) the number of local factors is large; (ii) the differences in cytokine activity could be due to changes in receptors or inhibitors as well as agonists; and (iii) it is difficult to quantitate these factors in human skeletal tissue.

Because of these difficulties, much of the research on local factors has been conducted using rodent models rather than studying human disease. However, rodent models also present difficulties, since there are marked differences in the structure, metabolic activity and response to hormones in different rodent strains, not unlike the differences seen in humans. Ultimately, these differences may be advantageous if it becomes possible to attribute some of the differences among strains to differences in local factors (Beamer et al., 1996; Rosen et al., 1997; Dimai et al., 1998). A full description of the local factors that have been identified as regulators of bone remodeling is beyond the scope of this chapter. Instead, we will try to summarize the data that suggest a role for these factors in menopausal and age-related bone loss.

Cytokines

IL-1, TNFα and IL-6 have all been implicated as pathogenetic factors in the bone loss that follows ovariectomy. In addition, IL-6 levels increase with age. IL-1 and TNFα are the most potent bone resorbers among the cytokines, but IL-6, in the presence of its soluble receptor, can enhance resorptive responses to other cytokines and increase prostaglandin production in bone. There is evidence for regulation of these factors by sex hormones (Horowitz, 1993; Mundy et al., 1996).

Other cytokines have been less well studied. IL-11 and IL-7 have been shown to stimulate bone resorption; IL-7 may act indirectly by stimulating B-cell production. IL-4 and IL-13 can inhibit resorption and decrease prostaglandin synthesis in bone. IL-18 inhibits bone resorption, probably by increasing the production of GM-CSF and diverting osteoclast precursors towards the macrophage pathway. Conversely, M-CSF increases osteoclastogenesis. However, there is, as yet, little evidence for a role for these factors in estrogen deficiency or aging (Canalis, 1996).

Cytokines, in particular IL-1 and TNFα, can also affect bone formation. In ovariectomized rats, treatment with IL-1 receptor antagonist or TNF binding protein not only prevents bone loss, but increases periosteal bone formation (Kimble et al., 1995). Knockout and over-expression animals have been used to test the cytokine hypothesis. Knockout of IL-6 gene was associated with a lack of bone loss after ovariectomy, but this may be related to the strain employed (Poli et al., 1994). Over-expression of TNFBP prevents ovariectomy bone loss, as does knockout of the IL-1 receptor type I gene (Ammann et al., 1997; Lorenzo et al., 1998). These results are most consistent with the involvement of a number of local cytokines, acting in concert, to produce increased bone resorption and decreased formation after ovariectomy.

Prostaglandins

Prostaglandins are complex multifunctional regulators of bone metabolism, but the major effect of prostaglandin E_2 is to stimulate both bone resorption and bone formation. Prostaglandins may play a role in ovariectomy-induced bone loss. Marrow supernatants from ovariectomized animals stimulate bone resorption in cultured mouse calvariae by a prostaglandin-dependent mechanism associated with an increase in the inducible cyclo-oxygenase, COX-2, which is the major regulator of prostaglandin synthesis in bone cells (Kawaguchi et al., 1995). Prostaglandins have also been implicated in the increase in bone resorption associated with immobilization.

Growth factors

Transforming growth factor beta (TGFI-β) and insulin-like growth factor I (IGF-I) are both produced by bone cells and stored in bone matrix. TGF-β is stored in an inactive form associated with a binding protein and is released during bone resorption; it can inhibit bone resorption as well as stimulate bone formation (Canalis et al., 1996). In osteoclast cultures, estrogen or tamoxifen increases apoptosis by a TGF-β-mediated mechanism (Hughes et al., 1996). Finally, reduced TGF-β concentrations were found in bone extracts from ovariectomized rats (Canalis, 1996).

The age-related decrease in growth hormone secretion could also be accompanied by an age-related decrease in local IGF-I production in the skeleton. In addition, changes in the IGF binding proteins have been described in osteoporotic patients and with aging. Other growth factors which may be important in the pathogenesis of osteoporosis include platelet-derived growth factor and fibroblast growth factor, both of which can act on bone and can be produced either by bone cells or adjacent hemotopoietic cells (Canalis, 1996).

Conclusion

Although we know a great deal about the regulation of bone remodeling, the specific changes that are responsible for the uncoupling of bone resorption and formation, and the resultant bone loss with menopause and aging have not been identified. It seems likely that many factors are acting in concert. Moreover, differences in hormonal response or local factor activity could be due to changes in receptors or signal transduction pathways, as well as to changes in the primary agonist. If we are to understand bone loss, new approaches will be needed. Measurements of local factors in bone by reverse transcriptase–polymerase chain reaction methodology, *in situ* hybridization, immunoassay and immunocyto- chemistry could help us to identify changes in specific factors. Another useful approach will be to identify additional genetic determinants of osteoporosis. Thus far, the study of candidate genes has been relatively disappointing, but genetic screening in animals may provide important clues to the relevant factors in humans.

REFERENCES

Abu, E. O., Horner, A., Kusec, V., Triffit, J. T., & Compston, J. E. (1997). The localization of andro- gen receptors in human bone. *J. Clin. Endocrinol. Metab.*, **82**(10), 3493–7.

Amano, H., Yamada, S., & Felix, R. (1998). Colony-stimulating factor-1 stimulates the fusion process in osteoclasts. *J. Bone Miner., Res.* **13**(5), 846–53.

Ammann, P., Rizzoli, R., Bonjour, J. P., Bourrin, S., Meyer, J. M., Vassalli, P., & Garcia, I. (1997). Transgenic mice expressing soluble tumor necrosis factor-receptor are protected against bone loss caused by estrogen deficiency. *J. Clin. Invest.*, **99**(7), 1699–703.

Anderson, F. H., Francis, R. M., Peaston, R. T., & Wastell, H. J. (1997). Androgen supplementa- tion in eugonadal men with osteoporosis: effects of six months' treatment on markers of bone formation and resorption. *J. Bone Miner. Res.*, **12**(3), 472–8.

Baron, R., Vignery, A., & Tran Van, P. (1980). The significance of lacunar erosion without osteo- clastis: studies on the reversal phase of the remodeling sequence. *Metab. Bone Dis. Relat. Res.*, **2S**, 35–40.

Beamer, W. G., Donahue, L. R., Rosen, C. J., & Baylink, D. J. (1996). Genetic variability in adult bone density among inbred strains of mice. *Bone*, **18**(5), 397–403.

Bilezikian, J. P., Morishima, A., Bell, J., & Grumbach, M. M. (1998). Increased bone mass as a result of estrogen therapy in a man with aromatase deficiency. *N. Engl. J. Med.*, **39**(9), 599–603.

Biskobing, D. M., Fan, X., & Rubin, J. (1995). Characterization of MCSF-induced proliferation and subsequent osteoclast formation in murine marrow culture. *J. Bone Miner. Res.*, **10**, 1025–32.

Canalis, E. (1996). Skeletal growth factors. In *Osteoporosis*, ed. R. Marcus, D. Feldman & J. Kelsey, pp. 261–79. San Diego, CA: Academic Press.

Canalis, E., McCarthy, T., & Centrella, M. (1988). Growth factors and the regulation of bone remodeling. *J. Clin. Invest.*, **81**, 277–81.

Carani, C., Qin, K., Simoni, M., Faustini-Fustini, M., Serpente, S., Boyd, J., Korach, K. S., & Simpson, E. R. (1997). Effect of testosterone and estradiol in a man with aromatase deficiency. *N. Eng. J. Med.*, **337**, 91–5.

Dempster, D. W. (1992). Bone remodeling. In *Disorders of Bone and Mineral Metabolism*, ed. F. L. Coe & M. J. Favus, pp. 355–80.

Dimai, H. P., Linkhart, T. A., Linkhart, S. G., Donahue, L. R., Beamer, W. G., Rosen, C. J., Farley, J. R., & Baylink, D. J. (1998). Alkaline phosphatase levels and osteoprogenitor cell numbers suggest bone formation may contribute to peak bone density differences between two inbred strains of mice. *Bone*, **22**(3), 211–16.

Frost, H. M. (1997). On our age-related bone loss: insights from a new paradigm. *J. Bone Miner. Res.*, **12**(10), 1539–46.

Horowitz, M. C. (1993). Cytokines and estrogen in bone: anti-osteoporotic effects. *Science*, **260**(5108), 626–7.

Hughes, D. E., Dai, A., Tiffee, J. C., Li, H. H., Mundy, G. R., & Boyce, B. F. (1996). Estrogen promotes apoptosis of murine osteoclasts mediated by TGF-beta. *Nat. Med.*, **2**(10), 1132–6.

Jilka, R. L., Weinstein, R. S., Takahashi, K., Parfitt, A. M., & Manolagas, S. G. (1996). Linkage of decreased bone mass with impaired osteoblastogenesis in a model of accelerated senescence. *J. Clin. Invest.*, **97**(7), 1732–40.

Kawaguchi, H., Pilbeam, C. C., Vargas, S. J., Morse, E. E., Lorenzo, J. A., & Raisz, L. G., (1995). Ovariectomy enhances and estrogen replacement inhibits the activity of bone marrow factors that stimulate prostaglandin production in cultured mouse calvariae. *J. Clin. Invest.*, **96**(1), 539–48.

Khosla, S., Melton, L. J., Atkinson, E. J., O'Fallon, W. M., Klee, G. G., & Riggs, B. L. (1998). Relationship of serum sex steroid levels and bone turnover markers with bone mineral density in men and women: a key role for bioavailable estrogen. *J. Clin. Endocrinol. Metab.*, **83**(7), 2266–74.

Kimble, R. B., Bain, S., & Pacifici, R. (1997). The functional block of TNF but not of IL-6 prevents bone loss in ovariectomized mice. *J. Bone Miner. Res.*, **12**(6), 935–41.

Kimble, R. B., Matayoshi, A. B., Vannice, J. L., Kung, V. T., Williams, C., & Pacifici, R. (1995). Simultaneous block of interleukin-1 and tumor necrosis factor is required to completely prevent bone loss in the early postovariectomy period. *Endocrinology*, **136**(7), 3054–61.

Longcope, C., Baker, R. S., Hui, S. L. & Johnson, C. C. Jr (1984). Androgen and estrogen dynamics in women with vertebral crush factors. *Maturitas*, **6**, 309–18.

Lorenzo, J., Naprta, A., Rao, Y., Alander, C., Glaccum, M., Wildmer, M., Gronowicz, G., Kalinowski, J., & Pilbeam, C. C. (1998). Mice lacking type I interleukin-1 receptor do not lose bone mass after ovariectomy. *Endocrinology*, **139**, 3022–5.

Manolagas, S. C. & Jilka, R. L. (1995). Bone Marrow, cytokines, and bone modeling. Emerging insights into the pathophysiology of osteoporosis. *N. Engl. J. Med.*, **332**, 305–11.

Matsuzaki, K., Udagawa, N., Takahashi, K., Yamaguchi, K., Yasuda, H., Shima, N., Morinaga, T., Toyama, Y., Yabe, Y., Higashio, K., & Suda, T. (1998). Osteoclast differentiation factor (ODF) induces osteoclast-like cell formation in human peripheral blood mononuclear cell cultures. *Biochem. Biophys. Res. Commun.*, **246**, 199–204.

Mundy, G. R., Boyce, B. F., Yoneda, T., Bonewald, L. F., & Roodman, G. D. (1996). Cytokines and bone remodeling. In *Osteoporosis*, ed. R. Marcus, D. Feldman & J. Kelsey, pp. 301–13. San Diego, CA: Academic Press Inc.

Parfitt, A. M., Matthews, C. H. E., Villaneuva, A. R., Kleerekoper, M., Frame, R., & Rao, D. S. (1983). Relationships between surface, volume, and thickness of iliac trabecular bone in aging and in osteoporosis: implications for the microanatomic and cellular mechanisms of bone. *J. Clin. Invest.*, **72**, 1396–409.

Poli, V., Balena, R., Fattori, E., Markatos, A., Yamamoto, M., Tanaka, H., Ciliberto, G., Rodan, G. A., & Constantini, F. (1994). Interleukin-6 deficient mice are protected from bone loss caused by estrogen depletion. *EMBO J.*, **13**(5), 1189–96.

Prestwood, K. M. & Kenny, A. M. (1998). Osteoporosis: pathogenesis, diagnosis and treatment in older adults. In *Clinics in Geriatric Medicine: Musculoskeletal and Connective Tissue Disorders*, ed. R. F. Loeser, Jr., vol. 14(3), pp. 577–99. Philadelphia: W. B. Saunders Co.

Raisz, L. G., Wiita, B., Artis, A., Bowen, A., Schwartz, S., Trahiotis, M., Shoukri, K., & Smith, J. (1996). Comparison of the effects of estrogen alone and estrogen plus androgen on biochemical markers of bone formation and resorption in post menopausal women. *J. Clin. Endocrinol. Metab.*, **81**(1), 37–43.

Riggs, B. L., Khosla, S., & Melton, L. J. (1998). A unitary model for involutional osteoporosis: estrogen deficiency causes both Type I and Type II osteoporosis in postmenopausal women and contributes to bone loss in aging men. *J. Bone Miner. Res.*, **13**(5), 763–73.

Rosen, C. J., Dimai, H. P., Vereault, D., Donahue, L. R., Beamer, W. G., Farley, J. Linkhart, S., Linkhart, T., Mohan, S., & Baylink, D. J. (1997). Circulating and skeletal insulin-like growth factor-I (IGF-I) concentrations in two inbred strains of mice with different bone mineral densities. *Bone*, **21**(3), 217–23.

Simonet, W. S., Lacey, D. L., Dunstan, C. R., Kelley, M., Chang, M.S., Luthy, R., Nguyen, H. Q., Wooden, S., Bennett, L., Boone, T., Shimamoto, G., DeRose, M., Elliott, R., Colombero, A., Tan, H. L., Trail, G., Sullivan, J., Davy, E., Bucay, N., Renshaw-Gegg, L., Hughes, T. M., Hill, D., Pattison, W., Campbell, P., Boyle, W. J. et al (1997). Osteoprotegerin: a novel secreted protein involved in the regulation of bone density. *Cell*, **89**, 309–19.

Smith, E.P., Boyd, J., Frank, G. R., Takahashi, H., Cohen, R. M., Specker, B., Williams, T. C., Lubahn, D. B., & Korach, K. S. (1995). Estrogen resistance caused by a mutation in the estrogen-receptor gene in a man. *N. Engl. J. Med.*, **332**(2), 131.

Tsukii, K., Shima, N., & Mochizuki, S. (1998). Osteoclast differentiation factor mediates an essential signal for bone resorption induced by 1 alpha, 25-dihydroxyvitamin D3, prostaglandin E2 or parathyroid hormone in the microenvironment of bone. *Biochem. Biophys. Res. Commun.*, **246**, 337–41.

Vega, E., Ghiringhelli, G., Mautalen, C., Rey, Valzacchi, G., Scaglia, H., & Zylberstein, C. (1998). Bone mineral density and bone size in men with primary osteoporosis and vertebral fractures. *Calcif. Tissue Int.*, **62**(5), 465–9.

Yao, G. Q., Sun, B. H., Hammond, E. E., Spencer, E. N., Horowitz, M. C., Insogna, K. L., &

Weir, E. C. (1998). The cell-surface form of colony-stimulating factor-I is regulated by osteotropic agents and supports formation of multinucleated osteoclast-like cells. *J. Biol. Chem.*, **273**, 4119–28.

Yasuda, H., Shima, N., Nakagawa, K., Yamaguchi, K., Kinosaki, M., Mochizuki, S., Tomoyasu, A., Yano, K., Goto, M., Murakami, A., Tsuda, E., Morinaga, T., Higashio, K., Udagawa, N., Takahashi, N., & Suda, T. (1998). Osteoclast differentiation factor is a ligand for osteoprotegerin/osteoclastogenesis-inhibitory factor and is identical to TRANCE/RANKL. *Proc. Natl Acad. Sci., USA*, **95**, 3597–602.

15

The role of parathyroid hormone and hyperparathyroidism in osteoporosis

Pierre D'Amour

Introduction

Indirect evidence for a permissive role of parathyroid hormone in osteoporosis

Parathyroid hormone (PTH) is essential to maintain normal calcium homeostasis (Chapter 6), bone turnover (Chapter 14) and vitamin D metabolism (cf. Chapter 7) under physiological conditions. It also appears as a significant permissive factor in most pathological conditions associated with osteoporosis. This is best illustrated by the fact that patients who have developed hypoparathyroidism following thyroid or parathyroid surgery have increased bone density at the radius, lumbar spine and hip compared to similar surgical patients without hypoparathyroidism (Abugassa et al., 1993; Fujiyama et al., 1995; Seeman et al., 1982). Hypoparathyroidism also prevents rapid bone loss associated with menopause (Fujiyama et al., 1995) and bone loss in patients with risk factors for osteoporosis (Touliatos et al., 1995). Furthermore, parathyroidectomy can minimize bone loss induced by a low calcium diet (Burkhart & Jowsey, 1967) or immobilization (Jowsey & Raisz, 1968) in experimental animals. This chapter will thus review how PTH and factors affecting PTH concentration and/or biological effects are involved in the development of primary and secondary osteoporosis.

Role of parathyroid hormone in osteoporosis

Role of PTH in primary osteoporosis

Two main factors have been implicated in the genesis of primary osteoporosis, the estrogen deficiency of menopause (type I osteoporosis) and a multifactorial secondary hyperparathyroidism associated with aging (type II osteoporosis).

Role of menopause in type I osteoporosis

Menopause is considered a central phenomenon in the development of type I osteoporosis because the associated rapid bone loss can greatly enhance fracture risk in susceptible women. Type I osteoporosis usually develops within 15 years of

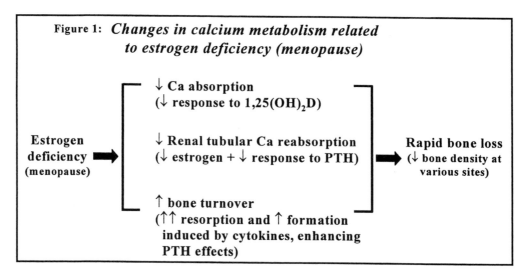

Figure 1: *Changes in calcium metabolism related to estrogen deficiency (menopause)*

Estrogen deficiency (menopause) ➡

- ↓ Ca absorption
  (↓ response to 1,25(OH)₂D)

- ↓ Renal tubular Ca reabsorption
  (↓ estrogen + ↓ response to PTH)

- ↑ bone turnover
  (↑↑ resorption and ↑ formation
  induced by cytokines, enhancing
  PTH effects)

➡ Rapid bone loss
(↓ bone density at
various sites)

Fig. 15.1   Changes in calcium metabolism related to estrogen deficiency (menopause).

menopause and affects predominantly cancellous bone (thoracic and lumbar vertebrae). Changes in phosphocalcic metabolism (Prince, 1994) and bone turnover (Turner et al., 1994) related to estrogen deficiency are central to this rapid bone loss. Estrogen deficiency induces a decrease in the intestinal absorption of calcium and reduces the biological activity of 1,25(OH)₂D (Gennari et al., 1990; Heaney et al., 1989). Calcium intake has to be increased from 1000 to 1500 mg/day to achieve a neutral balance (Heaney et al., 1978). It also enhances renal calcium excretion (Nordin et al., 1991) and affects the ability of PTH to reduce calciuria (McKane et al., 1995). Finally, it increases bone turnover with a higher level of bone resorption than bone formation (Garnero et al., 1996), leading to a reduced bone mass (Turner et al., 1994). Cytokines like IL-1, IL-6 and TNF, induced by estrogen deficiency, play a central role in inducing these changes in bone turnover (Pacifici, 1998). Calcium remains unchanged or is slightly increased and PTH remains unchanged or is slightly decreased, even if calcium absorption is reduced and renal calcium excretion is increased because more calcium is released from bone (Prince, 1994). Enhanced biological effectiveness of unchanged PTH levels induced by estrogen deficiency may be important for this last effect (Cosman et al., 1993). This may be particularly true at cancellous or trabecular bone sites, which are predominantly affected in type I osteoporosis. A schematic illustration of these events is provided in Fig. 15.1.

All these changes are reversed or prevented by estrogen-replacement therapy (Heaney et al., 1978, 1989; Gennari et al., 1990; Nordin et al., 1991; Cosman et al., 1993; McKane et al., 1995; Garnero et al., 1996), This includes preservation of bone mineral density at various sites, and a 50% decrease in the fracture rate with long-term therapy (Turner et al., 1994). Elimination of IL-1, IL-6 and/or TNF biological effects via inhibitors or in transgenic mice prevents bone loss induced by ovariectomy in mice (Pacifici, 1998). Similarly, hypoparathyroidism attenuates the rapid bone loss associated with menopause (Fujiyama et al., 1995), illustrating the permissive role of PTH.

Aging, secondary hyperparathyroidism and type II osteoporosis

Higher PTH concentrations and biological effects are observed in elderly people (Insogna et al., 1981; Forero et al., 1987, Young et al., 1987). They have been related to the increased bone turnover, decreased bone mineral density at various sites and type II osteoporosis observed in these people (Ledger et al., 1995; Garnero et al., 1996; Khosla et al., 1997, 1998). Type II osteoporosis is the clinical end point of age-related bone loss and is usually seen after age 70. It affects females more often than males. Secondary hyperparathyroidism is central to type II osteoporosis, and several factors have been implicated in this secondary hyperparathyroidism including estrogen deficiency, a decreasing renal function and calcium and vitamin D deficiencies.

Changes in phosphocalcic metabolism and in bone turnover induced by estrogen deficiency at menopause are still present in elderly women (Khosla et al., 1997) and possibly also in men, where circulating levels of bioactive testosterone and bioactive estrogen are also reduced (Khosla et al., 1998). These hormonal changes have been associated in both sexes with decreased bone density at various sites (Khosla et al., 1998). The ability of bone resorption to compensate for decreased intestinal calcium absorption and increased urinary calcium excretion may be partially impaired in elderly people, leading to higher circulating PTH levels. This is supported by the fact that estrogen-replacement therapy in older women not only decreases biochemical markers of bone turnover but also PTH levels (Khosla et al., 1998; Riggs et al., 1998).

Several studies have also related the higher PTH levels observed in older subjects to a decreased renal function (Freaney et al., 1993; Marcus et al., 1984; Orwoll & Meier, 1986; Tsai et al., 1984). This is particularly true for carboxyl-terminal PTH, which is cleared predominantly by the kidney (Freaney et al., 1993; Orwoll and Meier, 1986; Tsai et al., 1984) but also for intact-PTH (Marcus et al., 1984). The $1,25(OH)_2D$ and calcemic responses to exogenous hPTH(1–34) decrease with the GFR (Ritz et al., 1991; Tsai et al., 1984), and higher PTH levels are required to maintain normal levels of calcium, phosphate and $1,25(OH)_2D$. This is probably detrimental to bone, and creatinine clearance appears to be an important determinant of bone mineral density in older subjects (Orwoll & Meier, 1986; Yendt et al., 1991).

Several factors also contribute to decreased intestinal calcium absorption in

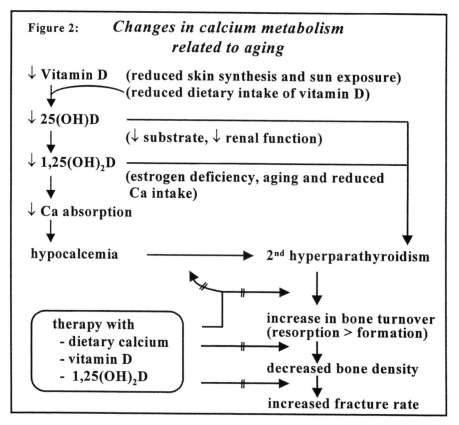

Fig. 15.2   Changes in calcium metabolism related to aging.

elderly people besides estrogen deficiency (Chapuy & Meunier, 1997; Eastell & Riggs, 1997). Vitamin D and calcium intake are below recommended average in many elderly persons (Carroll et al., 1983; McKenna, 1992). Aging of the skin and reduced sun exposure may decrease the endogenous production of vitamin D (MacLaughlin & Holick, 1985; Webb et al., 1990). All this leads to lower circulating levels of 25(OH)D and often 1,25(OH)$_2$D in elderly subjects (Chapuy & Meunier, 1997; Eastell & Riggs, 1997). In the latter case, decreasing renal function is also a contributory factor (Tsai et al., 1984; Ritz et al., 1991). This results in a decrease in intestinal calcium absorption which is enhanced by the direct effect of aging on the absorption process (Ebeling et al., 1992). Lower 25(OH)D circulating levels appear a major determinant of PTH level, bone resorption and formation marker levels and of measured bone mineral density at various sites in the elderly (Chapuy & Meunier, 1997; Eastell & Riggs, 1997).

Fig. 15.2 illustrates factors involved in the secondary hyperparathyroidism of aging. Many therapeutic trials to correct calcium, vitamin D and/or 1,25(OH)$_2$D deficiencies have been conducted in the elderly to observe the influence on circulating PTH level, bone mineral density measurements and fracture rate. Usually, but not always, these measures have led to an improved vitamin D status, decreased circulating PTH level, decreased level of bone resorption markers, improved bone mineral density at various sites and a decreased fracture rate (Chapuy & Meunier, 1997; Eastell & Riggs, 1997).

Role of PTH in secondary osteoporosis

The role of parathyroid hormone in secondary osteoporosis can be related to a primary increase in PTH levels observed in primary hyperparathyroidism or to a secondary increase in PTH levels observed with gastrointestinal or kidney diseases in relation to calcium and/or vitamin D deficiencies. These situations will be analyzed next.

Primary hyperparathyroidism (PHP)

The effects of PHP on bone are controversial and the relationship between PHP, osteoporosis and an increased fracture rate remains uncertain (Rao et al., 1988; Wilson et al., 1988). None the less, this topic is of great clinical importance, since the decision-making process in asymptomatic PHP is often influenced by bone mineral density measurements.

Primary hyperparathyroidism is a common disease, occurring predominantly in women over 50 (Heath, 1991) in the first decade after menopause. This means that estrogen deficiency is very often superimposed on a high circulating level of PTH in these patients. This complicates the analysis of their bone data. In these patients, 1,25(OH)$_2$D synthesis is enhanced by high PTH levels and calcium absorption is often increased. Calciuria is also greater, even if tubular calcium reabsorption is increased by high PTH levels because of the increased filtered load of calcium. Finally, bone turnover is also enhanced. All this leads to hypercalcemia, the biochemical hallmark of the disease (Heath, 1991).

Under exceptional circumstances, patients can present with an extreme form of bone disease called osteitis fibrosa cystica (Heath, 1996). Diffuse or focal bone pain and pathological fracture through an osteoclastoma ('brown tumor') are present most of the time. Subperiosteal resorption of the distal phalanges is present on high resolution radiographs of the hands. Osteolytic lesions of bone may be mistaken for metastasis (Joyce et al., 1994). Bone density at various sites would be expected to be low, but this is not always the case (Heath III, 1996). PTH values in these patients are very high as is the calcium concentration. 1,25(OH)$_2$D concentration is often suppressed even though PTH is elevated, because calcium is very high

(Brossard et al., 1993). This probably contributes to the severity of the bone disease. Correction of the calcemia with a biphosphonate in one patient was associated with an important increase in 1,25(OH)$_2$D levels, a decrease of PTH values, even though the calcemia had decreased, and evidence of bone healing prior to surgery of the parathyroid lesion (Brossard et al., 1993). Great gains in bone mineral density at various sites over a relatively short time period have been observed after surgery of the parathyroid lesion in some of these patients (Brossard et al., 1993).

In most patients with primary hyperparathyroidism, a less severe form of bone disease is present. Bone density is decreased in the total skeleton and at various sites (Silverberg et al., 1995a). Many publications have suggested that cortical sites (radius and to a lesser extend the hip) are more often affected than trabecular ones (vertebrae) (Parisien et al., 1990, 1992; Silverberg et al., 1995a). Bone biopsies of the iliac crest have shown reduced cortical thickness, preserved or even increased trabecular bone volume and connectivity and increased bone turnover (Parisien et al., 1990, 1992). Why patients with primary hyperparathyroidism appear to have a certain degree of preservation of cancellous or trabecular bone over cortical bone remains uncertain. The same situation is often prevalent in secondary hyperparathyroidism. PTH can be anabolic for bone particularly when it is injected intermittently rather than continuously, a situation different from PHP (Marcus, 1994). Other factors, such as patient's calcium and vitamin status and estrogen deficiency, may be important determinants of bone response to PTH. This is suggested by the fact that patients with primary hyperparathyroidism and the lowest calcium absorption also had the lowest bone mineral density at various sites (Peacock et al., 1984).

The decrease in bone mineral density is usually modest in primary hyperparathyroidism, being less than 10%. Even though an increased fracture rate has been found in some patients with PHP (Peacock et al., 1984), recent studies do not suggest that this is always the case (Melton et al., 1992; Silverberg et al., 1995a; Wilson et al., 1988). Surgical correction of the PHP in these patients can result in a 10 to 15% increase in lumbar spine and femoral neck bone mineral density over 4 years (Silverberg et al., 1995b). Estrogen therapy in postmenopausal women with asymptomatic primary hyperparathyroidism also appears to have the same beneficial effects on bone mineral density at various sites than as observed in women without primary hyperparathyroidism even if their measured values remain lower than those of normal women on estrogen therapy (McDermott et al., 1994). Estrogen therapy causes a small decrease in calcium concentration, reduces the concentration of bone resorption markers and does not change PTH levels in women with PHP. This has been interpreted as further proof of the modulatory effect of estrogen on PTH biological effects.

Table 15.1. Gastrointestinal disorders associated with acquired bone disease

Postgastrectomy
Celiac disease
Pancreatic disease
Inflammatory bowel disease
  • Crohn's disease
  • Ulcerative colitis
Jejunoileal bypass
Total parenteral nutrition
Liver conditions
  • Biliary cirrhosis
  • Alcoholic liver disease
  • Liver transplantation
  • Intake of enzyme inductors

Secondary hyperparathyroidism (SHP)

Gastrointestinal diseases

Although it has been found that osteomalacia, or unmineralized bone, is occasionally associated with various gastrointestinal diseases, it is only recently that the incidence of osteoporosis in the same medical conditions has been appreciated. Table 15.1 provides a list of gastrointestinal and hepatic conditions associated with osteoporosis. A detailed analysis of each cause is beyond the scope of this chapter, and is provided in two recent reviews (Bikle, 1996; Mawer & Davies, 1997). The physiopathology of bone disease in these situations is sufficiently similar for me to provide an overall approach, since SHP is often but not invariably present. With or without SHP other nutritional deficiencies may also prove important for the development of osteoporosis (Parfitt, 1983).

Experimentally, it is possible to create secondary hyperparathyroidism in dogs by feeding them a diet deficient in calcium and vitamin D (Cloutier et al., 1992), a situation similar to the one created by most gastrointestinal diseases where calcium and/or vitamin D absorption is impaired by lack of acidity, steatorrhea, destroyed or abnormal gut cells, bypass of critical regions of the gut, lack of bile salts, malnutrition, etc. (Bikle, 1996; Mawer & Davies, 1997). This is further complicated by the use of corticosteroids in some of these conditions, with their adverse effect on calcium absorption and bone formation (Lukert, 1996). Calcium does not need to decrease for PTH to initially increase in this model, and the initial decrease in 25(OH)D, even if 1,25(OH)$_2$D remains normal or even increases, explains rising PTH levels (Cloutier et al., 1992). Eventually, calcium concentration will also decrease when 1,25(OH)$_2$D levels start to decrease in relation to the extensive 25(OH)D deficit (Cloutier et al., 1992). This situation probably prevails in most gastrointestinal and liver diseases, and the initial deficit in 25(OH)D, accelerated by a faster turnover in presence of secondary hyperparathyroidism (Clemens et al., 1987), is probably the initial critical step. At this stage, increased bone turnover which may lead to osteoporosis is present. Later on, hypocalcemia is often seen and will contribute with the decreasing 1,25(OH)$_2$D levels to the progression of secondary hyperparathyroidism (Cloutier et al., 1992). Very low levels of 25(OH)D and calcium will impair bone mineralization, leading to osteomalacia, a more severe and advanced form of bone disease.

Appropriate therapy of the primary gastrointestinal disorder with or without the addition of vitamin D and calcium supplements will generally reverse the secondary hyperparathyroidism and improve bone mass density measurements after a while (Bikle 1996; Mawer & Davies, 1997). Correction of the secondary hyperparathyroidism may not be complete, due to the increased mass of parathyroid tissue (Cloutier et al., 1994). There is evidence in dogs (Cloutier et al., 1994) and in man (D'Amour et al., 1996) that normal but higher than original intact PTH levels will be achieved at the expense of very high carboxyl-terminal PTH levels. Is this detrimental to bone and the treatment of osteoporosis? The role of carboxyl-terminal receptors to PTH on bone cells (Murray et al., 1994) and of increased PTH carboxylterminal fragment levels on the bone response to any osteoporotic treatment remains an unexplored issue.

Renal failure

Renal failure is associated with secondary hyperparathyroidism, and parathyroid hormone has always been an important determinant of bone disease associated with renal insufficiency (renal osteodystrophy). Bone biopsy has been the preferred tool to evaluate uremic bone disease (Coburn & Salusky, 1994) and less information is available on bone mineral density at various sites in the same conditions. Osteoporosis has been an occasional problem in advanced renal failure, but a more systematic one following renal transplantation (Julian et al., 1991).

In early and moderate renal failure (GFR > 30 ml/1.73 m^2 min^{-1}), peripheral resistance to PTH (Bover et al., 1994; Massry et al., 1973), possibly of parathyroid gland origin (Rodriguez et al., 1991) and lower but still normal levels of 1,25(OH)$_2$D (St John et al., 1992) are responsible for the secondary hyperparathyroidism. Higher PTH levels are required to maintain normal levels of calcium, phosphate and 1,25(OH)$_2$D. A lower bone mineral density at various sites may be present and GFR appears as an important determinant of bone mass in early and moderate renal failure (Orwoll & Meier, 1986; Yendt et al., 1991). In advanced renal failure (GFR < 30 ml/1.73 m^2 min^{-1}) very low levels of 1,25(OH)$_2$D, high levels of serum phosphate and low levels of calcium become additional factors in increasing the parathyroid function and parathyroid gland mass (Martin & Slatopolsky, 1994). Although it is difficult to predict which patient will develop which type of bone disease, PTH levels remain helpful in that regard (Coburn & Salusky, 1994).

Osteitis fibrosa cystica is generally seen in patients with the highest PTH values. Their bone disease is similar to the one described for primary hyperparathyroidism. On bone biopsy, both bone formation and bone resorption parameters are greatly increased and peritrabecular fibrosis is important (Coburn & Salusky, 1994; Martin & Slatopolsky, 1994). Hypercalcemic patients, who have, in fact, developed primary hyperparathyroidism on hyperplastic glands (tertiary hyperparathyroidism), are best treated by surgical parathyroidectomy. Hypocalcemic patients may be treated with oral or IV $1\alpha(OH)D$ or $1,25(OH)_2D$, while controlling their serum phosphate with diet and calcium carbonate. This may lower PTH levels by 50% or more and improve the bone disease with at least partial healing (Coburn & Salusky, 1994; Martin & Slatopolsky, 1994). A milder form of the same bone disease is seen in patients with less severe secondary hyperparathyroidism. Bone remodeling is slightly increased and peritrabecular fibrosis is minimal. These patients are generally better controlled than the preceding group with the same medical approach (Coburn & Salusky, 1994; Martin & Slatopolsky, 1994).

An adynamic form of bone disease has been diagnosed more frequently on bone biopsy specimens obtained in the last 20 years. Inappropriately low levels of PTH are usually seen in these patients (less than three times the upper limit of normal). Bone surfaces are hypocellular and there is no remodeling. This situation has been related to overtreatment with calcium carbonate, $1\alpha(OH)D$ or $1,25(OH)_2D$, high calcium dialysate and is seen more often in patients with diabetes mellitus and those on ambulatory peritoneal dialysis (Coburn & Salusky, 1994). More experience with the long-term evolution of this form of bone disease is required. Measures to increase PTH level, such as lower calcium dialysate concentrations, can indeed increase PTH levels (Coburn & Salusky, 1994) and possibly bone turnover. Other forms of bone disease, such as osteomalacia and mixed bone disease (osteomalacia + osteitis fibrosa cystica), have been related to aluminum deposition in bone or other unidentified factors in patients with or without prior severe SHP. Removal of the factor when possible may improve the condition (Coburn & Salusky, 1994; Martin & Slatopolsky, 1994).

The last condition to be addressed is the loss of bone mineral density associated with renal transplantation. Bone fractures is a more prevalent problem in this group of patients (Elmstedt & Svahn, 1981). Glucocorticoids and cyclosporine as immunosuppressive agents have both been implicated in the pathogenesis of osteoporosis (Epstein & Shane, 1996). There is also a possibility that residual secondary hyperparathyroidism may be of importance in the pathogenesis of this type of bone loss, particularly after renal transplantation. More studies are required to investigate this issue. Bisphosphonates, with their inhibitory effect on bone resorption, appear to be promising agents in preventing this type of osteoporosis where bone formation may be stimulated by cyclosporine or cyclosporine-like drugs (Epstein & Shane, 1996).

Conclusion

PTH inhibition in the treatment of osteoporosis

The present review has brought out the fact that PTH is involved in the genesis of both primary and secondary forms of osteoporosis. Lowering circulating PTH levels by the administration of calcium, vitamin D, $1\alpha(OH)D$, $1,25(OH)_2D$, by parathyroidectomy or decreasing the peripheral response to PTH through estrogen therapy has been associated with improvement in bone mineral density at various sites and also with a decreased fracture rate, at least in primary forms of osteoporosis. These facts demonstrate that PTH is an important determinant of the osteoporotic process. This is further sustained by the protective effect of hypoparathyroidism on the development of primary and secondary osteoporosis. Therapeutic approaches to reduce the parathyroid function, such as the use of calcimimetics, to decrease the biological response to PTH may become, in the future, further options in the treatment of osteoporosis.

REFERENCES

Abugassa, S., Nordenström, J., Erikson, S., & Sjöden, G. (1993). Bone mineral density in patients with chronic hypoparathyroidism. *J. Clin. Endocrinol. Metab.*, **76**, 1617–21.

Bikle, D. D. (1996). Osteoporosis in gastrointestinal, pancreatic, and hepatic diseases. In *Osteoporosis*, ed. R. Marcus, D. Feldman, & J. Kelsey, Chap. 44, pp. 863–84. San Diego, CA: Academic Press.

Bover, J., Rodriguez, M., Trinidad, P., Jara, A., Martinez, M. E., Machado, L., Llach, F., & Felsenfeld, A.J. (1994). Factors in the development of secondary hyperparathyroidism during graded renal failure in the rat. *Kidney Int.*, **45**, 953–61.

Brossard, J. H., Garon, J., Lepage, R., Gascon-Barré, M., & D'Amour, P. (1993). Inhibition of $1,25(OH)_2D$ production by hypercalcemia in osteitis fibrosa cystica: influence on parathyroid hormone secretion and hungry bone disease. *Bone Miner.*, **23**, 15–26.

Burkhart, J. M. & Jowsey, J. (1967). Parathyroid and thyroid hormones in the development of immobilization osteoporosis. *Endocrinology*, **81**, 1053–62.

Carroll, M. D., Abraham, S., & Dresser, C. M. (1983). Dietary intake source data: United States, 1976–80. *Vital and Health Statistics*. Series II, No. 231, DHHS Publ. No (PHS) 83–1681.

Chapuy, M. C. & Meunier, P. J. (1997). Vitamin D insufficiency in adults and the elderly. In

Vitamin D, ed. D. Feldman, F. H. Glorieux, & J. W. Pike, Chap. 43, pp. 679–93. San Diego, CA: Academic Press.

Clemens, M. R., Johnson, L., & Fraser, D. R. (1987). A new mechanism for induced vitamin D deficiency in calcium deprivation. *Nature*, **325**, 62–5.

Cloutier, M., Brossard, J. H., Gascon-Barré, M., & D'Amour, P. (1994). Lack of involution of hyperplastic parathyroid glands in dogs. Adaptation via a decrease in the calcium stimulation set point and a change in secretion profile. *J. Bone Miner. Res.*, **9**, 621–9.

Cloutier, M., Gascon-Barré, M., & D'Amour, P. (1992). Chronic adaptation of dog parathyroid function to a low-calcium-high-sodium-vitamin D-deficient diet. *J. Bone Miner. Res.*, **7**, 1021–8.

Coburn, J. W. & Salusky, I. B. (1994). Hyperparathyroidism in renal failure. Clinical features, diagnosis, and management. In *The Parathyroids*, ed. J. P. Bilezikian, M. A. Levine, & R. Marcus, Chap. 42, pp. 721–45. New York, USA: Raven Press.

Cosman, F., Shen, V., Xie, F., Seibel, M., Ratcliffe, A., & Lindsay, R. (1993). Estrogen protection against bone resorbing effects of parathyroid hormone infusion. *Ann. Int. Med.*, **118**, 337–43.

D'Amour, P., Faughnan, M., Paradis, E., Lepage, R., Ste-Marie, L. G., Glorieux, F., Rousseau, L., & Brossard, J. H. (1996). An increased C-PTH level in a normocalcemic individual may reflect an adaptation to an increased parathyroid function. *J. Bone Min. Res.*, **11**, S483 (abst. T736).

Eastell, R. & Riggs, B. L. (1997). Vitamin D and osteoporosis. In *Vitamin D*, ed. D. Feldman, F. H. Glorieux, & J. W. Pike, Chap. 44, pp. 695–711. San Diego, CA: Academic Press.

Ebeling, P. R., Sandgren, M. E., Dimagno, E. P., Lane, A. W., DeLuca, H. F., & Riggs, B. L. (1992). Evidence of an age-related decrease in intestinal responsiveness to vitamin D: Relationship between serum 1,25-dihydroxyvitamin D_3 and intestinal vitamin D receptor concentrations in normal women. *J. Clin. Endocrinol. Metab.*, **75**, 176–82.

Elmstedt, E. & Svahn, T. (1981). Skeletal complications following renal transplantation. *Acta Orthop Scand.*, **52**, 279–86.

Epstein, S. & Shane, E. (1996). Transplantation osteoporosis. In *Osteoporosis*, ed. R. Marcus, D. Feldman, & J. Kelsey, Chap. 48, pp. 947–57. San Diego, CA: Academic Press.

Forero, M. S., Klein, R. F., Nissenson, R. A., Nelson, K., Heath, H., Arnaud, C. D., & Riggs, L. (1987). Effect of age on circulating immunoreactive and bioactive parathyroid hormone levels in women. *J. Bone Miner. Res.*, **2**, 363–6.

Freaney, R., McBrinn, Y., & Mc Kenna, M. J. (1993). Secondary hyperparathyroidism in elderly people: combined effect of renal insufficiency and vitamin D deficiency. *Am. J. Clin. Nutr.*, **58**, 187–91.

Fujiyama, K., Kiriyama, T., Ito, M., Nakata, K., Yamashita, S., Yokoyama, N., & Nagataki, S. (1995). Attenuation of post menopausal high turnover bone loss in patients with hypoparathyroidism. *J. Clin. Endocrinol. Metab.*, **80**, 2135–8.

Garnero, P., Sornay-Rendu, E., Chapuy, M., & Delmas, P. D. (1996). Increased bone turnover in late post menopausal women is a major determinant of osteoporosis. *J. Bone Miner. Res.*, **11**, 337–49.

Gennari, C., Agnusdei, I. D., Nardi, P., & Civitelli, R. (1990). Estrogen preserves a normal intestinal responsiveness to 1,25-dihydroxyvitamin D_3 in nephrectomized women. *J. Clin. Endocrinol. Metab.*, **71**, 1288–93.

Heaney, R. P., Recker, R. R., & Saville, P. D. (1978). Menopausal changes in calcium balance performance. J. *Lab. Clin. Med.*, **99**, 953–63.

Heaney, R. P., Recker, R. R., Stegman, M. R., & Moy, A. J. (1989). Calcium absorption in women: Relationships to calcium intake, estrogen status, and age. *J. Bone Miner. Res.*, **4**, 469–75.

Heath, H. (1991). Clinical spectrum of primary hyperparathyroidism: evolution with changes in medical practice and technology. *J. Bone Miner. Res.*, **6**, S63–S70.

Heath, H. (1996). Primary hyperparathyroidism, hyperparathyroid bone disease, and osteoporosis. In *Osteoporosis*, ed. R. Marcus, D. Feldman, & J. Kelsey, Chap. 45, pp. 885–94. San Diego, CA: Academic Press.

Insogna, K. L., Lewis, A. M., Lipinski, B. A., Bryant, C., & Baran, D. T. (1981). Effect of age on serum immunoreactive parathyroid hormone and its biological effects. *J. Clin. Endocrinol. Metab.*, **53**, 1072–5.

Jowsey, J. & Raisz, L. G. (1968). Experimental osteoporosis and parathyroid activity. *Endocrinology*, **82**, 384–96.

Joyce, J. M., Idea, R. J., Grossman, S. J., Liss R. G., & Lyons, J. B. (1994). Multiple brown tumors in unsuspected primary hyperparathyroidism mimicking metastatic disease on radiograph and bone scan. *Clin. Nucl. Med.*, **19**, 630–5.

Julian, B. A., Laskow, D. A., Duborsky, J., Duborsky, E. V., Curtis, J. J., & Quarles, L. D. (1991). Rapid loss of vertebral mineral density after renal transplantation. *N. Engl. J. Med.*, **325**, 544–550.

Khosla, S., Atkinson, E. J., Melton, L. J., & Riggs, B. L. (1997). Effects of age and estrogen status on serum parathyroid hormone levels and biochemical markers of bone turnover in women: a population-based study. *J. Clin. Endocrinol. Metab.*, **82**, 1522–7.

Khosla, S., Melton, L.J., Atkinson, E. J., O'Fallon, W. M., Klee, G. G., & Riggs, B. L. (1998). Relationship of serum sex steroid levels and bone turnover markers with bone mineral density in men and women: A key role for bio-available estrogen. *J. Clin. Endocrinol. Metab.*, **83**, 2266–74.

Ledger, G. A., Burritt, M. F., Kao, P. C., O'Fallon, W. M., Riggs, B. L., & Khosla, S. (1995). Role of parathyroid hormone in mediating nocturnal and age-related increases in bone resorption. *J. Clin. Endocrinol. Metab.*, **80**, 3304–10.

Lukert, B. (1996). Glucocorticoid-induced osteoporosis. In *Osteoporosis*, ed. R. Marcus, D. Feldman, & J. Kelsey, Chap. 40, pp. 801–13. San Diego, CA: Academic Press.

McDermott, M. T., Perloff, J. J., & Kidd, G. S. (1994). Effects of mild asymptomatic primary hyperparathyroidism on bone mass in women with and without estrogen replacement therapy. *J. Bone Miner. Res.*, **9**, 509–14.

McKane, W. R., Khosla, S., Burritt, M. F., Pai, C. K., Wilson, D. M., Ory, S. J., & Riggs, L. (1995). Mechanism of renal calcium conservation with estrogen replacement therapy in women in early menopause. A clinical research center study. *J. Clin. Endocrinol. Metab.*, **80**, 3458–64.

McKenna, M. J. (1992). Differences in vitamin-D status between countries in young adults and the elderly. *Am. J. Med.*, **93**, 69–77.

MacLaughlin, J. & Holick, M. F. (1985). Aging decreases the capacity of human skin to produce vitamin D_3. *J. Clin. Invest.*, **76**, 1536–8.

Marcus, R. (1994). Parathyroid hormone and growth hormone in the treatment of osteoporosis.

In *The Parathyroids*, ed. J. Bilezikian, M. A. Levine, & R. Marcus, Chap. 49, pp. 813–21. New York, USA: Raven Press.

Marcus, R., Madvig, P., & Young, G. (1984). Age-related changes in parathyroid hormone and parathyroid hormone action in normal humans. *J. Clin. Endocrinol. Metab.*, **58**, 223–30.

Martin, K. J. & Slatopolsky, E. (1994). The parathyroids in renal disease. Pathophysiology. In *The Parathyroids*, ed. J. B. Bilezikian, M. A. Levine, & R. Marcus, Chap. 41, pp. 711–19. New York, USA: Raven Press.

Massry, S. G., Lee, D. B. N., & Kleeman, C. R. (1973). Skeletal resistance to parathyroid hormone in renal failure. Studies in 105 human subjects. *Ann. Int. Med.*, **78**, 357–64.

Mawer, E. B. & Davies, M. (1997). Bone disorders associated with gastrointestinal and hepatobiliary disease. In *Vitamin D*, ed. D. Feldman, F. H. Glorieux, & J. W. Pike, Chap. 51, pp. 831–47. San Diego, CA: Academic Press.

Melton, L. J. III., Atkinson, E. J., O'Fallon, W. M., & Heath III, H. (1992). Risk of age-related fractures in patients with primary hyperparathyroidism. *Arch. Intern. Med.*, **152**, 2269–73.

Murray, T. M., Rao, L. G., & Rizolli, R. E. (1994). Interactions of parathyroid hormone-related protein, and their fragments with conventional and non-conventional receptor sites. In *The Parathyroids. Basic and Clinical Concepts*, ed. R. Marcus & M. A. Levine, Chap. 13, pp. 185–212. New York, USA: Raven Press.

Nordin, B. E. C., Need, A. G., Morris, H. A., Horowitz, M., & Robertson, W. G. (1991). Evidence for a renal calcium leak in postmenopausal women. *J. Clin. Endocrinol. Metab.*, **72**, 401–7.

Orwoll, E. S. & Meier, D. E. (1986). Alterations in calcium, vitamin D and parathyroid hormone physiology in normal men with aging: Relationship to the development of senile osteopenia. *J. Clin. Endocrinol. Metab.*, **63**, 1262–9.

Pacifici, R. (1998). Cytokines, estrogen, and postmenopausal osteoporosis. The second decade (editorial). *Endocrinology*, **139**, 2659–61.

Parfitt, A. M. (1983). Dietary risk factors for age related bone loss and fractures. *Lancet*, **ii**, 1181–4.

Parisien, M., Mellish, R. W. E., Silverberg, S. J., Shane, E., Lindsay, R., Bilezikian, J. P., & Dempster, D. (1992). Maintenance of cancellous bone connectivity in primary hyperparathyroidism: Trabecular strut analysis. *J. Bone Miner. Res.*, **7**, 913–19.

Parisien, M., Silverberg, S. J., Shane, E., de la Cruz, L., Lindsay, R., Bilezikian, J. P., & Dempster, D. W. (1990). The histomorphometry of bone in primary hyperparathyroidism: Preservation of cancellous bone. *J. Clin. Endocrinol. Metab.*, **70**, 930–8.

Peacock, M., Horsman, A., Aaron, J. E., Marshall, D. H., Selby, P. L., & Simpson, M. (1984). The role of parathyroid hormone in bone loss. In *Osteoporosis I*, ed. Christiansen et al., pp. 463–7. Denmark: Department of Clinical Chemistry, Glostrups Hospital.

Prince, R. L. (1994). Estrogen effects on calciotropic hormones and calcium homeostasis. *Endocrine Rev.*, **15**, 301–9.

Rao, D. S., Wilson, R. J., Kleerekoper, M., & Parfitt, A. M. (1988). Lack of biochemical progression or continuation of accelerated bone loss in mild asymptomatic primary hyperparathyroidism. Evidence for biphasic disease course. *J. Clin. Endocrinol. Metab.*, **67**, 1294–8.

Riggs, B. L., Khosla, S., & Melton, L. J. (1998). A unitary model for involutional osteoporosis:

Estrogen deficiency causes both type I and type II osteoporosis in postmenopausal women and contributes to bone loss in aging men. *J. Bone Miner. Res.*, **13**, 763–73.

Ritz, E., Seidel, A., Ramisch, H., Szabo, A., & Bouillon, R. (1991). Attenuated rise of 1,25(OH)$_2$ vitamin D in response to parathyroid hormone in patients with incipient renal failure. *Nephron*, **57**, 314–18.

Rodriguez, M., Felsenfeld, A. J., & Llach, F. (1991). Calcemic response to parathyroid hormone in renal failure: Role of calcitriol and the effect of parathyroidectomy. *Kidney Int.*, **40**, 1063–8.

Seeman, E., Wahner, H. W., Offord, K. P., Kumar, R., Johnson, W. J., & Riggs, B. L. (1982). Differential effects of endocrine dysfunction on the axial and the appendicular skeleton. *J. Clin. Invest.*, **69**, 1302–9.

Silverberg, S. J., Gartenberg, F., Jacobs, T. P., Shane, E., Siris, E., Staron, R. B., & Bilezikian, J. P. (1995a). Longitudinal measurements of bone density and biochemical induces in untreated primary hyperparathyroidism. *J. Clin. Endocrinol. Metab.*, **80**, 723–8.

Silverberg, S. J., Gartenberg, F., Jacobs, T. P., Shane, E., Siris, E., Staron, R. B., McMalson, D. J., & Bilezikian, J. P. (1995b). Increased bone mineral density after parathyroidectomy in primary hyperparathyroidism. *J. Clin. Endocrinol. Metab.*, **80**, 729–34.

St. John, A., Thomas, M. B., Davies, P. C., Mullan, B., Dick, I., Hutchison, B., Van der Schaff, A., & Prince, R. L. (1992). Determinants of intact parathyroid hormone and free 1,25-dihydroxy-vitamin D levels in mild and moderate renal failure. *Nephron*, **61**, 422–7.

Touliatos, J. S., Sebes, J. I., Hinton, A., Mc Common, D., Karas, J. G., & Palmieri, G. M. A. (1995). Hypoparathyroidism counteracts risk factors for osteoporosis. *Am. J. Med. Sci.*, **310**, 56–60.

Tsai, K. S., Heath, H., Kumar, R., & Riggs, B. L. (1984). Impaired vitamin D metabolism with aging in women. Possible role in the pathogenesis of senile osteoporosis. *J. Clin. Invest.*, **73**, 1668–72.

Turner, R. T., Riggs, B. L., & Spelsberg, T. C. (1994). Skeletal effects of estrogen. *Endocrine Rev.*, **15**, 275–300.

Webb, A. R, Pilbeam, C., Hanafin, N., & Holick, M. F. (1990). An evaluation of the relative contributions of exposure to sunlight and of diet to the circulating concentrations of 25-hydroxyvitamin D in an elderly nursing-home population in Boston. *Am. J. Clin. Nutr.*, **51**, 1075–81.

Wilson, R. J., Rao, D. S., Ellis, B., Kleerekoper, M., & Parfitt, M. (1988). Mild asymptomatic primary hyperparathyroidism is not a risk factor for vertebral fractures. *Ann. Intern. Med.*, **109**, 959–62.

Yendt, E. R., Cohanim, M., Jarzylo, S., Jones, G., & Rosenberg, G. (1991). Bone mass is related to creatinine clearance in normal elderly women. *J. Bone Miner. Res.*, **6**, 1043–50.

Young, G., Marcus, R., Minkoff, J. R., Lance, Y. K., & Segre, G. V. (1987). Age-related rise in parathyroid hormone in man: the use of intact and midmolecule antisera to distinguish hormone secretion from retention. *J. Bone Miner. Res.*, **2**, 367–74.

16

Senile Osteoporosis

Patrick M. Doran and Sundeep Khosla

Introduction

Senile osteoporosis consists of a metabolic bone disease characterized by low bone mass and microarchitectural deterioration of the skeleton, leading to enhanced bone fragility and a consequent increase in fracture risk. It is estimated that 1.5 million fractures attributable to osteoporosis occur annually in the United States, incurring a total cost estimated at 13.8 billion dollars in 1995 alone (Ray et al., 1997). Hip fracture is the most costly and catastrophic of the osteoporotic complications; about 25% of these patients have a fatal outcome, half of the survivors are unable to walk unassisted, and a quarter become confined to a long-term care institution. However, other types of osteoporotic fractures can also cause considerable functional impairment (Ray et al., 1997).

Although osteoporosis is more common in women, men also sustain substantial bone loss with aging (Riggs & Melton, 1986), and elderly men have age-specific hip and vertebral fracture rates that are at least half those in women (Melton, 1995). Thus, senile osteoporosis has significant clinical and economic consequences in both men and women, and the seriousness of this problem is being further magnified by the aging of the postwar generation. This chapter describes the role played by bone resorption and its relationship to reduced levels of sex steroids in both male and female osteoporosis.

Patterns of bone loss over time

Women undergo two phases of involutional bone loss, whereas men undergo a single one (Riggs & Melton, 1986), as shown schematically in Fig. 16.1. Peak bone mass is achieved in young adulthood and determined by multiple environmental and genetic factors, as discussed in a previous chapter. Subsequently, bone mineral density remains relatively constant in both genders until middle life. At menopause, women undergo an accelerated, transient phase of bone loss that is most apparent over the subsequent 10 to 15 years and accounts for cancellous bone losses of 20–30% and cortical bone losses of 5–10% (Riggs & Melton, 1986). Clinically, these

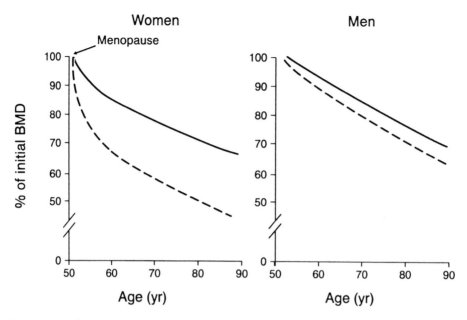

Fig. 16.1   Schematic representation of changes in bone mass over life in cancellous (broken line) and cortical (solid line) bone in women and men from age 50 onward. See text for details. Reproduced with permission from Riggs et al. (1998).

losses characteristically translate into fractures that occur at sites rich in cancellous bone, such as painful 'crush fractures' of the vertebrae, Colles' fracture of the distal forearm, and fractures of the ankle (Riggs & Melton, 1983, 1990).

This accelerated phase is superimposed on, and merges asymptotically with, an underlying phase of slow bone loss that continues indefinitely. In aging men, the slow, continuous phase of bone loss resembles the late slow phase in postmenopausal women. Over life, this slow phase accounts for losses of about 20–30% of cancellous bone and 20–30% of cortical bone in both genders (Riggs & Melton, 1986). It is characterized by fractures at sites containing substantial proportions of both cortical and cancellous bone (Riggs & Melton, 1983, 1990), namely the hip, proximal humerus, proximal tibia, and pelvis. Vertebral fractures also occur during the slow phase of bone loss and are often of the multiple wedge type, leading to painless dorsal kyphosis (sometimes referred to as 'dowager's hump').

Mechanisms of bone loss in women

Bone is limited in the ways it can respond to disease states, and bone loss is the final common pathway to a number of different pathophysiologic processes, as illustrated by the following.

Accelerated, transient phase of bone loss

This transient phase of bone loss clearly results from estrogen deficiency, since it coincides with the onset of menopause, ovariectomy, or any other form of ovarian failure, and since it can be prevented by estrogen replacement. Estrogen acts via high affinity estrogen receptors in osteoblasts (Eriksen et al., 1988; Komm et al., 1988) and osteoclasts (Oursler et al., 1991b) to tonically restrain bone turnover. When estrogen levels fall, this restraint is lost and overall bone turnover increases. Moreover, the associated increase in bone resorption is greater than that of bone formation, as illustrated by both radiocalcium kinetics and bone marker studies (Eastell et al., 1988; Garnero et al., 1996). At the cellular level, estrogen deficiency is characterized by a simultaneous increase in frequency of activation of bone remodeling units, and a loss of balance between osteoblastic and osteoclastic activity in favor of the latter at each of these units. Cancellous bone has a greater surface area than cortical bone, making it more vulnerable to increased osteoclastic activity. The deeper osteoclastic resorption cavities lead to trabecular plate perforation and loss of cancellous bone structural integrity. This process eventually increases bone fragility and ultimately leads to the above-mentioned acute collapse, most typically of the vertebrae.

In addition to its direct effects on bone cells, estrogen deficiency has also been associated with increased local skeletal production of a number of bone-resorbing mediators such as interleukin-1, interleukin-6, tumor necrosis factor-alpha, macrophage-colony stimulating factor, and prostaglandins (Manolagas & Jilka, 1995; Pacifici, 1992). Also, estrogen normally increases transforming growth factor-beta (TGF-β) production by osteoclasts and osteoblasts, which may inhibit osteoclastic bone resorption in an autocrine and paracrine fashion, respectively (Oursler et al., 1991a; Robinson et al., 1996). Recent studies also indicate that estrogen promotes apoptosis of osteoclasts, and that this effect may be also mediated by TGF-β (Hughes et al., 1996). Thus, estrogen deficiency may augment bone turnover and resorption by the stimulation of the release of osteoclast activating factors and/or by the inhibition of the production of osteoclast inhibiting factors. Further, lack of estrogen also increases bone sensitivity to parathyroid hormone (PTH) and, possibly, to other resorption-inducing agents that further enhance the net resorption effect.

Compensatory increases in urinary calcium excretion and decreases in intestinal calcium absorption (Heany et al., 1978), prevent the resultant skeletal outflow of calcium into the extracellular fluids from producing hypercalcemia. Consequently, serum intact PTH levels remain within normal limits in early postmenopausal women, although there is a trend toward slightly decreased levels. Some studies have shown that institution of estrogen replacement results in a relative increase in serum PTH levels, suggesting that there was a small compensatory drop in PTH secretion at steady state (McKane et al., 1995). This decrease in PTH production results in reduced circulating levels of 1,25-dihydroxyvitamin D (1,25(OH)$_2$D), which itself may impair calcium absorption and further accentuate bone loss (Gallagher et al., 1982).

The mechanisms behind the transient nature of the accelerated phase are still incompletely understood. One conceptual model holds that, because of the high rate of cancellous bone loss during this early phase, this bone compartment becomes rapidly depleted. Once the amount of cancellous bone falls below some threshold, biochemical forces prevail in limiting the rate of further cancellous loss. Alternatively, another explanation uses a two-compartment model of bone loss, where cancellous loss may follow first-order kinetics because of its greater surface-to-volume ratio than that of cortical bone, while the latter may follow simple linear kinetics because of this difference. Computer simulations have indicated that such a model would closely resemble the bone loss curves shown in Fig. 16.1.

Only a relatively small proportion of postmenopausal women, 10–20%, develop significant osteoporosis during the accelerated phase of bone loss, even though all postmenopausal women are relatively estrogen deficient. Serum sex steroid levels are similar, at 10–20% of premenopausal levels, in postmenopausal women with and without significant bone loss. Thus, one or more additional causal factors are present in postmenopausal osteoporotic women that interact with estrogen deficiency to determine individual susceptibility. The possible additional factors include impaired coupling of formation with resorption, increased local production of cytokines or other factors that increase bone resorption, prolongation of the phase of accelerated bone loss, low bone density at the inception of menopause, or some combination thereof (Riggs & Melton, 1990).

Slow, protracted phase of bone loss

In contrast to its accelerated counterpart, this phase of bone loss affects all women, produces equal losses of cancellous and cortical bone, and if left untreated progresses inexorably through the remainder of life. It is also characterized by being predominantly caused by changes in extraskeletal calcium metabolism with secondary hyperparathyroidism, as opposed to the direct disinhibition of bone turnover and consequent lower PTH levels noted during the accelerated phase.

Renal function tends to decline with aging, but not to levels that would increase parathyroid function. The pathogenic mechanisms behind the secondary hyperparathyroidism include a significant reduction in renal calcium conservation (Ledger et al., 1995) and in intestinal calcium absorption in elderly women (Gallagher et al., 1979). The decreases in calcium absorption with aging have been attributed variously to impaired hydroxylation of vitamin D to 1,25 (OH)$_2$D, primary impairment of calcium absorption, or decreased concentrations of intestinal vitamin D receptors (Ebeling et al., 1992). Finally, some elderly women, especially those who are housebound and reside in countries that do not fortify milk products with vitamin D, have exogenous vitamin D deficiency that may contribute to the secondary hyperparathyroidism (Chapuy et al., 1992).

Serum intact PTH levels and indices of bone turnover increase in parallel in aging women, and these increases correlate directly with each other, even after adjusting for the effects of age (Riggs et al., 1998). The suppression of PTH secretion by intravenous calcium infusion abolishes the differences in bone resorption markers between young and elderly women, strongly suggesting that the increase in bone resorption in aging women is PTH-dependent. Furthermore, a number of randomized trials have shown that dietary calcium and vitamin D supplementation in elderly women reverses age-associated hyperparathyroidism and reduces bone loss (McKane et al., 1996; Reid et al., 1995) and fracture rates (Dawson-Hughes et al., 1997).

It is widely agreed that estrogen deficiency causes the accelerated transient phase of bone loss in early postmenopausal women. However, what role does estrogen deficiency play in the pathogenesis of the secondary hyperparathyroidism and increased bone turnover that underlie the slow bone loss in late postmenopausal women? Recent studies indicate that this role is a critical one. Thus, while intestinal calcium absorption is reduced in elderly women, estrogen replacement therapy (ERT) in postmenopausal women with osteoporosis has been shown to increase both serum total and free $1,25(OH)_2D$ levels, as well as intestinal calcium absorption (Cheema et al., 1989; Gallagher et al., 1979). In addition, in perimenopausal before and 6 months after oophorectomy, the expected increase in calcium absorption in response to $1,25(OH)_2D$ was blunted in the presence of estrogen deficiency, suggesting also a direct enhancing effect of estrogen on intestinal calcium absorption, possibly through a preservation of mucosal $1,25(OH)_2D$ receptor density (Horst et al., 1990).

In addition to effects on intestinal calcium absorption, estrogen may also have significant effects on renal calcium handling, resulting in improved calcium balance. McKane et al. (1995), for example, assessed renal calcium transport directly at baseline and during administration of a saturating dose of PTH in postmenopausal women before and after 6 months of ERT. They demonstrated a PTH-independent increase in tubular calcium absorption in the estrogen replete compared with the estrogen-deficient women, whereas tubular reabsorption of other cations was unaffected, observations that are consistent with a direct effect of estrogen on renal calcium conservation.

Estrogen may also have direct effects on PTH secretion. Thus, it was found that ERT in postmenopausal women decreased PTH secretion in response to EDTA-induced hypocalcemia (Cosman et al., 1994), suggesting that estrogen also acts directly on the parathyroid gland to reduce PTH secretion. Supporting this conclu-

Table 16.1. Comparative effects of age and estrogen status in women

Variable	Premenopausal	Postmenopausal untreated	Postmenopausal treated
n	30	30	30
Age (years)	32.0 ± 0.5	74.2 ± 0.6	73.8 ± 0.6
Serum			
PTH (pmol/l)	2.7 ± 0.2	3.6 ± 0.3^{a}	2.5 ± 0.2
Urine			
NTx (nmol/mmol Cr)	28.8 ± 2.3	42.9 ± 3.5^{b}	24.6 ± 2.3
PYD	45.6 ± 2.3	61.2 ± 3.2^{b}	40.7 ± 1.1
DPD	11.9 ± 0.5	16.2 ± 1.0^{b}	9.4 ± 0.5

Notes:
Serum intact PTH was fasting morning value. Bone resorption markers were measured by
ELISA kit for N-telopeptide of type I collagen (NTx) and by fluorometric detection after HPLC
for pyridinoline (PYD) and deoxypyridinoline (DPD). All results are mean $\pm$ SE.
For difference from premenopausal [a]$P<0.05$, [b]$P<0.005$.
From Riggs, B. L. et al. (1998), with permission.

sion, the parathyroid gland has been found to contain estrogen receptors by some
(Navey-Many et al., 1992), albeit not by others (Prince et al., 1991).

These multiple extraskeletal effects of estrogen thus appear to prevent age-
related secondary hyperparathyroidism in elderly postmenopausal women by
improving overall calcium homeostasis in favor of a less negative calcium balance.
Corroborating this, recent studies comparing young adult premenopausal women,
untreated older women, and older women on ERT have found that once estrogen
deficiency is corrected, serum PTH and bone resorption markers are similar in
elderly, estrogen-treated and young women (Khosla et al., 1997; Riggs et al., 1998)
(Table 16.1). Moreover, short-term ERT of women over 80 years of age reduced
bone turnover markers significantly (Prestwood et al., 1994). Finally, a prospective
study comparing endogenous sex steroid levels in untreated postmenopausal
women over 65 showed that individuals with estradiol levels below the limit of
detection of a sensitive assay (<18 pmol/l) had hip and vertebral fracture risks that
were significantly greater than those of women of the same age with endogenous
estradiol levels above this threshold (Cummings et al., 1998).

In summary, estrogen deficiency at the time of menopause accounts for the
accelerated, transient phase of bone loss through the loss of restraint on bone turnover rate, while favoring resorption over formation. The slow bone loss that occurs

later in menopause seems to be predominantly caused by hyperparathyroidism secondary to multiple changes in extraskeletal calcium homeostasis. In turn these changes also appear tightly associated with estrogen deficiency, can be reversed with ERT, and bone-preserving effects of ERT appear to reach well into the ninth decade, possibly even later. Although postmenopausal bone loss is caused mainly by increased bone resorption, the net resorptive effect is amplified in both early and late phases by impaired compensatory osteoblastic function, as discussed in another chapter.

Mechanisms of bone loss in men

During their lifetimes, despite the absence of a menopause equivalent, men still undergo two-thirds of the bone loss sustained by women. Also, after accounting for the absence of an accelerated phase, the slow, continuous bone loss and accompanying increase in PTH and bone resorption markers incurred by aging men are virtually superimposable on those previously described in aging women, both in pattern and in prevalence (Khosla et al., 1998).

Conventional wisdom holds that bone mass is maintained mainly by estrogen in women and mainly by testosterone in men, given the similar rapid bone loss that follows oophorectomy and orchiectomy (Stepan et al., 1989), respectively. Only a few aging men develop overt hypogonadism, however, and serum total testosterone decreases only slightly with aging in men. Thus, previous epidemiologic studies assessing serum total testosterone levels and bone density in aging men have found no relationship. Furthermore, because the testes produce both sex steroids and because testosterone can be converted to estrogen by aromatization in peripheral tissues, a deficiency of either or both could mediate postorchiectomy bone loss.

Data from several so-called 'experiments of nature' have suggested that estrogen may play a major role in maintaining bone mass in men. In 1994, Smith et al. (1994) described a 28-year-old man with homozygous null mutations of the estrogen receptor gene who was eunuchoid with unfused epiphyses, marked osteopenia and elevated bone turnover indices, despite normal serum testosterone and elevated serum estrogen levels. Subsequently, a similar skeletal phenotype was described in two males with homozygous null mutations of the gene for aromatase (Carani et al., 1997; Morishima et al., 1995), which is required for conversion of androgens to estrogens. In both instances, bone mineral density (BMD) was severely reduced despite normal androgen levels. Although testosterone treatment in one patient did not significantly affect bone turnover (Carani et al., 1997), estrogen replacement markedly increased BMD in both patients. These individuals and their response to treatment suggest that, also in males, estrogen is an essential mediator of epiphyseal closure, attainment of maximal bone mass, as well as maintenance of the equilibrium between bone formation and resorption.

Even though earlier reports had been negative, recent epidemiologic evidence supports the concept that estrogen is a critical mediator of skeletal metabolism in aging men. Four population-based, observational studies (Center et al., 1997; Greendale et al., 1997; Khosla et al., 1998; Slemenda et al., 1997) involving an aggregate total of 1410 men from young adulthood to old age have demonstrated by multivariate analysis that free serum estrogen rather than free serum testosterone was the main predictor of bone mass at all measured sites, except at some cortical bone sites in the appendicular skeleton. Also, whereas serum total testosterone and estrogen decreased only modestly with age in these studies, there were large decreases in serum-free testosterone and estrogen, as well as in bioavailable testosterone and estrogen (free and bound to albumin). These decreases were partially due to elevations in the levels of sex hormone binding globulin, which decrease the availability of testosterone and estrogen to peripheral tissues. Another study (Bernecker et al., 1995) found that mean levels of serum estrogen rather than testosterone were significantly reduced in 56 men with established idiopathic osteoporosis. Finally, even these findings may be conservative, given that some or even most of the effects of circulating testosterone on bone cells may still be mediated by estrogen after local aromatization of testosterone to estrogen in bone (Purohit et al., 1992).

Collectively, these data support the hypothesis that estrogen deficiency plays a major role in involutional bone loss in men as well as in women. However, osteoblasts contain androgen receptors (Colvard et al., 1989), and testosterone clearly accounts for the sexual dimorphism of the skeleton that develops following puberty and probably also stimulates periosteal accretion of cortical bone.

Conclusion

Estrogen deficiency accounts for the early accelerated and late slow phases of bone loss in women and for an important proportion of the continuous phase of bone loss in men, and acts through different mechanisms to produce its various manifestations on the skeleton. These preliminary data suggesting the importance of estrogen in men, coupled with the ever-expanding array of selective estrogen receptor modulating agents, gives rise to a new and exciting approach to the treatment of male osteoporosis. Although we have already made great strides in our understanding of bone homeostasis, future work will undoubtedly shed much needed light on the relative contributions of estrogen and androgen deficiencies in both male and female osteoporosis.

REFERENCES

Bernecker, P. M., Willvonseder, R., & Resch, H. (1995). Decreased estrogen levels in male patients with primary osteoporosis. *J. Bone Miner. Res.,* **10**, S445.

Carani, C., Qin, K., Simoni, M., Faustini-Fustini, M., Serpente, S., Boyd, J., Korach, K. S., & Simpson, E. R. (1997). Effects of testosterone and estradiol in a man with aromatase deficiency. *N. Engl. J. Med.,* **337**, 91–5.

Center, J. R., Nguyen, T. V., White, C. P., & Eisman, J. A. (1997). Male osteoporosis predictors: sex hormones and calcitropic hormones. *J. Bone Miner. Res.,* **12**, S368.

Chapuy, M. C., Arlot, M. E., Duboeuf, F., Brun, J., Crouzet, B., Arnaud, S., Delmas, P. D., & Meunier, P. J. (1992). Vitamin D_3 and calcium to prevent hip fractures in elderly women. *N. Engl. J. Med.,* **327**, 1637–42.

Cheema, C., Grant, B. F., & Marcus, R. (1989). Effects of estrogen circulating 'free' and total 1,25-dihydroxyvitamin D and on the parathyroid-vitamin D axis in postmenopausal women. *J. Clin., Invest.,* **83**, 527–42.

Colvard, D. S., Eriksen, E. F., Keeting, P. E., Wilson, E. M., Lubahn, D. B., French, F. S., Riggs, B. L., & Spelsberg, T. C. (1989). Identification of androgen receptors in normal human osteoblast-like cells. *Proc. Natl Acad. Sci., USA,* **86**, 854–7.

Cosman, F., Nieves, J., Horton, J., Shen, V., & Lindsay, R. (1994). Effects of estrogen on response to edetic acid infusion in postmenopausal osteoporotic women. *J. Clin. Endocrinol. Metab.,* **78**, 939–43.

Cummings, S. R., Browner, W. S., Bauer, D., Stone, K., Ensrud, K., Jamal, S., & Ettinger, B. (1998). Endogenous hormones and the risk of hip and vertebral fractures among older women. *N. Engl. J. Med.,* **339**, 733–8.

Dawson-Hughes, B., Harris, S. S., Krall, E. A., & Dallal, G. E. (1997). Effects of calcium and vitamin D on bone density in men and women 65 years of age or older. *N. Engl. J. Med.,* **337**, 670–6.

Eastell, R., Delmas, P. D., Hodgson, S. F., Eriksen, E. F., Mann, K. G., & Riggs, B. L. (1988). Bone formation rate in older normal women: concurrent assessment with bone histomorphometry calcium kinetics, and biochemical markers. *J. Clin. Endocrinol. Metab.,* **67**, 741–8.

Ebeling, P. R., Sandgren, M. E., DiMagno, E. P., Lane, A. W., De Luca, H. F., & Riggs, B. L. (1992). Evidence of an age-related decrease in intestinal responsiveness to vitamin D: relationship between serum 1,25-dihydroxyvitamin D_3 and intestinal vitamin D receptor concentrations in normal women. *J. Clin. Endocrinol. Metab.,* **75**, 176–82.

Eriksen, E. F., Colvard, D. S., Berg, N. J., Graham, M. L., Mann, K. G., Spelsberg, T. C., & Riggs, B. L. (1988). Evidence of estrogen receptors in normal human osteoblast-like cells. *Science,* **241**, 84–6.

Gallagher, J. C., Jerpbak, C. M., Jee, W. S. S., Johnson, K. A., DeLuca, H. F., & Riggs, B. L. (1982). 1,25-dihydroxyvitamin D_3: short- and long-term effects on bone and calcium metabolism in patients with postmenopausal osteoporosis. *Proc. Natl Acad. Sci., USA,* **79**, 3325–9.

Gallagher, J. C., Riggs, B. L., Eisman, J., Hamstra, A., Arnaud, S. B., & DeLuca, H. F. (1979).

Intestinal calcium absorption and serum vitamin D metabolites in normal subjects and osteo-porotic patients: effects of age and dietary calcium. *J. Clin. Invest.*, **64**, 729–36.

Garnero, P., Sornay-Rendu, E., Chapuy, M., & Delmas, P. D. (1996). Increased bone turnover in late postmenopausal women is a major determinant of osteoporosis. *J. Bone Miner. Res.*, **11**, 337–49.

Greendale, G. A., Edelstein, S., & Barrett-Connor, E. (1997). Endogenous sex steroids and bone mineral density in older women and men 'The Rancho Bernado study'. *J. Bone Miner. Res.*, **12**, 1833–43.

Heany, R. P., Recker, R. R., & Saville, P. D. (1978). Menopausal changes in calcium balance performance. *J. Lab. Clin. Med.*, **92**, 953–63.

Horst, R. L., Goff, J. P., & Reinhardt, T. A. (1990). Advancing age results in reduction of intestinal and bone 1,25-dihydroxyvitamin D receptor. *Endocrinology*, **126**, 1053–7.

Hughes, D. E., Dai, A., Tiffee, J. C., Li, H. H., Mundy, G. R., & Boyce, B. F. (1996). Estrogen promotes apoptosis of murine osteoclasts mediated by TGF-beta. *Nature Med.*, **2**, 1132–6.

Khosla, S., Atkinson, E. J., Melton, L. J., & Riggs, B. L. (1997). Effects of age and estrogen status on serum parathyroid hormone levels and biochemical markers of bone turnover in women: a population-based study. *J. Clin. Endocrinol. Metab.*, **82**, 1522–7.

Khosla, S., Melton, L. J., Atkinson, E. J., O.Fallon, W. M., Klee, G. G., & Riggs, B. L. (1998). Relationship of serum sex steroid levels with bone mineral density in aging women and men: a key role for bioavailable estrogen. *J. Clin. Endocrinol. Metab.*, **83**, 2266–74.

Komm, B. S., Terpening, C. M., Benz, D. J., Graeme, K. A., O'Malley, B. W., & Haussler, M. R. (1988). Estrogen binding receptor mRNA, and biologic response in osteoblast-like osteosarcoma cells. *Science*, **241**, 81–4.

Ledger, G. A., Burritt, M. F., Kao, P. C., O'Fallon, W. M., Riggs, B. L., & Khosla, S. (1995). Role of parathyroid hormone in mediating nocturnal and age-related increases in bone resorption. *J. Clin. Endocrinol. Metab.*, **80**, 33304–10.

McKane, W. R., Khosla, S., Burritt, M. F., Kao, P. C., Wilson, D. M., Ory, S. J., & Riggs, B. L. (1995). Mechanism of renal calcium conservation with estrogen replacement therapy in women in early postmenopause – a clinical research center study. *J. Clin. Endocrinol. Metab.*, **80**, 3458–64.

McKane, W. R., Khosla, S., Egan, K. S., Robins, S. P., Burritt, M. F., & Riggs, B. L. (1996). Role of calcium intake in modulating age-related increases in parathyroid function and bone resorption. *J. Clin. Endocrinol. Metab.*, **81**, 1699–703.

Manolagas, S. C. & Jilka, R. L. (1995). Bone marrow, cytokines, and bone remodeling: emerging insights into the pathophysiology of osteoporosis. *N. Engl. J. Med.*, **332**, 305–11.

Melton, L. J. (1995). Epidemiology of fractures. In *Osteoporosis. Etiology, Diagnosis, and Management*, 2nd edn, ed. B. L. Riggs & L. J. Melton, III, pp. 225–47. Philadelphia: Lippincott-Raven.

Morishima, A., Grumbach, M. M., Simpson, E. R., Fisher, C., & Qin, K. (1995). Aromatase deficiency in male and female siblings caused by a novel mutation and the physiological role of estrogens. *J. Clin. Endocrinol Metab.*, **80**, 3689–98.

Navey-Many, T., Almogi, G., Livni, N., & Silver, J. (1992). Estrogen receptors and biologic response in rat parathyroid tissue and C cells. *J. Clin. Invest.*, **90**, 2434–8.

Oursler, M. J., Cortese, C., Keeting, P., Anderson, M. A., Bonde, S. K., Riggs, B. L., & Spelsberg,

T. C. (1991a). Modulation of transforming growth factor-beta production in normal human osteoblast-like cells by 17 beta-estradiol and parathyroid hormone. *Endocrinology*, **129**, 3313–20.

Oursler, M. J., Osbody, P., Pyfferoen, J., Riggs, B. L., & Spelsberg, T. C. (1991b). Avian osteoclasts as estrogen target cells. *Proc. Natl Acad. Sci., USA*, **88**, 6613–17.

Pacifici, R. (1992). Is there a causal role for IL-1 in postmenopausal bone loss? *Calcif. Tissue Int.*, **50**, 295–9.

Prestwood, K. M., Pilbream, C. C., Burleson, J. A., Woodiel, F. N., Delmas, P. D., Deftos, L. J., & Raisz, L. G. (1994). The short-term effects of conjugated estrogens on bone turnover in older women. *J. Clin. Endocrinol. Metab.*, **79**, 366–71.

Prince, R. L., MacLaughlin, D. T., Gaz, R. D., & Neer, R. M. (1991). Lack of evidence for estrogen receptors in human and bovine parathyroid tissue. *J. Clin. Endocrinol. Metab.*, **72**, 1226–8.

Purohit, A., Flanagan, A. M., & Reed, M. J. (1992). Estrogen synthesis by osteoblast cell lines. *Endocrinology*, **131**, 2027–9.

Ray, N. F., Chan, J. K., Thamer, M., & Melton, L. J. (1997). Medical expenditures for the treatment of osteoporotic fractures in the United States in 1995: report from the National Osteoporosis Foundation. *J. Boner Miner. Res.*, **12**, 24–35.

Reid, I. R., James, R. W., Evans, M. C., Gamble, G. D., & Sharpe, S. J., (1995). Long-term effects of calcium supplementation on bone and fractures in postmenopausal women: a randomized controlled trial. *Am. J. Med.*, **98**, 331–5.

Riggs, B. L. & Melton, L. J. (1983). Evidence for two distinct syndromes of involutional osteoporosis. *Am. J. Med.*, **75**, 899–901.

Riggs, B. L. & Melton, L. J. (1986). Medical progress series: involutional osteoporosis. *N. Engl. J. Med.*, **314**, 1676–86.

Riggs, B. L. & Melton, L. J. (1990). Clinical heterogeneity of involutional osteoporosis: implications for prevention and therapy. *J. Clin. Endocrinol. Metab.*, **70**, 1229–32.

Riggs, B. L., Khosla, S., & Melton, L. J. (1998). A unitary model for involutional osteoporosis: estrogen deficiency causes both type I and type II osteoporosis in postmenopausal women and contributes to bone loss in aging men. *J. Bone Miner. Res.*, **13**, 763–73.

Robinson, J. A., Riggs, B. L., Spelsberg, T. C., & Oursler, M. J. (1996). Osteoclasts and transforming growth factor-β: estrogen-mediated isoform-specific regulation of production. *Endocrinology*, **137**, 615–21.

Slemenda, C. W., Longcope, C., Zhou, L., Hui, S. L., Peacock, M., & Johnston, C. (1997). Sex steroids and bone mass in older men: positive associations with serum estrogens and negative associations with androgens. *J. Clin. Invest.*, **100**, 1755–9.

Smith, E. P., Boyd, J., Frank, G. R., Takahashi, H., Cohen, R. M., Specker, B., Williams, T. C., Lubahn, D. B., & Korach, K. S. (1994). Estrogen resistance caused by a mutation in the estrogen-receptor gene in a man. *N. Engl. J. Med.*, **331**, 1056–61.

Stepan, J. J., Lachjman, M., Zverina, J., & Pacovsky, V. (1989). Castrated men exhibit bone loss: effects of calcitonin treatment on biochemical indices of bone remodeling. *J. Clin. Endocrinol. Metab.*, **69**, 523–7.

Part IV

Clinical aspects of osteoporosis

17

Biochemical markers of bone turnover

David A. Hanley

The 1980s and 1990s have seen major advances in the understanding of regulation of bone metabolism. The section on cellular and hormonal environment of bone reviews the basics of biochemistry and cell biology of bone. With the elucidation of the synthesis and post-translational modification of bone collagen, has come the ability to measure markers of both collagen synthesis and its breakdown. In the formation of new bone, and the breakdown or resorption of old bone, components of the non-collagen matrix of bone are also released by the cells that are synthesizing these products or remodeling the bone matrix. Because these components are released from bone into the circulation, their measurement may provide a window for clinical assessment of the process of bone resorption and formation.

The normal adult human skeleton is constantly remodeling. This is illustrated diagrammatically in Fig. 17.1. The skeleton may be regarded as being made up of millions of basic multicellular units (BMUs) or bone remodeling units (abbreviated in some publications as BRU). At any given time, most BMUs are in a resting stage. In a response to a variety of stimuli (mechanical stress, parathyroid hormone, withdrawal of estrogen, local release of growth factors and cytokines, etc.) a resting BMU can be stimulated into activity. Cells of the osteoblast lineage release factors which stimulate the differentiation of precursor cells into osteoclasts and the process of bone resorption begins. Resorption proceeds over a period of 2 to 4 weeks, with release of bone mineral, matrix proteins, and their breakdown products. It is not known what causes the process of resorption to stop, but after a preset resorption depth is achieved, the osteoclasts lift off the resorption service. Then a new group of cells enter the area, laying down a cement line, and osteoblasts begin the process of laying down new collagen which is slowly mineralized. The process of new bone formation can vary in length from under 3 months to more than a year (Fig. 17.2). Bone resorption and formation in a BMU are tightly coupled. Normally, bone resorption is always followed by bone formation, and in a BMU in the young adult skeleton the newly formed bone essentially replaces all the bone lost through the resorption phase. With physical stress, and under certain hormonal or growth factor stimuli, the process of bone formation can exceed resorption (a positive bone

Bone remodeling

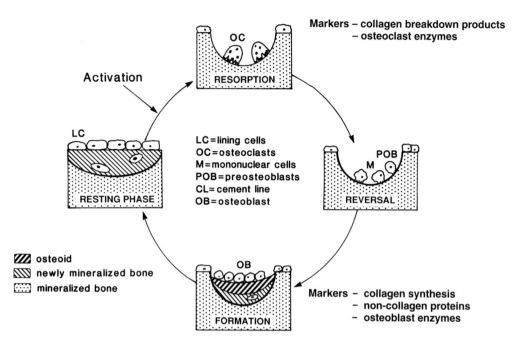

Fig. 17.1   The bone remodeling cycle of a basic multicellular unit (BMU) of trabecular bone. This figure depicts a net bone balance of zero (complete replacement of the resorbed bone).

balance). After mid-adulthood, bone resorption always slightly exceeds formation, contributing to the gradual loss of bone mass with aging (negative bone balance).

After withdrawal of gonadal hormones (e.g., menopause) the number of BMUs undergoing remodeling is markedly increased. Since by this age, women have entered the stage of gradual decline in skeletal mass, an increase in bone turnover would be expected to be associated with accelerated loss of bone. Markers of bone resorption and formation would both be expected to be increased. This is certainly what is seen clinically around the time of menopause and for the first 5 to 10 years after menopause (Fig. 17.3).

Other clinical disorders can increase the rate of bone turnover, and increased bone turnover is usually associated with negative bone balance in these conditions, as well. The most common clinical disorders that are associated with a general increase in bone turnover and resultant bone loss are primary hyperparathyroidism and hyperthyroidism.

Paget's disease of bone, a regional bone disorder featuring runaway bone remodeling and the deposition of markedly abnormal bone, still follows the normal sequence of bone formation following resorption (Roodman, 1999). In Paget's

Bone remodeling

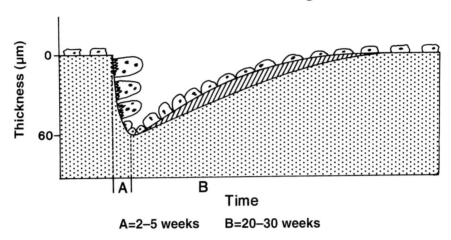

Fig. 17.2   The time sequence of remodeling of a BMU.

disease, the resorption and formation are so excessive that the resulting new bone is not of normal organization and strength.

Certain clinical conditions are particularly devastating for bone, as they seem to be associated with increased bone resorption but decreased bone formation. This is sometimes referred to as uncoupling of bone resorption from formation. Cushing's disease, or long-term (more than three months) glucocorticoid therapy would probably be the best example of this kind of excessive bone loss (Lane & Lukert, 1998). Hypercalcemia of malignancy mediated by humoral factors such as parathyroid hormone related peptide (PTHrP) or cytokines, may also cause a marked excess of bone resorption over formation (Stewart et al., 1982). In contrast, often metastatic prostate cancer and occasionally metastatic breast cancer will be termed 'osteoblastic', as the metastases cause exuberant new bone formation in the region of metastasis (Goltzman, 1997).

A variety of laboratory methods of assessing bone turnover have been developed. An exhaustive review of this topic would be beyond the scope of this chapter, and the discussion will be focused upon markers which have found some clinical application. Several excellent reviews of biochemical markers of bone turnover have been published recently (Bikle, 1997; Calvo et al., 1996; Garnero & Delmas, 1998; Knott & Bailey, 1998). The review by Calvo et al., is particularly thorough for readers interested in more details of the biochemistry of biochemical markers. If references are not given in the text of this chapter, they will be found in one of these reviews.

To gain clinical application, biochemical markers of bone turnover must be validated by other techniques that directly quantitate bone turnover. The markers

Menopause

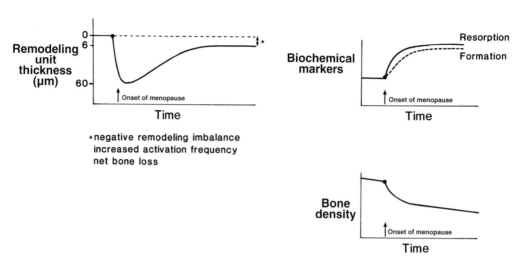

Fig. 17.3   Increased bone remodeling at the time of menopause features a normal depth of resorption, but a net negative bone balance due to incomplete replacement of resorbed bone. There is an increased number of active BMUs, so that biochemical markers of both resorption and formation increase, and there is accelerated bone loss seen with bone density measurement over time.

discussed here have all been shown to correlate well with bone formation or resorption, as measured by bone biopsy or radioactive calcium kinetics. Further, most have been shown to be elevated in conditions known to increase or decrease bone formation or resorption and to respond appropriately to effective treatment of these clinical conditions.

Most of the markers of resorption and one of the markers of formation are related to the structure of collagen. When collagen is degraded, the markers of resorption which we measure (hydroxyproline, hydroxylysine, pyridinolines and telopeptides) are not recycled into newly formed bone. Pertinent points of collagen synthesis will be reviewed in the discussion of the individual markers. Biochemical markers of bone turnover that are in fairly common use in clinical studies or in clinical practice are listed in Table 17.1.

Biochemical markers of bone resorption

Collagen cross-link markers: pyridinolines and telopeptides (urine or serum)

When collagen molecules are secreted by osteoblasts into the extracellular matrix, they are stabilized by the formation of pyridinium (pyridinoline and deoxypyridinoline) cross-links from the action of lysyl hydroxylase on the lysine and hydroxyly-

Table 17.1. Biochemical markers of bone turnover

Bone resorption	Bone formation
Blood:	*Blood:*
Tartrate-resistant acid phosphatase	Total or bone-specific alkaline phosphatase
Free pyridinoline or deoxypyridinoline	Osteocalcin
N- or C-telopeptide of type I collagen	Procollagen I C- and N-terminal extension peptides
Cross-links	
Urine:	
Fasting urine calcium-to-creatinine ratio	
Hydrocyproline	
Glycosides of hydroxylysine	
Pyridinoline and deoxypyridinoline	
N- and C-telopeptide of type I collagen	

sine residues in the amino (N-) and carboxy (C-) terminal domains of the type I collagen fibrils (telopeptides). Pyridinoline is formed by the combination of three hydroxylysines, while deoxypyridinoline is formed by combination of two hydroxylysines with one lysine. The pyridinium cross-links occur between the N- or C-telopeptide of a collagen molecule and the helical portion of an adjacent collagen molecule, about 90 amino acids from either end. When collagen is degraded, the pyridinoline moiety is released, either as a 'free' pyridinoline, or in association with its telopeptide. Although type I collagen is not unique to bone, the pyridinium cross-linking of collagen tends to be more tissue specific. The type I collagen of bone has a higher proportion of deoxypyridinoline in the cross-linking than does the collagen in (for example) articular cartilage, so the measurement of free deoxypyridinoline seems to reflect bone resorption better than free pyridinoline.

Probably the biochemical marker which has gained the most widespread acceptance as a sensitive indicator of bone resorption would be one of the telopeptides of the pyridinoline cross-links. Measured changes in the urinary excretion of the N- and C-telopeptides seem to be more pronounced than changes in the secretion of the free deoxypyridinoline or pyridinoline entities, but the individual variability is also greater for the telopeptides. Bone resorption follows a diurnal variation, and for telopeptides, this can result in much higher levels measured in the morning than in the afternoon or evening. Urine sampling for these compounds should either be done as 24-hour urine collection, or as a timed collection aimed at measuring these metabolites at the peak of their daily levels (early morning). The advantages of the pyridinoline-related measurements over hydroxyproline (see below) are that they are not affected by diet, and they are more specific for the type I collagen of bone.

Hydroxyproline and hydroxylysine glycosides

The collagen molecule is extremely rich in hydroxylated lysine and proline. When collagen is synthesized, the hydroxylation of proline and lysine is followed by glycosylation of the collagen molecule, and the ratio of galactosylhydroxylysine to glucosyl-galactosylhydroxylysine is fairly tissue specific (e.g., 1.6 to 1 in skin and 1 to 7 in bone) (Krane et al., 1977). Hydroxyproline was the earliest marker of bone resorption to receive wide clinical use. Unfortunately, hydroxyproline is significantly affected by diet. In the monitoring of diseases like Paget's disease of bone, in which bone resorption is extremely accelerated, the dietary influence on hydroxyproline excretion is probably not that important, and hydroxyproline may still may be an effective marker of the progression or treatment of the Paget's disease. However, for the N- and C-telopeptides and free deoxypyridinoline, there is a reasonably clear separation between free- and postmenopausal levels (low vs. higher turnover) such that some clinicians are now using these markers to monitor response to pharmacologic therapy of osteoporosis.

Urinary calcium-to-creatinine ratio

A fasting early morning urine specimen for calcium-to-creatinine ratio should reflect calcium released into the circulation from bone resorption, as the dietary contribution to urinary calcium should be low when the measurement is made on a fasting morning specimen. However, urinary calcium excretion depends largely on the actions of parathyroid hormone, and can be influenced by drugs such as diuretics, or vitamin D supplementation.

Tartrate-resistant acid phosphatase (TRAP)

TRAP is a lysosomal enzyme that is not entirely specific to bone, but is highly prevalent in osteoclasts and its measurement in bone biopsies is one of the keys to identifying osteoclast activity. TRAP occurs in many tissues, and because it is present in platelets, it must be measured in plasma rather than serum. In plasma, much of the circulating TRAP is derived from osteoclasts, but its lack of specificity for bone has meant that it will not gain widespread clinical use. Assays are being developed for the bone isoenzyme of TRAP.

Biochemical markers of bone formation

Alkaline phosphatase – total and bone specific

Serum total alkaline phosphatase is an enzyme that is widely distributed in the body, and particularly prominent in bone and liver. Although total alkaline phosphatase is not specific for bone, when measured in Paget's disease it is usually markedly elevated, and is a good indicator of disease activity. For studies of bone formation in clinical trials, however, more specific assays of bone alkaline phosphatase have been developed. The actual chemical difference between the alkaline phosphatases from different sources are not great, and there is still some cross-reactivity between the so-called bone-specific alkaline phosphatase measurements and the liver isoenzyme which is so prominent in the circulation. However, there are other more liver-specific enzymes, which can usually help to determine whether an elevated alkaline phosphatase originates from liver disease or bone.

Total alkaline phosphatase is measured in biological activity (hydrolysis of *p*-nitrophenyl phosphate). It is readily measured on automated systems available in virtually all commercial clinical laboratories. Newer bone-specific alkaline phosphatase measurements are by immunoassay techniques, although some are still assays of biological activity.

Osteocalcin

Probably the most widely used marker of bone formation in clinical and physiologic studies after alkaline phosphatase would be the serum osteocalcin. Osteocalcin is a small peptide of 49 amino acids, and is also called bone Gla-protein or BGP, because it contains three residues of γ-carboxyglutamic acid. These glutamic acid residues are carboxylated in the gamma position of its glutamic acid residues posttranslationally, through the action of vitamin K. The recent association of vitamin K deficiency with osteopenia may be related to these effects on osteocalcin. A lower proportion of γ-carboxylated osteocalcin to the fully carboxylated species has been noted in elderly patients, and this can be corrected with vitamin K supplementation (Garnero & Delmas, 1998).

Like alkaline phosphatase, osteocalcin is a protein that is secreted by osteoblasts, and is widely distributed in bone. It probably plays a major role in the regulation of mineral deposition into collagen. It is incorporated into the extracellular matrix of bone, and is released during bone resorption, so its presence in plasma is really a marker of bone turnover as well as of bone formation due to osteoblast activity.

Although alkaline phosphatase does not display a very significant diurnal variation, this is not the case for osteocalcin and other commonly measured biochemical markers. Osteocalcin has a very wide circadian rhythm, with a peak in the early morning and a trough around 5:00 pm. In clinical trials, it is important to measure osteocalcin at the same time of day in order to make comparisons of changes in levels of circulating osteocalcin. It is also markedly affected by renal function, relying on the kidney for its secretion. The molecule also has a variety of circulating fragments which some methods of measurement recognize and some do not. Because of the vagaries in the measurement of the peptide, the marked diurnal variation, its instability in stored blood samples, and its dependence upon normal renal function, osteocalcin measurements are not recommended for general clinical use at this time.

Serum procollagen extension peptides

The third marker of bone formation which has seen some use in clinical trials is the N- or C-terminal extension peptide of type I procollagen. A brief review of type I collagen synthesis is in order at this point. Within the osteoblast, type I procollagen a chains are synthesized, the lysines and prolines are hydroxylated, and the process of glycosylation begins. The procollagen α chains are assembled into a triple helix that is initially stabilized by disulfide bonds between the C-terminal propeptides, and the molecule is then transported to the Golgi, in preparation for secretion. After the procollagen triple-helical molecule is secreted by osteoblasts, it undergoes further cleavage to remove the N-terminal and C-terminal extension peptides (often abbreviated PINP and PICP), most of which are then released into the circulation. These extension peptides can now be measured in plasma. However, further improvements are required in the measurement techniques before clinical utility is established. At present, they do not appear to be as sensitive indicators of changes in bone turnover as alkaline phosphatase, osteocalcin, or most of the resorption markers. They are not used in routine clinical practice.

Use of biochemical markers in metabolic bone disease

Paget's disease of bone

Most of the biochemical markers are elevated in active Paget's disease. In clinical practice, it is usual for a marker of bone formation (alkaline phosphatase) and a marker of bone resorption (hydroxyproline or N- or C-telopeptide) to be measured. Because non-specific alkaline phosphatase is inexpensive and falls dramatically with appropriate therapy of Paget's disease, it is probably the most appropriate biochemical marker to follow in this disorder. Although most clinical assessment recommendations include markers of both formation and resorption, there is no evidence that anything more than the alkaline phosphatase is needed in the monitoring of most patients' response to therapy. Serum measurements of procollagen extension peptides and osteocalcin are unreliable as markers of Paget's disease activity. The reason for this problem is not clear. Collagen and osteocalcin gene expression and secretion are characteristic of a different stage of osteoblast maturity than alkaline phosphatase, and there is speculation that Paget's disease may feature abnormalities of osteoblast maturation (Bikle, 1997).

Malignant bone disease

The biochemical markers are not particularly diagnostic of the nature of malignant bone disease, but a few have notable characteristics.

(i) Multiple myeloma features lytic bone lesions without an increased bone formation, and alkaline phosphatase is usually not elevated. Similarly, bone scans do not show the lytic lesions well, as bone scan positivity reflects osteoblast activity. Markers of bone resorption are elevated.

(ii) Prostate carcinoma and breast carcinoma, when associated with osteoblastic metastases, will show an increase in alkaline phosphatase, and other markers of bone formation.

(iii) In most skeletal metastases, alkaline phosphatase and resorption markers are both elevated. A recent study suggested that pyridinoline and deoxypyridinoline were more sensitive than alkaline phosphatase in identifying patients with bone metastases (Pecherstorfer et al., 1995). However, biochemical markers other than alkaline phosphatase and acid phosphatase (prostate cancer) have not found general clinical use in monitoring patients with cancer.

Osteomalacia

In osteomalacia, there is a general increase in bone turnover, although bone formation and in particular, mineralization, is ineffective. All of the biochemical markers are usually increased. Alkaline phosphatase is the only marker that has gained acceptance in monitoring the response to therapy.

Hyperthyroidism

General increased bone turnover is seen in hyperthyroidism, and hyperthyroidism is considered a major risk factor for later development of osteoporosis (Cummings et al., 1995). There is biochemical evidence for a marked excess of bone resorption (free pyridinoline) over formation (osteocalcin) in patients with hyperthyroidism (Garnero et al., 1994). Although biochemical markers have helped provide answers in our study of the pathophysiology of the bone disease associated with hyperthyroidism, they are not part of the routine clinical investigation of this disorder.

Hyperparathyroidism

This is a disorder which features increased bone resorption and formation, but the biochemical markers are not considered to be of great clinical value in evaluating patients with primary hyperparathyroidism. The presence of an elevated alkaline phosphatase may signify the patient has more active parathyroid hormone-related bone disease. However, a low bone density measurement would be more specific in identifying patients with otherwise mild, asymptomatic hyperparathyroidism, who might be sent for surgery to protect against further bone loss (Bilezikian, 1994).

Osteoporosis

In the assessment of patients with osteoporosis, there does not yet appear to be a well-defined role for biochemical markers of bone turnover in general clinical

Osteoporosis treatment with antiresorptive agent

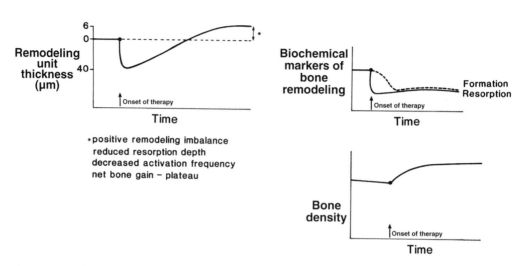

Fig. 17.4   When an antiresorptive agent is given, there is a net positive bone balance, due to reduced activation of resorption and (especially in the case of bisphosphonates) reduced depth of resorption. The markers of bone turnover fall, but the effect on formation lags behind the effect on resorption. Until a balance of resorption and formation is re-established, there is a transient increase in bone density.

practice. However, it is becoming apparent that the biochemical markers can be used in clinical trials to monitor the response to various pharmacologic agents used in the treatment of osteoporosis. Similarly, there is growing evidence that markers of bone resorption are of particular value as predictors of overall fracture risk. The EPIDOS Study, a multicentre epidemiologic study of osteoporosis incidence in healthy women in France, identified two biochemical markers of bone turnover that are independent predictors of risk of hip fracture. These were C-telopeptide and free deoxypyridinoline (Garnero et al., 1996). An elevated level of these markers above the normal range was associated with approximately a doubling in the risk of hip fracture, and this increased risk was unchanged after adjusting for other known risk factors for hip fractures such as bone density.

A possible use of biochemical markers in the assessment of patients with osteoporosis would be to identify those women at the time of menopause who are undergoing a rapid rate of bone turnover and might be better candidates for pharmacologic intervention such as hormone replacement therapy. Few studies have been done to test this hypothesis, but one 12-year prospective study very impressively showed that a combination of bone density, urinary calcium, and calcium excretion could predict the change in bone density from 1997 to 1989 with extremely high accuracy (Hansen et al., 1991).

Treatment with glucocorticoids

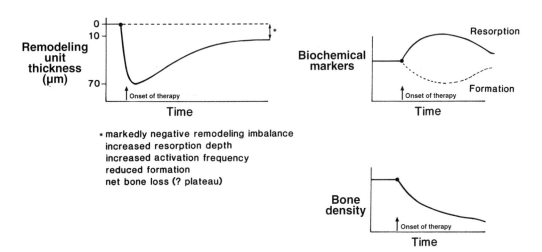

* markedly negative remodeling imbalance
  increased resorption depth
  increased activation frequency
  reduced formation
  net bone loss (? plateau)

Fig. 17.5   Glucocorticoid therapy places the skeleton in double jeopardy, with increased resorption and reduced bone formation. There is a separation of the biochemical markers, reflecting the uncoupling of resorption and formation, and a dramatic loss of bone.

It is very clear from all of the recent studies of pharmacologic agents being used in the treatment of osteoporosis that biochemical markers of bone formation and resorption respond dramatically to the therapeutic intervention. In particular, in the case of antiresorptive therapies (Fig. 17.4), there is a rapid decline in the bone resorption markers in the first month or two of therapy, and a later decline in bone formation. This is the biochemical marker reflection of an imbalance in bone remodeling, such that the suppression of bone resorption precedes and exceeds the suppression of bone formation. There is a net positive bone balance, resulting in a modest increase in bone mass, which later reaches a plateau as bone resorption and bone formation come back into balance. This pattern of biochemical marker and bone density response can be seen in the published clinical trials of estrogen, bisphosphonates, calcitonin, raloxifene, and other antiresorptive agents.

In glucocorticoid-induced osteoporosis, a combination of increased bone resorption and reduced bone formation results in a rapid and severe loss of bone (Fig. 17.5). This is reflected in a modest increase in markers of bone resorption and a decrease in osteocalcin, as a marker of bone formation.

Treatment of osteoporosis with an agent like sodium fluoride which has no effect on bone resorption, results in no change in the biochemical markers of bone resorption, but an increased level of biochemical markers of bone formation. The response to sodium fluoride is depicted in Fig. 17.6.

Osteoporosis treatment with fluoride

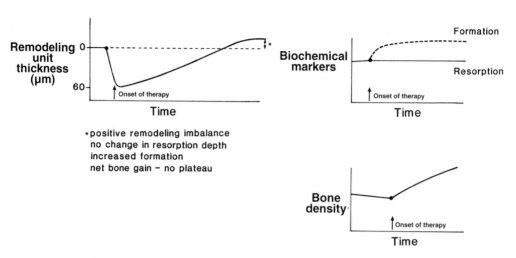

Fig. 17.6   Fluoride is the only agent available which directly stimulates bone formation. It is associated with dramatic increases in bone density, of up to 30% in 4 years (Riggs et al., 1990). Unfortunately, there is concern about the quality of the mineralized bone resulting from fluoride therapy of osteoporosis. Biochemical markers reflect increased bone formation with no change in resorption.

Although the biochemical markers have demonstrated their value in clinical trials and epidemiologic studies, the utility of these measurements in following an individual patient with osteoporosis remains controversial. In addition to significant intra- and interassay variability for some of these markers, there is significant day-to-day individual variation in the levels of the markers. Although they tend to be of more predictive value than bone formation markers in patients with osteoporosis, the resorption markers also have a significant diurnal variation. Because of all these problems, the likelihood that an average clinical practitioner can find value in measuring a marker in routine monitoring of an individual patient's response to therapy becomes questionable.

Some bone specialists have begun using biochemical markers in certain clinical situations. When a patient is continuing to lose bone while receiving a pharmacologic therapy of osteoporosis, an elevated resorption marker might indicate that the therapy needs adjustment or a change of drugs. A theoretical approach to the use of biochemical markers in combination with bone density measurements to help make a decision about treating a postmenopausal woman with a pharmacologic agent such as estrogen is outlined in Fig. 17.7.

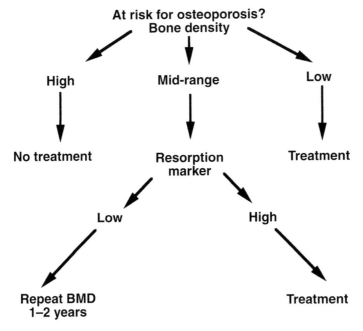

Fig. 17.7   An algorithm for use of biochemical markers in the management of patients who might be candidates for osteoporosis prevention therapy at, or after, menopause.

Conclusions

In this brief review, the aim has been to introduce the reader to a newly developing area of study of metabolic bone disease. Biochemical markers hold great promise for clinical laboratory investigation of patients, and in some areas (e.g., Paget's disease) they have gained a position in the routine investigation and management of patients. In osteoporosis investigation and management, certain markers (particularly resorption markers such as the telopeptides) have some utility. With improvements in the measurements, they may become more widely used in monitoring response to therapy and as an aid in encouraging patients' adherence to prescribed therapy.

REFERENCES

Bikle, D. D. (1997). Biochemical markers in the assessment of bone disease. *Am. J. Med.*, **103**, 427–36.

Bilezikian J.P. (1994) Guidelines for the medical or surgical management of primary hyperparathyroidism. In *The Parathyroids*, ed. J. P. Bilezikian, M. A. Levine, & R. Marcus, pp. 567–74. New York: Raven Press.

Calvo, M. S., Eyre, D. R., & Gundberg, C. M. (1996). Molecular basis and clinical application of biological markers of bone turnover. *Endocr. Rev.*, 17, 333–68.

Cummings, S. R., Nevitt, M. C., Browner, W. S., Stone, K., Fox, K. M., Ensrud, K. E., Cauley, J., Black, D., & Vogt, T. M. (1995). Risk factors for hip fracture in white women. *N. Engl. J. Med.*, 332, 767–73.

Garnero, P. & Delmas, P. D. (1998). Biochemical markers of bone turnover: applications for osteoporosis. *Endocrinol. Metab. Clin. N. Am.*, 27: 303–23.

Garnero, P., Sornay-Rendu, E., Chapuy, M. C., & Delmas, P. D. (1996). Increased bone turnover in late postmenopausal women is a major determinant of osteoporosis. *J. Bone Miner. Res.*, 11, 337–49.

Garnero P., Vassy V., Bertholin A., Riou, J. P., & Delmas, P. D. (1994). Markers of bone turnover in hyperthyroidism and the effects of treatment. *J. Clin. Endocrinol. Metab.*, 78, 955–9.

Goltzman, D. (1997). Mechanisms of the development of osteoblastic metastases. *Cancer*, 80(8 Suppl.), 1581–7.

Hansen, M. A., Overgaard, K., Riis, B. J., & Christiansen, C. (1991). Role of peak bone mass and bone loss in postmenopausal osteoporosis: twelve year study. *Br. Med. J.*, 303, 961–4.

Knott, L. & Bailey, A. J. (1998). Collagen cross-links in mineralizing tissues: A review of their chemistry function and clinical relevance. *Bone*, 22, 181–7.

Krane, S. M., Kantrowytz, F. G., Byrne, M., Pinnell, S. R., & Singer, F. R. (1977). Urinary secretion of hydroxylysine and its glycosides as an index of collagen degradation. *J. Clin. Invest.*, 59: 819–27.

Lane, N. E. & Lukert, B. (1998). The science and therapy of glucocorticoid-induced bone loss. *Endocrinol. Metab. Clin. N. Am.*, 27, 465–83.

Pecherstorfer, M., Zimmer-Roth, I., Schilling, T., Woitge, H. W., Schmidt, H., Baumgartner, G., Thiebaud, D., Ludwig, H., & Seibel, M. J. (1995). The diagnostic value of urinary pyridinium cross-links of collagen, serum total alkaline phosphatase, and urinary calcium excretion in neoplastic bone disease. *J. Clin. Endocrinol. Metab.*, 80, 97–103.

Riggs, B. L., Hodgson, S. F., O'Fallon, W. M., Chao, E. Y., Wahner, H. W., Muhs, J. M., Cedel, S. L., & Melton, L. J. (1990). Effect of fluoride treatment on the fracture rate in postmenopausal women with osteoporosis. *N. Engl. J. Med.*, 22(322), 802–9.

Roodman, D. G. (1999). Mechanisms of abnormal bone turnover in Paget's disease. *Bone*, 24(5 suppl.), 39S-40S.

Stewart, A. F., Vignery, A., Silverglate, A., Ravin, N. D., LiVolsi, V., Broadus, A. E., & Baron, R. (1982). Quantitative bone histomorphometry in humoral hypercalcemia of malignancy: uncoupling of bone cell activity. *J. Clin. Endocrinol. Metab.*, 55, 19–27.

18

Radiologic assessment of osteoporosis

Jacqueline C. Hodge.

Introduction

Osteoporosis (OP) is probably the most common metabolic disorder of the musculoskeletal system, affecting more than 200 million people (Whitcroft & Stevenson, 1992). Because the sequelae of OP, namely hip, vertebral, and distal radial fractures, result in considerable morbidity and mortality, OP has become a significant healthcare problem.

OP, a disorder of both cortical (compact) and trabecular (cancellous) bone, is characterized by a paucity of qualitatively normal bone. It is thought to be due to increased bone resorption rather than deficient bone formation (Aguado et al., 1997). Although advanced stages of OP are frequently detected by radiography, plain radiography is insensitive to early and intermediate stages of OP. Twenty-five to 50% of bone loss must occur before radiographic detection is possible (Resnick & Niwayama, 1998). Furthermore, plain radiographs are unable to precisely quantify OP. Thus plain radiography's role is primarily to distinguish OP from osteomalacia and other etiologies of OP, and to assess the progression and sequelae of OP.

Quantification of osteoporosis

Well-established techniques allowing quantification of bone mineral density include X-ray absorptiometry, photon absorptiometry, and quantitative computerized tomography. More recently, ultrasound and magnetic resonance imaging have also demonstrated some utility in assessment of bone mineral density.

X-ray absorptiometry employs an X-ray source to determine bone mineral density in the spine and peripheral skeleton. Photon absorptiometry, used primarily in the spine and hip, utilizes a gamma-ray source and detector to calculate combined trabecular and cortical bone mineral density (BMD). Quantitative computerized tomography (QCT) uses an X-ray source to measure BMD in the spine. Because of its cross-sectional imaging capability, QCT is the only modality to calculate the BMD of trabecular bone exclusively. For this reason, QCT is a better predictor of OP vertebral fractures than X-ray absorptiometry, as is expected given the disproportionate loss of trabecular bone with OP (Pacifici et al., 1990).

Ultrasound has been utilized to measure BMD of the calcaneus. BMD measurements calculated by this method show a significant correlation with the risk of OP-related spine and hip fractures (La Fianza et al., 1997; Sastry et al., 1994). Most recently, a relationship has been observed between bone density, the structure of the trabecular network, and marrow relaxation times on magnetic resonance imaging (MRI) (Majumdar & Genant, 1995). However, preliminary studies have demonstrated a large amount of regional variability of marrow relaxation times within a given bone, limiting the accuracy and precision of MRI in the determination of OP (Guglielmi et al., 1996).

Plain radiography and osteoporosis

The criteria utilized to suggest the presence of OP on skeletal radiographs include increased radiolucency, prominence of vertical trabeculae due to disproportionate resorption of horizontal trabeculae, the presence of reinforcement lines, and thinning of the vertebral endplates. However, these qualitative criteria are imprecise and may be frankly misleading on occasion. In assessing the skeleton for OP, it is important to note that bone resorption is site dependent, appearing first in the axial and then subsequently in the appendicular skeleton (Resnick & Niwayama, 1988). This is based on the fact that OP results in relatively more loss of trabecular bone as compared with cortical bone. The implication of this is that calculations of BMD acquired in the appendicular skeleton are insensitive to spinal OP. Therefore, the ideal test is one which is able to measure both axial and appendicular BMD.

Within the axial skeleton, the vertebral compression fracture, initially thought to be a more objective expression of osteoporosis, has also proven to be indiscriminate in identifying those patients with OP (Adami et al., 1992; Ryan & Fogelman, 1994) (Fig. 18.1). The criteria used to determine wedge or biconcave ('fish vertebra') compression fractures are based on the ratio between the posterior vertebral body height and that of the anterior or middle vertebra, respectively. However, analysis has shown that there is typically a large degree of overlap between normal and compressed vertebra. Additionally, the Cupid's bow contour of the vertebra, somewhat similar in appearance to the 'fish vertebra' of OP, is a developmental phenomenon unrelated to OP (Chan et al., 1997). None the less, vertebral compression fractures may still serve as a useful method for following the progression of OP in those with known OP.

Within the appendicular skeleton, OP may be suggested by the presence of trabecular, intracortical, or endosteal resorption. In general, subperiosteal resorption

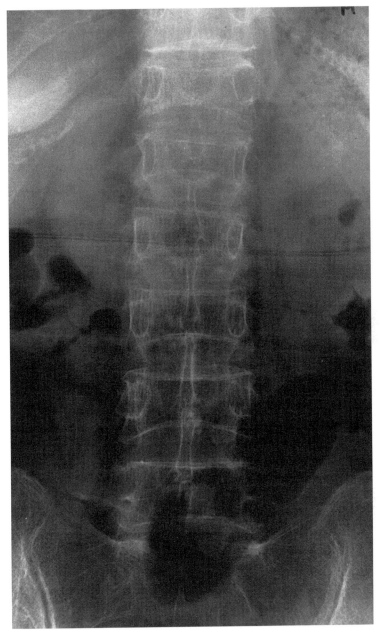

Fig 18.1   (*a*) Anteroposterior and (*b*) lateral radiographs of the lumbosacral spine in a patient with known senile osteoporosis. There is uniform deminineralization with prominent vertical trabeculae. Compression fractures are noted from T$_{12}$ to L$_4$, inclusive.

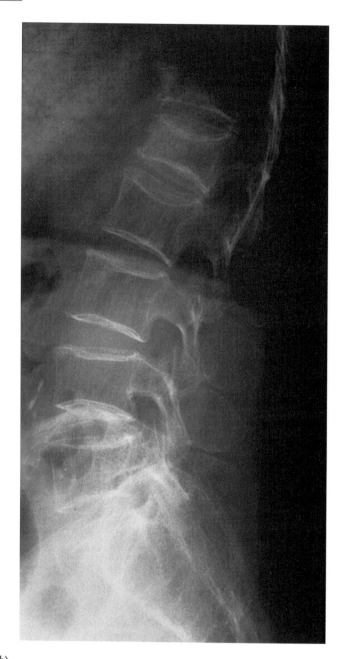

Fig 18.1(*b*)

is almost pathognomonic for hyperparathyroidism and is not a feature of OP. The presence of reinforcement lines, dense lines that occur perpendicular to the cortex of tubular bones, supports the diagnosis of chronic OP.

To detect relatively early radiographic signs of OP, several methods, including magnification radiography and radiogrammetry, have been utilized in the appendicular skeleton (Meema, 1991; Resnick & Niwayama, 1988). Magnification radiography, also known as microradioscopy, is a technique utilized to obtain fine-detail radiographs of the hands. Detection of OP is earlier by this technique as compared with its detection by conventional radiographs. However, magnification radiography is still relatively insensitive in the early stages of OP. Radiogrammetry, usually performed within the metacarpals, is a reproducible method of determining the cortical thickness of a bone as compared with its entire thickness. This method is inexpensive and readily obtained, but it too is insensitive to early OP (Weissman, 1987).

In the proximal femur, the Singh index has been used as a crude indicator of OP. Five anatomic groups of trabeculae are defined within the proximal femur: principal and secondary compressive groups, principal and secondary tensile groups, and the greater trochanteric group. Singh et al. defined the severity of OP based on the increased prominence of some groups of trabeculae and the resorption of other trabecular groups. However, the reliability of the Singh index is in question given the high degree of intraobserver and interobserver variability (Koot et al., 1996).

The equivalent of the Singh index, the calcaneal index, determined from a lateral radiograph of the calcaneus, was intended to be used as an indicator of BMD within calcaneus. Although some have found it to be a valid predictor of the risk of hip fracture, others have shown virtually no correlation between the calcaneal index and BMD (Ahl et al., 1993; Sastry et al., 1994).

Osteopenia

Increased radiolucency is often referred to as OP, although to be precise this condition is defined as osteopenia, a state of too little bone. OP is far more common than osteomalacia, a condition in which the quality of bone is altered. Osteomalacic bone, like rachitic bone, is characterized by a normal amount of bone matrix but insufficient mineralization laid down upon the matrix. Radiographically, it is often quite difficult to distinguish osteomalacia from OP. Indistinctness of bony trabeculae, and loss of corticomedullary distinction are features of osteomalacia. The presence of protrusio acetabulae, a bell-shaped thorax, and/or pseudofractures of the femoral neck, pubic rami, ribs or axillary margins of the scapulae support the diagnosis of osteomalacia (Fig. 18.2).

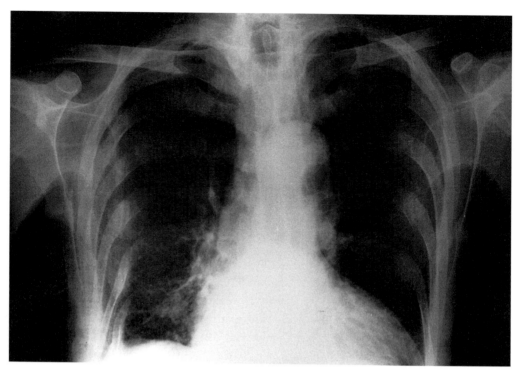

Fig 18.2   Frontal radiograph of the chest. Multiple healing rib fractures are identified bilaterally. Radiolucent fracture lines, perpendicular to the long axis of the lateral scapular margin, are identified. These represent Looser's zones which are pathognomonic for osteomalacia. This patient also had bilateral inferior pubic rami fractures and a fracture of the medial femoral calcar (not shown).

Differential diagnosis of osteoporosis

Sudeck's atrophy, disuse OP, transient OP, and regional migratory OP are readily distinguished from generalized OP because of their focality. Furthermore, a history of prior trauma can usually be elicited from those with Sudeck's atrophy or disuse OP.

Among the etiologies of generalized OP, senile, also known as postmenopausal, OP is the most common cause. However, senile OP is a diagnosis of exclusion. A careful medication history must be obtained to exclude drug-induced OP, an entity which is radiologically identical to senile OP. Corticosteroids, utilized in the treatment of asthma, chronic lung diseases, systemic lupus erythematosis, and posttransplantation, are the most frequently implicated medications contributing to OP (Epstein et al., 1995; Picado & Luengo, 1996). Interestingly, renal transplant recipients are less susceptible to overt OP than are cardiac or liver transplant recipients

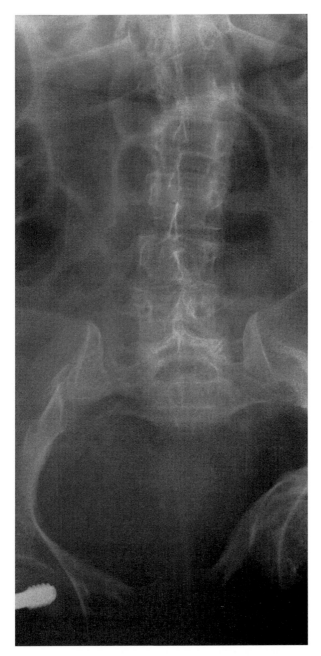

Fig 18.3   Anteroposterior radiograph of the lumbosacral spine in a patient with known osteogenesis imperfecta. There is apex-levoscoliosis centered at the thoracolumbar junction, and generalized decreased mineralization. Pelvic deformity due to protrusio acetabulae is present on the left. A Richard's screw transfixes a proximal femoral shaft fracture. Healed fracture deformities of both pubic rami are noted.

(Epstein et al., 1995). In the transplant population, bone loss is most critical during the first 6 months following transplantation. Heparin has been well established as a cause of OP (Ginsberg et al., 1990). Nutritional impairment, including malnutrition and calcium deficiency, chronic liver disease, and excessive alcohol intake may also result in OP. Cessation of responsible medication or improvement in nutritional status reverses the OP attributed to drugs and malnutrition, respectively.

Ancillary radiographic findings help to distinguish senile OP from less common causes of OP, among them hyperparathyroidism, hyperthyroidism, anemias, and osteogenesis imperfecta. The presence of subperiosteal resorption, resorption of the distal tufts, rugger jersey spine, brown tumors, and/or soft tissue calcification support the diagnosis of hyperparathyroidism. Cranial vault thickening, under-pneumatization of the sinuses, and/or soft tissue extramedullary hematopoiesis are pathognomonic for severe anemias. Short stature, multiple fractures in varying states of healing, and profound OP indicate the presence of osteogenesis imperfecta (Fig. 18.3).

Idiopathic juvenile OP, radiographically identical to senile OP, is also a diagnosis of exclusion. This self-limited disorder undergoes spontaneous recovery and is distinguished from senile OP on the basis of patient age.

REFERENCES

Adami, S., Gatti, D., Rossini, M., Adamoli, A., James, G., Girardello, S., & Zamberlan, N. (1992). The radiological assessment of vertebral osteoporosis. *Bone*, **2**, S33–6.

Aguado, F., Revilla, M., Villa, L. F., & Rico, H. (1997). Cortical bone resorption in osteoporosis. *Calcif. Tissue Int.*, **60**, 323–6.

Ahl, T., Dalen, N., Nilsson, H., & Dahlborn, M. (1993). Trabecular patterns of the calcaneum as an index of osteoporosis. A comparison using gamma-absorptiometry. *Int. Orthop.*, **17**, 266–8.

Chan, K. K., Sartoris, D. J., Haghighi, P., Sledge, P., Barrett-Connor, E., Trudell, D. T., & Resnick, D. (1997). Cupid's bow contour of the vertebral body: evaluation of pathogenesis with bone densitometry and imaging–histopathologic correlation. *Radiology*, **202**, 253–6.

Epstein, S., Shane, E., & Bilezikian, J. P. (1995). Organ transplantation and osteoporosis. *Curr. Opin. Rheum.*, **7**, 255–61.

Ginsberg, J. S., Kowalchuk, G., Hirsh, J., Brill-Edwards, P., Burrows, R., Coates, G., & Webber, C. (1990). Heparin effect on bone density. *Thromb. Haemost.*, **64**, 286–9.

Guglielmi, G., Selby, K., Blunt, B. A., Jergas, M., Newitt, D. C., Genant, H. K., & Majumdar, S. (1996). Magnetic resonance of the calcaneus: preliminary assessment of trabecular bone-dependent regional variations in marrow relaxation time compared with dual X-ray absorptiometry. *Acad. Radiol.*, **3**, 336–43.

Koot, V. C., Kesselaer, S. M., Clevers, G. J., de Hooge, P., Weits, T., & van der Werken, C. (1996). Evaluation of the Singh index for measuring osteoporosis. *J. Bone Joint Surg.*, **78B**, 831–4.

La Fianza, A., Taverna, E., Pistorio, A., Pallavicini, D., Preda, L., Di Maggio, E. M., Caprotti, A., Candiani, T., Parrini, M., & Campani, R. (1997). Speed of calcaneal ultrasound attenuation in the identification of vertebral fractures in patients with senile osteoporosis. *Radiol. Med.*, **93**, 51–5.

Majumdar, S. & Genant, H. K. (1995). A review of the recent advances in magnetic resonance imaging in the assessment of osteoporosis. *Osteoporos. Int.*, **5**, 79–92.

Meema, H. E. (1991). Radiologic study of endosteal, intracortical, and periosteal surfaces of hand bones in metabolic bone diseases. *Hand Clin.*, **7**, 37–51.

Pacifici, R., Rupich, R., Griffin, M., Chines, A., Susman, N., & Avioli, L. V. (1990). Dual energy radiography versus quantitative computer tomography for the diagnosis of osteoporosis. *J. Clin. Endocrinol. Metab.*, **70**, 705–10.

Picado, C. & Luengo, M. (1996). Corticosteroid-induced bone loss. Prevention and management. *Drug Safety*, **15**, 347–59.

Resnick, D. & Niwayama, G. (1988). Diagnosis of bone and joint disorders. In *Osteoporosis*, ed. D. Resnick & G. Niwayama, pp. 2023–85. W. B. Saunders,

Ryan, P. J. & Fogelman, I. (1994). Osteoporotic vertebral fractures: diagnosis with radiography and bone scintigraphy. *Radiology*, **190**, 669–72.

Sastry, N. V., Sridhar, G. R., Reddy, G. N., Davidraju, S., Madhavi, G. V., & Nagamani, G. (1994). Evaluation of osteoporosis in patients with fracture neck of femur using conventional radiography. *J. Assoc. Phys. India.*, **42**, 209–11.

Weissman, B. N (1987). Osteoporosis: radiologic and nuclear medicine procedures. *Public Health Rep.*, **S**, 127–31.

Whitcroft, S. & Stevenson, J. C. (1992). Osteoporosis. *Curr. Opin. Orthop.*, **3**, 77–81.

19

Bone mineral density measurements

Paul D. Miller and Carol Zapalowski

Bone densitometry is accepted as a useful quantitative measurement technique for assessing skeletal status (Miller et al., 1996) and predicting the risk of fragility fractures. Low bone mineral density (BMD) is the most important risk factor for fracture. BMD testing is an objective measurement supported by extensive data showing that low bone mass and future fracture risk are inversely related. Low bone mass is as valuable a predictor of fracture as high cholesterol or high blood pressure are as predictors of their respective clinical outcomes of myocardial infarction and stroke (The WHO Study Group, 1994). Historical risk factors cannot identify the individual patient with low bone mass with adequate certainty (Pouilles et al., 1991). This does not discount the importance of assessing other risk factors for fracture. In conjunction with BMD, risk factors add valuable information required for decisions related to which patients should be treated. Also, some risk factors can be modified to help reduce fracture risk (Cummings, 1996). This is particularly true in the perimenopausal population, or in patients with secondary conditions associated with bone loss.

Diagnosis of osteoporosis using bone densitometry: the WHO criteria

In order for bone densitometry to be utilized for the purpose of identifying asymptomatic individuals at risk for fracture, a paradigm shift in the definition of osteoporosis had to occur. Even though the new definition includes the terms BMD, systemic microarchitectural deterioration, and increased bone fragility, only BMD can be objectively measured at the current time. Prior to the previous consensus statement defining osteoporosis, a diagnosis was made on the basis of the presence of a fragility fracture. Now osteoporosis can be defined on the basis of a certain reduced level of BMD. This definition was implemented in 1991 by the Consensus Development Conference on Osteoporosis and was completed in 1994 by a highly regarded committee of the World Health Organization (WHO) (The WHO Study Group, 1994). The major justification for changing the diagnostic criteria for osteoporosis from one of prevalent fragility fractures to one of low BMD is data estab-

Table 19.1. World Health Organization criteria for the diagnosis of osteopenia and osteoporosis

Osteopenia = T-score <-1.0 and >-2.5
Osteoporosis = T-score <-2.5

lishing the higher risk of a second fracture once the first fracture has occurred. There is a greater risk of additional vertebral fractures as well as hip fracture following the first vertebral fracture. This risk is far greater than the increased risk of a first fracture in elderly individuals who have low bone mass alone (Ross et al., 1991). The logical corollary of this data is the need to identify individuals with low bone mass prior to the occurrence of the first fracture. The WHO criteria for the diagnosis of osteopenia and osteoporosis (Table 19.1) are based on a patient's comparison to peak adult bone mass (PABM) and use standardized scores (T-score). The WHO working group chose to categorize individuals using the number of standard deviations (SD) a patient's bone mass is below the mean of a young normal reference population bone mass. This removes the differences in actual BMD related to machine calibration observed using different manufacturers' equipment. The cutoff point of 2.5 SD below PABM is based on epidemiological data derived from a population of postmenopausal Caucasian women, 50% of whom had already suffered a fragility fracture. Since fracture risk is a gradient, increasing with declining levels of bone mass (Huang et al., 1998), the WHO created a second diagnostic category of osteopenia (low bone mass, T-score >-2.5 but <-1.0 SD) to alert the clinician that individuals with smaller reductions in bone mass merit attention, particularly if they are postmenopausal or have secondary conditions associated with bone loss. Postmenopausal women who are not receiving hormonal replacement therapy (HRT) will predictably lose bone, as will most men and women receiving medications or diagnosed with medical conditions associated with bone loss. As the emphasis on skeletal health shifts from treatment to prevention, the diagnostic category of osteopenia may take on increasing importance. Osteopenic postmenopausal women, not receiving therapy to prevent bone loss may unknowingly continue to lose bone, thereby progressively increasing their fracture risk. Hence, postmenopausal women identified as osteopenic may be targeted for prevention strategies to preserve their skeletal mass. Individuals with osteopenia may also experience fragility fractures, particularly when risk factors for factors are present (Riis et al., 1996). Such factors include increased rates of bone turnover, advancing age, increased likelihood of falling, etc. It is not surprising, therefore, that some of these patients with small reductions in BMD and other risk factors may have fragility fractures.

Table 19.2. World Health Organization criteria for the diagnosis of osteopenia/osteoporosis

Pros and cons
Pro
(i) Provides a simple objective diagnostic number for practitioners to use.
(ii) Recognizes that osteoporosis should be diagnosed prior to the first fragility fracture.
Con
(i) Limited data relating WHO criteria to fracture risk in other races or genders.
(ii) Dependent on peak adult bone mass reference databases.
(iii) Not all low bone mass is osteoporosis.
(iv) Fracture risk is a gradient, not a threshold, and -2.5 SD may be used as a threshold cutoff.
(v) Application to healthy premenopausal, estrogen-replete women and young men is inappropriate.

Like all diagnostic criteria, there are strengths and limitations in the WHO criteria for the diagnosis of osteoporosis. These are listed in Table 19.2. The WHO criteria provide a practitioner with an objective number to be used for the diagnosis of osteoporosis, akin to a blood pressure level of 140/90 for the diagnosis of hypertension. Practitioners are now provided with objective criteria that initiate the cognitive process of assessment leading to intervention. In addition, the WHO criteria stress the importance of making a diagnosis of low bone mass (osteopenia) or osteoporosis before the first fracture occurs.

The limitations presented in Table 19.2 appear to outnumber the strengths. However, this belies the beneficial impact the WHO criteria have had in the prevention and management of osteoporosis. The WHO criteria have facilitated the widespread measurement of bone mass for the identification of individuals at risk for fracture.

One of the limitations of the WHO criteria is the lack of applicability to women of other races and to men. The WHO criteria are based on fracture prevalence in postmenopausal Caucasian women. Similar data in men and women of other racial groups are not well established. Two initial studies have shown that fracture rates in Caucasian men per standard deviation (SD) reduction in BMD parallel that seen in Caucasian women (Lunt et al., 1997; Mussolino et al., 1998). It may, therefore, be reasonable to apply WHO criteria to elderly Caucasian men as well. As prospective fracture data are obtained for other races, the applicability of the WHO criteria can accurately be judged. WHO criteria were never intended to be applied to healthy premenopausal women of any race.

BMD data for the total hip and femoral neck were analyzed from the National Health and Nutrition Examination Survey III (NHANES III), in men and women of different races. These data have helped determine the prevalence of osteoporosis at the hip in men and women of different races, using the WHO criteria (Looker et al., 1995). The incorporation of this common reference database into the three major manufacturers' central dual energy X-ray absorptiometry (DXA) equipment has eliminated the potential for machine-specific misdiagnoses of osteoporosis or osteopenia at the hip (Faulkner et al., 1996). However, as previously mentioned, the relationship between the WHO diagnostic categories and hip fracture risk is unknown except in elderly Caucasian women. Nevertheless, low bone mass in any individual is still the most important factor in the determination of fragility fracture risk.

Skeletal sites other than the hip still use non-uniform reference databases. This is an issue in the field of bone densitometry since one of the basic principles of statistics is that each sample derived from a given population yields a different mean and potentially a different SD. The PABM mean and SD from that mean form the basis of the calculation of the T-score: T-score = (Measured BMD in g/cm^2 − PABM mean in g/cm^2) / PABM SD in g/cm^2. As a consequence, an individual may be classified quite differently if different young normal sample populations are used to create the reference database to which the patient is compared (Ahmed et al., 1997). This presents problems clinically since a patient may be classified differently by various bone mass measurement devices, if each device uses a different young normal reference population. It has been suggested that different T-scores in the same patient measured on various devices are due to the technology or bone type being measured and that different WHO criteria might be needed (i.e., different T-score cutoff levels) according to the bone mass measurement device used. While this hypothesis might be true, these differences might also be related to differences in the SD of the different young normal reference groups used. Such a device-dependent T-score, which classifies individuals differently, will lead to bone mass measurement credibility issues, and patient misclassification. These issues could be resolved by the creation of a standardized uniform reference database for each skeletal site and technique which could be adapted by all the major manufacturers. It has been shown, in postmenopausal women, that bone mass measured by various heel measuring devices (ultrasound and DXA) and hip DXA have similar T-scores when the T-score is calculated using the same young normal reference population (Greenspan et al., 1997). This finding supports the hypothesis that differences in T-scores may be related more to different young normal reference populations than to technology or skeletal site differences. A uniform database could become the gold standard to which future databases could be compared as new techniques emerge. Presently, this uniform database does not exist.

The lack of a standardized reference database not withstanding, the various devices themselves measure bone mineral content per unit volume of bone with extraordinary accuracy and precision (Genant et al., 1996; Grampp et al., 1997). Therefore, comparing a patient's BMC/BMD to the BMC/BMD of a young reference group, as a tool for the assessment of fracture risk rather than the T-score as a diagnostic tool, could minimize discrepancies observed in individual patients measured on different equipment. Absolute fracture risk may be similar, regardless of the technique used if BMC/BMD (or its ultrasound equivalent) is used.

The WHO chose to define osteoporosis on the basis of the T-score, the comparison to the PABM rather than the Z-score, the comparison to age-matched bone mass. Although bone mass declines with advancing age (Arlot et al., 1997), it is illogical to assume that bone loss is desirable or inevitable. If only those individuals who lose more bone than predicted for their age are termed 'diseased,' then many individuals with increased risk of fracture will go unrecognized and untreated. Therefore, even though the bone mass may be at a level that is expected for the patient's age, the risk of fracture is increased and it would be illogical to classify such a bone mass as 'normal.' If the prevalence of osteoporosis was defined using age-matched BMD data, it would not increase with age. This is an illogical approach, since declining bone mass increases the risk for fracture and fracture is the outcome of the disease osteoporosis. Using age-matched Z-scores would result in the under-diagnosis of osteoporosis (The Who Study Group, 1994). This would damage the credibility of bone densitometry by the incorrect reporting 'normal for age' in elderly patients with fragile skeletons or possibly even prevalent fragility fractures. Even if 70% of Caucasian women over the age of 80 years have osteoporosis using the WHO criteria, this is not an over-diagnosis since 50% of these women will suffer a fragility fracture if left untreated (Cummings et al., 1989). Using PABM as the diagnostic level for comparisons recognizes the true magnitude of the osteoporotic problem. Age-matched data is appropriate for comparisons in the growing child or adolescent; however, once PABM is achieved, the desirable clinical goal is to maintain the bone density at that level, not accept losses in excess of those predicted with age. It has been suggested that age-matched Z-scores which are less than -2.0 SD may indicate the presence of a metabolic process causing bone loss other than aging or estrogen deficiency in the postmenopausal population. Though intuitively correct, this suggestion remains an untested hypothesis.

As mentioned previously, the WHO criteria were never meant to be applied to healthy, estrogen-replete premenopausal women. The inappropriate use of these diagnostic criteria may cause undue fear regarding fracture risk and the initiation of inappropriate or excessive therapy. The majority of longitudinal data suggest that healthy, estrogen-replete premenopausal women are not losing bone mass (Riis, 1994). Healthy premenopausal women with low bone mass may not have any

Table 19.3. Techniques for bone mass measurement

Central skeleton
DXA – spine (AP or lateral), or hip
QCT – spine or hip
Peripheral skeleton
DXA – wrist, heel, finger
QCT – wrist
Ultrasound – calcaneus, finger, tibia

greater current fracture risk than their age-matched peers with normal BMD. The scant fracture data available in young people is cross-sectional, assessed small numbers or have wide confidence intervals (Marshall et al., 1996). Healthy young individuals may be inappropriately restricted in their activities or have reduced quality of life by the inappropriate application of the WHO criteria. Since PABM follows a normal distribution, the discovery of low bone mass in healthy premenopausal women does not necessarily mean that bone loss has occurred. It may simply represent a genetically determined low PABM. Such individuals require assessment to exclude secondary causes of potential bone loss, conservative prevention advice, a repeat bone mass measurement in 2 years to assure that bone loss is not occurring, and prompt protection of their skeleton at the menopause. There are presently no data to suggest that additional pharmacological intervention with bisphosphonates, calcitonin, or estrogen analogs has any value in the premenopausal, estrogen-replete woman.

Why are bone mass measurements performed?

There are three clinical applications for bone mass measurement. Each has a distinct value in clinical decision-making. The three applications are:
  (i) diagnosis of osteopenia or osteoporosis;
  (ii) fracture risk prediction;
  (iii) serial monitoring to measure response to intervention(s) or diseases/medications that effect bone.
Clinicians have at their disposal various devices that measure bone mineral density. These devices are characterized as central or peripheral. Central devices measure the spine or the hip and peripheral devices measure the wrist, heel, or finger. These devices are listed in Table 19.3.

For each of the three applications of bone density measurement listed above, the central and peripheral devices have advantages and disadvantages (Miller & McClung, 1996; Baran et al., 1997).

The diagnosis of osteopenia and osteoporosis

The diagnosis of osteopenia (T-score of < -1.0 but > -2.5) is clinically important independent of fracture risk assessment. This diagnostic category represents the range of bone density for which prevention strategies for early postmenopausal bone loss are designed. It has been shown that the recognition of low bone mass in early postmenopausal women facilitates the acceptance of hormone replacement therapy (HRT) (Rubin & Cummings, 1992). It will most likely be the same for the other FDA-approved interventions for the prevention of early postmenopausal bone loss such as bisphosphonates and the selective estrogen receptor modulators (SERMs). These agents are recommended for the prevention of bone loss in post-menopausal women with T-scores < -1.0 who are unwilling or unable to utilize HRT.

The utility of central or peripheral sites in detecting osteopenia is dependent upon the age of the patient and on the particular skeletal site measured. BMD is discordant throughout the skeleton, and this discordance is greater in the early menopausal population than in the elderly (> 65 years) population (Arlot et al., 1997; Pouilles et al., 1993). In the elderly, the greater concordance in BMD at various skeletal sites reduces the likelihood of missing a diagnosis of osteopenia or osteoporosis when only one skeletal site is measured. However, in the elderly, if only the AP spine is measured by DXA, osteophytes and/or facet sclerosis of the posterior elements may falsely increase the value causing misdiagnosis (Greenspan et al., 1995). In the elderly, central measurements except the AP spine and all peripheral measurements have equivalent value for diagnosing osteopenia or osteoporosis. The lack of prospective fracture data for lateral spine DXA measurements is a major obstacle to its utilization for diagnosis. However, the very strong correlation between lateral spine DXA-BMD and QCT-BMD, the latter of which has adequate fracture predictive data, would strongly suggest that, in the elderly, low lateral spine DXA values should predict increased fracture risk (Finkelstein et al., 1994).

Although central and peripheral BMD sites appear to have equal diagnostic utility in elderly women, this may not be true for perimenopausal women due to skeletal discordance in BMD. There are at least three potential explanations for this discordance:

(i) differences in development of PABM at various sites (Bonnick et al., 1997);

(ii) differences in rates of bone loss between cancellous bone and cortical bone;

(iii) differences in the accuracy of measuring BMC using various techniques.

Yet, data suggests that, in early menopausal women, if one skeletal site is osteo-porotic (T-score < -2.5 SD), then there is less than a 10% chance that any other skeletal site will be normal (Arlot et al., 1997; Nelson et al., 1998). Published studies have not yet clarified how many early postmenopausal women have normal BMD at one site and osteopenia at another. These numbers may not be insignificant.

Table 19.4. Patients with a normal peripheral bone mass who may need additional bone mass testing

---

(i) Postmenopausal patients concerned about osteoporosis, not receiving HRT, but would accept HRT, bisphosphonates or SERMs if BMD is found to be low.

(ii) Patients at high risk for hip fracture, who have a maternal history of hip fracture, who are >5′7″ tall, who weigh <127 lb., or who smoke.

(iii) Patients receiving medications associated with bone loss (e.g., glucocorticoids, antiseizure medications, chronic heparin, etc.).

(iv) Patients with secondary conditions associated with low bone mass or bone loss (e.g., hyperparathyroidism, malabsorption, hemigastrectomy, hyperthyroidism, etc.).

(v) Patients found to have high urinary collagen cross-links (>1.0 SD above the upper limit for premenopausal women), where more rapid bone loss may be present.

(vi) Patients with a history of fragility fractures.

Hence, many early menopausal women may need additional BMD testing if a single skeletal site measurement is normal in order to diagnose osteopenia. This is particularly true if the woman has additional risk factors for low BMD or if a diagnosis of osteopenia would change the pharmacological preventive intervention. Patients with a normal single skeletal site BMD who may need additional BMD tests are described in Table 19.4. These guidelines are required to minimize the potential for misdiagnosis (Miller et al., 1998).

There are other patient populations in which a diagnosis of osteopenia may lead to changes in intervention strategies. The prevention of bone loss associated with glucocorticoid therapy is recommended in patients with T-scores <−1.0 (Reid, 1998). It may also be appropriate to intervene in other medical conditions associated with bone loss (i.e., hyperthyroidism, hyperparathyroidism, post-transplantation, etc.) based on a finding of osteopenia.

The prediction of fracture risk

There is little debate that low bone mass is the most important predictor of fragility fracture. Approximately 80% of the variance in bone strength and resistance of bone to fracture in animal models is explained by the bone mineral content per unit volume of bone. Other risk factors are predictive of fracture but some are not as objectively quantifiable as bone mass and some are not modifiable (Cummings et al., 1995). Risk factors such as increased height (>5′7″), low body weight (<127 lb.), smoking or maternal history of hip fracture are strong predictors of hip fracture. However, BMD is an objective, quantifiable measurement that offers clinical value akin to showing patients their blood pressure or cholesterol measurement on a printed sheet. Bone loss can now be halted, and gains in bone density can be achieved. Increased height or maternal history of hip fracture independently increase fracture risk but there is no way to modify these risk factors.

The relationship between fracture risk and bone density is best described as a gradient rather than as a threshold. The diagnostic category of osteopenia can be used to initiate preventive interventions in early menopausal women, in order to reduce lifetime fracture risk and as a predictor of current fragility fracture risk in elderly women. A 1.0 SD reduction in BMD is associated with increased fracture risk and is greater at the same level of BMD as age increases (Hui et al., 1988). Since bone loss is an asymptomatic process, identifying small reductions in bone mass in the early menopausal patients is important to allow early intervention to halt bone loss, since fracture risk will continue to increase as BMD decreases and age increases. Some patients will fracture with BMD which is only minimally reduced (osteopenia) due to the effects of other factors that lead to bone fragility. In some of these patients, the rate of bone turnover, or the nature of a fall may lead to fracture with only minimal reduction in BMD (Garnero et al., 1996; Greenspan et al., 1994; Riis et al., 1996).

Fracture prediction can be expressed as current fracture risk or lifetime fracture risk. Current risk is the risk of fracture within 3–5 years of the bone mass measurement. Current fracture risk can be expressed as relative risk (RR), absolute risk or incidence, or annual risk. Relative risk, the ratio of two absolute risks, is increased 1.5–3 times for each 1.0 SD reduction in BMD (Cummings et al., 1993; Ross et al., 1991). All the data available in the elderly suggest that fracture prediction is not dependent upon the skeletal site measured or on the technique (central or peripheral) used (Cummings et al., 1993; Yates et al., 1995). This observation is probably related to the concordance of bone mass at different skeletal sites in the elderly population. Thus, in this elderly population, low BMD measured at one site is more likely to represent a global reduction in BMD. The only exception is the prediction of hip fracture risk, which appears to be better if the BMD at the proximal femoral sites are used (Cummings et al., 1993). This observation does not, however, diminish the strong predictive value that peripheral bone mass measurement has for the prediction of hip fracture. Data on current fracture risk have been obtained only in elderly Caucasian women due to the fact that younger women fracture infrequently and are not therefore, included in studies designed to determine current fracture risk.

Current fracture risk data should not be applied to younger perimenopausal women or premenopausal women with low PABM. Even though one prospective and a few cross-sectional studies suggest that low BMD in adolescents or premenopausal women is associated with higher current fracture risk (Duppe et al., 1997; Goulding et al., 1998), the number of patients included in such studies is small or the confidence intervals so wide that conclusions are difficult to reach. Clearly, advancing age, over 60 years, is an independent predictor of fracture. For discussion, it is correct to state that the current fracture risk of a 50-year-old woman at a given level of BMD is substantially lower than the current fracture risk of a 70-year-old woman with the same BMD (Hui et al., 1988). However, the 50-year-old woman with low BMD may have a greater lifetime fracture risk than her 50-year-old counterpart with a normal BMD (Black et al., 1992; Kanis, 1997). However, no direct data exists to support this conclusion. Certainly, if the 50-year-old woman with low bone mass is postmenopausal, she should be strongly advised to instigate options to maintain her BMD, without altering her normal life activities.

Intuitively, a 50-year-old woman with low bone mass may have a higher lifetime fracture risk than her peer with a normal BMD. Most postmenopausal women lose bone mass after the menopause without intervention. Therefore, untreated post-menopausal women are expected to lose bone mass as they age, and this will be associated with an increased current fracture risk. However, all lifetime fracture prediction models are hypothetical, and have not yet been validated by direct longitudinal data (Cummings et al., 1989; Huang et al., 1998; Kanis, 1997). Clinically, however, it is useful to discuss the implications of low bone mass at the menopause relative to probable lifetime fracture risk, since it may facilitate the acceptance of HRT or other pharmacological prevention interventions.

Serial assessments of bone mass

Bone densitometry can be used for serial monitoring of the natural progression of disease processes (such as primary hyperparathyroidism) or for monitoring the response of bone to pharmacological interventions. There is currently a clear advantage of the central skeleton over the peripheral skeleton for serial monitoring. In monitoring the response of bone to estrogens, SERMs, bisphosphonates, or calcitonin the axial skeleton consistently demonstrates the greatest magnitude of change in the shortest period of time (Lufkin et al., 1992; Watts et al., 1990). The femur tends to demonstrate changes in response to pharmacological interventions, though at rates lower than the spine, while little or no change is observed at the wrist, finger or heel. The reason peripheral skeletal sites have a limited response to pharmacological intervention is unclear. It is not due to the precision of the measurement of peripheral techniques, which is excellent (1.0%). Several hypotheses have been suggested to explain this observation, such as differences in the bone marrow environment of the peripheral skeleton vs. the central skeleton, differences in surface area of bone, and differences in blood flow between the two bone compartments. No matter which hypothesis is correct, the reality is that the bone mass of the spine and hip is more responsive to pharmacological intervention. There is some limited data, suggesting that forearm bone mass measurements may be useful in monitoring the response to HRT in individual patients (Christiansen & Lindsay,

1990) and that calcaneal ultrasound may show changes to pharmacological inter-ventions as well. These studies need to be repeated and confirmed.

The forearm appears to be the best skeletal site to monitor the effects of excess parathyroid hormone activity (Silverberg et al., 1989). It may also be valuable in decisions regarding the timing of surgical parathyroidectomy.

The change observed between serial BMD measurements can be expressed as a percentage change (% change) between two measurements or absolute change (in g/cm^2) between two measurements. Change expressed in either format is accept-able, providing the precision of the measurement is available from the testing facil-ity. Individual DXA manufacturers may publish precision errors of 1% or less at the AP spine, when in fact, their precision error may be 3–4% in the elderly population with low BMD values (Faulkner & McClung, 1995). This is due to an increased pre-cision error (coefficient of variation) as the BMD declines at each skeletal site. In addition, variability may be introduced by the technologist during positioning or analysis which will increase the precision error even in individuals with normal BMD. Once the precision error is known, then the significance of a change in serial BMD may be determined. At the 95% confidence level, a significant change in two serial BMD values is at least 2.77 times the precision error. For example, if the pre-cision error is 1.5%, then a 4.16% change (magnitude of change necessary for 95% confidence $= 1.5\% \times 2.77$ or 4.16%) is required between two BMD measurements to be significant at the 95% confidence level. However, if the precision error is 3%, then it would require almost a 9% change (magnitude of change necessary for 95% confidence $= 3\% \times 2.77$ or 8.31%) to be 95% confident that a true change in BMD has occurred. Misleading conclusions may be drawn, based on non-significant serial changes, with attending inappropriate alterations in treatments, if precision errors are not known.

In contrast, absolute change in serial BMD has a small margin of error because the SD of BMD is reasonably constant over a wide range of BMD. Any change in BMD greater than $0.04 \ g/cm^2$ at the AP spine or $0.05 \ g/cm^2$ at the femoral neck will generally be significant at the 95% confidence level. Absolute change is calculated by subtracting the second BMD measurement from the baseline measurement. In the medical literature serial change has generally been expressed as a percentage; however, either method described above is valid. BMD testing for serial monitor-ing is generally performed no more often than every 12–24 months, depending upon the disease process or therapeutic intervention being monitored. In patients who have a documented response to pharmacological intervention, which may be defined as either a gain or no loss in BMD, annual BMD measurements may not be necessary. In patients with a documented response to HRT, repeat BMD measure-ments every 3–5 years may improve the poor long-term compliance to therapy.

Even in elderly women who have been previously documented to be estrogen responders, a 3–5 year BMD testing interval may be used to document continued response and compliance to therapy, since age-related bone loss may induce BMD loss even with continual estrogen use (Cauley et al., 1995).

It is very difficult to compare serial changes in BMD when the measurements are performed on different manufacturers' machines. It is often difficult to compare values obtained from different machines from the same manufacturer. It would be ideal if patients had serial measurements performed on the same machine by the same technician. However, this is unrealistic in today's world. Given the proprietary design of the various devices and the differences in calibration, the absolute BMD values from different machines in an individual patient will not be the same. Even when the machines are made by the same manufacturer, slight differences in calibration or differences in technique during data acquisition will introduce error. The establishment of the standardized BMD (sBMD), by the International Bone Densitometry Standards Committee, allows for better comparisons to be made between BMD values obtained on different manufacturers' equipment. Utilizing the calculated sBMD of the spine and hip for serial comparison reduces, but does not eliminate the variance in the measurements. As a general rule, even using sBMD, an additional 1% precision error should be added to the calculation of percentage change.

Conclusions

Bone densitometry has revolutionized the clinical approach to osteoporosis. Much as the sphygmomanometer changed the field of hypertension and the prediction of the risk of stroke, bone densitometry provides a direct measurement of bone mineral density which is directly related to fracture risk. If the results of bone densitometry are used responsibly and competently, patient care will be enhanced. The measurement of bone mineral density enables physicians and their patients to make informed decisions regarding preventive and therapeutic strategies. It also allows the physician to monitor the longitudinal efficacy of these interventions.

REFERENCES

Ahmed, A. I. H., Blake, G. M., Rymer, J. M., & Fogelman, I. (1997). Screening for osteopenia and osteoporosis: do the accepted normal ranges lead to overdiagnosis? *Osteoporos. Int.*, 7, 432–8.

Arlot, M. E., Sornay-Rendu, E., Garnero, P., Vey-Marty, B., & Delmas, P. D. (1997). Apparent pre- and postmenopausal bone loss evaluated by DXA at different skeletal sites in women: the OLEFY cohort. *J. Bone Miner. Res.*, 12, 683–90.

Baran, D. T., Faulkner, K. G., Genant, H. K., Miller, P. D., & Pacifici, R. (1997). Diagnosis and management of osteoporosis: guidelines for the utilization of bone densitometry. *Calcif. Tissue Int.*, **61**, 433–40.

Black, D. M., Cummings, S. R., & Melton, L. J. (1992). Appendicular bone mineral and a woman's lifetime risk of hip fracture. *J. Bone Miner. Res.*, 7, 639–45.

Bonnick, S. L., Nichols, D. L., Sanborn, C. F., Lloyd, K., Payne, S. G., Lewis, L., & Reed, C. A. (1997). Dissimilar spine and femoral Z-scores in premenopausal women. *Calcif. Tissue Int.*, **61**, 263–5.

Cauley, J. A., Seeley, D. G., Ensrud, K., Ettinger, B., Black, D., & Cummings, S. R. (1995). Estrogen replacement therapy and fracture in older women. *Ann. Intern. Med.*, **122**, 9–16.

Christiansen, C. & Lindsay, R. (1990). Estrogens, bone loss and preservation. *Osteoporos. Int.*, 1, 7–12.

Cummings, S. R. (1996). Treatable and untreatable risk factors for hip fracture. *Bone*, **18**, 165S–7S.

Cummings, S. R., Black, D. M., Nevitt, M. C., Browner, W., Cauley, J., Ensrud, K., Genant, H. K., Palermo, L., Scott, J., & Vogt, T. M. (1993). Bone density at various sites for prediction of hip fracture. *Lancet*, **341**, 72–5.

Cummings, S. R., Black, D. M., & Rubin, S. M. (1989). Lifetime risks of hip, Colles' or vertebral fracture and coronary heart disease among White postmenopausal women. *Arch. Int. Med.*, **149**, 2445–8.

Cummings, S. R., Nevitt, M. C., Browner, W. S., Stone, K., Fox, K. M., Ensrud, K. E., Cauley, J., Black, D., & Vogt, T. M. (1995). Risk factors for hip fracture in White women. *N. Engl. J. Med.*, **332**, 767–73.

Duppe, H., Gardsell, P., Nilsson, B., & Johnell, O. (1997). A single bone density measurement can predict fractures over 25 years. *Calcif. Tissue Int.*, **60**, 171–4.

Faulkner, K. G. & McClung, M. R. (1995). Quality control of DXA instruments in multicenter trials. *Osteoporos. Int.*, **5**, 218–27.

Faulkner, K. G., Roberts, L. A., & McClung, M. R. (1996). Discrepancies in normative data between Lunar and Hologic DXA system. *Osteoporos. Int.*, **6**, 432–6.

Finkelstein, J. S., Cleary, R. L., Butler, J. P., Antonelli, R., Mitlak, B. H., Deraska, D. J., Zamora-Quezada, J. C., & Neer, R. M. (1994). A comparison of lateral versus anterior-posterior spine dual energy X-ray absorptiometry for the diagnosis of osteopenia. *J. Clin. Endocrinol. Metab.*, **78**, 724–30.

Garnero, P., Hausherr, E., Chapuy, M-C., Marcelli, C., Grandjean, H., Muller, C., Cornier, C., Breart, G., Meunier, P. J., & Delmas, P. D. (1996). Markers of bone resorption predict hip fracture in elderly women: the EPIDOS prospective study. *J. Bone Miner. Res.*, **11**, 1531–7.

Genant, H. K., Engelke, K., Furst, T., Gluer, C. C., Gramp, S., Harris, S. T., Jergas, M., Lang, T., Lu, V., Majumdar, S., Mathur, A., & Takeda, M. (1996). Noninvasive assessment of bone mineral and structure: state of the art. *J. Bone Miner. Res.*, **11**, 707–30.

Goulding, A., Cannan, R., Williams, S. M., Gold, E. J., Taylor, R. W., & Lewis-Barned, N. J. (1998). Bone mineral density in girls with forearm fractures. *J. Bone Miner. Res.*, **13**, 143–8.

Grampp, S., Genant, H. K., Mathur, A., Lang, P., Jergas, M., Takada, M., Gluer, C-C., Lu, Y., & Chavez, M. (1997). Comparisons of noninvasive bone mineral measurements is assessing age-related loss, fracture discrimination, and diagnostic classification. *J. Bone Miner. Res.*, 12, 697–711.

Greenspan, S. L., Bouxsein, M. L., Melton, M. E., Kolodny, A. H., Clair, J. H., Delucca, P. T., Stek, M. Jr., Faulkner, K. G., & Orwoll, E. S. (1997). Precision and discriminatory ability of calcaneal bone assessment technlogies. *J. Bone Miner. Res.*, 12, 1303–13.

Greenspan, S. L., Maitland-Ramsey, L., & Myers, E. (1995). Classification of osteoporosis in the elderly is dependent on site-specific analysis. *Calcif. Tissue Int.*, 58, 409–14.

Greenspan, S. L., Myers, E. R., Maitland, L. A., Resnick, N. M., & Hayes, W. C. (1994). Fall severity and bone mineral density as risk factors for hip fracture in ambulatory elderly. *JAMA*, 271, 128–33.

Huang, C., Ross, P. D., & Wasnich, R. D. (1998). Short-term and long-term fracture prediction by bone mass measurements: a prospective study. *J. Bone Miner. Res.*, 13, 107–13.

Hui, S. L., Slemenda, C. W., & Johnston, C. C. Jr. (1988). Age and bone mass as predictors of fracture in a prospective study. *J. Clin. Invest.*, 81, 1804–9.

Kanis, J. A. (1997). Diagnosis of osteoporosis. *Osteoporos. Int.*, 7(S3),S108–16.

Looker, A. C., Wahner, H. W., Dunn, W. L., Calvo, M. E., Harris, T. B., Heyse, S. P., Johnson, C. C. Jr., & Lindsay, R. L. (1995). Proximal femur bone mineral levels of US adults. *Osteoporos. Int.*, 5, 389–409.

Lufkin, E. G., Wahner, H. W., O'Fallon, W. M., Hodgson, S. F., Kotowicz, M. A., Lane, A. W., Judd, H. L., Caplan, R. H., & Riggs, B. L. (1992). Treatment of postmenopausal osteoporosis with transdermal estrogen. *Ann. Intern. Med.*, 117, 1–9.

Lunt, M., Felsenberg, D., Reeve, J., Benevolenskaya, J., Cannata, J., Dequeker, J., Dodenhof, C., Falch, J. A., Masaryk, P., Pols, H. A. P., Poor, G., Reid, D. M., Scheidt-Nave, C., Weber, K., Varlow, J., Kanis, J. A., O'Neill, T. W., & Silman, A. J. (1997). Bone density variation and its effect on risk of vertebral deformity in men and women studied in thirteen European centers: the EVOS study. *J. Bone Miner. Res.*, 12, 1883–94.

Marshall, D., Johnell, O., & Wedel, H. (1996). Meta-analysis of how well measures of bone mineral density predict occurrence of osteoporotic fractures. *Br. Med. J.*, 312, 1254–9.

Miller, P. D. & McClung, M. (1996). Prediction of fracture risk I: bone density. *Am. J. Med. Sci.*, 312, 257–9.

Miller, P. D., Bonnick, S. L., Johnston, C. C. Jr., Kleerekoper, M., Lindsay, R. L., Sherwood, L. M., and Siris, E. S. (1998). The challenges of peripheral bone density testing. *J. Clin. Densitometry*, 1, 1–7.

Miller, P. D., Bonnick, S. L., & Rosen, C. J. (1996). Clinical utility of bone mass measurements in adults: consensus of an international panel. *Semin. Arthritis Rheum.*, 25, 361–72.

Mussolino, M. E., Looker, A. C., Madans, J. H., Langlois, J. A., & Orwoll, E. S. (1998). Risk factors for hip fracture in White men: the NHANES I epidemiological follow-up study. *J. Bone Miner. Res.*, 13, 918–25.

Nelson, D. A., Molloy, R., & Kleerekoper, M. (1998). Prevalence of osteoporosis in women referred for bone density testing: utility of multiple skeletal sites. *J. Clin. Densitometry*, 1, 5–12.

Pouilles, J. M., Ribot, C., & Tremollieres, F. (1991). Risk factors of vertebral osteoporosis: results of a study of 2279 women referred to a menopause clinic. *Rev. Rheum. Mal. Osteoarth.*, 58, 169–77.

Pouilles, J. M., Tremollieres, F., & Ribot, C. (1993). Spine and femur densitometry at the meno-pause: are both sites necessary in the assessment of the risk of osteoporosis? *Calcif. Tissue Int.*, 52, 344–7.

Reid, I. (1998). Glucocorticoid-induced osteoporosis: assessment and treatment. *J. Clin. Densitometry*, 1, 55–65.

Riis, B. J. (1994). Premenopausal bone loss: fact or artifact? *Osteoporos. Int.*, S1, S35–7.

Riis, B. J., Hansen, M. A., Jensen, A. M., Overgaard, K., & Christiansen, C. (1996). Low bone mass and fast rate of bone loss at menopause: equal risk factors for future fracture: a 15-year follow-up study. *Bone*, 19, 9–12.

Ross, P. D., Davis, J. W., Epstein, R. S., & Wasnich, R. D. (1991). Pre-existing fractures and bone mass predict vertebral fracture incidence in women. *Ann. Intern. Med.*, 114, 919–23.

Rubin, S. M. & Cummings, S. R. (1992). Results of bone densitometry affect women's decisions about taking measures to prevent fractures. *Ann. Intern. Med.*, 116, 990–5.

Silverberg, S. J., Shane, E., de la Cruz, L., Dempster, D. W., Feldman, F., Seldin, D., Jacobs, T. P., Siris, E. S., Cafferty, M., Parisien, M. V., Lindsay, R., Clemens, T. L., & Bilezikian, J. P. (1989). Skeletal disease in primary hyperparathyroidism. *J. Bone Miner. Res.*, 4, 283–91.

The WHO Study Group (1994). *Assessment of Fracture Risk and its Application to Screening for Postmenopausal Osteoporosis*. Geneva: World Health Organization.

Watts, N. B., Harris, S. T., Genant, H. K., Wasnich, R. D., Miller, P. D., Jackson, R. D., Licata, A. A., Ross, P., Woodson, G. C., Yanover, M. J., Mysiw, W. J., Kohse, L., Rao, M. B., Steiger, P., Richmond, B., & Chesnut, C. H. III (1990). Intermittent cyclic etidronate treatment of post-menopausal osteoporosis. *N. Engl. J. Med.*, 323, 73–9.

Yates, A. J., Ross, P. D., Lydick, E., & Epstein, R. S. (1995). Radiographic absorptiometry in the diagnosis of osteoporosis. *Am. J. Med.*, 98(S2A),41S–7S.

20

Hormone replacement therapy

Jonathan D. Adachi and Alexandra Papaioannou

The effects of hormone replacement therapy (HRT) on bone cannot be discussed in isolation, and the risks and benefits of therapy must be addressed as they relate to each individual. Hormone replacement therapy has been shown to have a positive impact on bone mineral density (BMD) in all areas of the skeleton that have been studied and has been shown to reduce the risk of osteoporotic fractures. Positive effects of estrogen on the cardiovascular system have also been reported; however, more recently there is evidence to the contrary. The association of unopposed estrogen therapy to uterine cancer is established and it is felt that the addition of a progestational agent reduces that risk. The potential association of estrogen therapy with increased risk of breast cancer remains an area of controversy. However, it is likely that there is a slight increase in risk. HRT unequivocally aids with menopausal symptoms and is the reason most women consider it. Hot flashes, flushes, and urogenital symptoms may be improved with HRT. Recent suggestions that associate improved memory with HRT are encouraging, but require further study. As is evident, the amount of information that needs to be assimilated by both patient and physician is formidable, making the decision to commence HRT a difficult one. This chapter is an attempt to summarize a very complex and changing area.

Effects of hormone replacement therapy on bone

Cellular effects

The cellular hallmark of bone loss caused by estrogen deficiency is increased bone remodeling and is characterized by an imbalance of bone resorption over bone formation. The osteoclast plays a crucial role in the imbalance seen with estrogen deficiency. An increase in the proliferation and differentiation of hematopoietic osteoclast progenitors, an increase in stromal/osteoblastic cell number and support of osteoclast formation and a decrease in the incidence of osteoclast apoptosis is seen with ovariectomy (Jilka, 1998).

An increase in interleukin-1 (IL-1), interleukin-6 (IL-6) and tumor necrosis factor (TNF) occurs with the loss of estrogen. IL-1, IL-6 and TNF stimulate osteo-clast progenitor replication and differentiation. An important characteristic of these cytokines that regulate osteoclast formation is their ability to stimulate their own and each other's synthesis in an autocrine and synergistic fashion. Not only do IL-1, IL-6, and TNF induce their own synthesis, but TNF acts synergistically with IL-1 to stimulate both TNF and IL-6. Parathyroid hormone also acts synergistically with TNF to stimulate IL-6 production. Consistent with evidence that IL-6 medi-ates the increase in osteoclast formation caused by estrogen deficiency, estrogen suppresses production of IL-6, by inhibiting the IL-1- and TNF-stimulated biosyn-thesis of IL-6 in stromal/osteoblastic cells (Jilka, 1998).

The differentiation into functional osteoclasts depends on factors that are pro-duced by stromal/osteoblastic cells. Physical contact between the progenitors and the support cells is thought to be required. It is likely that stromal/osteoblastic cells represent a subset of the marrow stromal cells that support hematopoiesis. They are in intimate contact with the endocortical and cancellous bone surfaces, as well as with marrow monocytes, hematopoietic progenitors, and the endothelial cells lining the blood vessels of the extravascular intersinusoidal space. Thus, they are ideally poised to respond to endocrine factors such as sex steroids and PTH, that are present in the circulation, as well as to the cytokines and growth factors that are made in the bone marrow. Together with increased cytokine production, changes in the number and activity of stromal/osteoblastic cells appear to play a key role in the increased osteoclast formation caused by estrogen deficiency. Ovariectomy stimulates osteoblast formation, as indicated by the finding of an increased number of osteoblast progenitors in the murine bone marrow (Jilka et al., 1998). In view of the close relationship of stromal/osteoblastic cells to the osteoblast lineage, it is likely that the number of cells capable of supporting osteoclast formation is also increased in estrogen deficiency.

Recent findings indicate that apoptosis is stimulated by estrogen either directly or indirectly, via the regulation of cytokines that influence osteoclast apoptosis. In vitro studies have demonstrated that TGF stimulates osteoclast apoptosis, while IL-1, TNF, and IL-6 inhibit it (Jilka, 1998). Thus, it is highly likely that an ovariectomy-induced increase in the latter cytokines, together with decreased levels of TGF, prolongs the lifespan of osteoclasts.

The effects of HRT on bone mineral density

A number of RCTs have demonstrated that HRT has a beneficial effect on bone mineral density (BMD). (Adami et al., 1989; Blake et al., 1993; Komulainen et al., 1997; Lufkin et al., 1992; Nachtigall et al., 1979; Speroff et al., 1996; The Writing Group for the PEPI Trial, 1996)

The PEPI study was a 3-year randomized controlled trial (RCT) comparing a variety of estrogen treatment regimens to placebo looking at spine and hip BMD as outcome measures (The Writing Group for the PEPI Trial, 1996). Those assigned to the placebo group lost an average of 1.8% of spine BMD and 1.7% of hip BMD by the 3-year visit, while those assigned to active regimens gained BMD at both sites, ranging from 3.5% to 5.0% mean total increases in spinal BMD and a mean total increase of 1.7% of BMD in the hip measurements. Older women, women with low initial BMD, and those with no previous hormone use gained significantly more bone than younger women, women with higher initial BMD, and those who had used hormones previously. They concluded that estrogen replacement therapy increases BMD at clinically important sites.

Withdrawal of estrogen results in the loss of bone at rates similar to those seen in patients who are not on treatment (Christiansen et al., 1981).

There is evidence that long-term estrogen therapy is of benefit in the prevention of bone loss. One 10-year, double-blind prospective study was undertaken to evaluate the effects of estrogen replacement therapy (Nachtigall et al., 1979). Estrogen-treated patients whose therapy started within 3 years of menopause showed improvement or no increase in osteoporosis. A second 10-year study found that lumbar spine BMD was significantly higher in HRT-treated women than in those who remained untreated with an increase of 13.1% from baseline values on HRT compared with a reduction of 4.7% without therapy (Eiken et al., 1996). Forearm bone mineral content decreased by 0.7% over the 10-year period in the HRT group compared with a reduction of 17.6% in untreated women ($P<0.001$). These results confirm that long-term HRT exerts a continuous effect against bone loss in postmenopausal women.

The protective effect of HRT against bone loss appears to be of greater benefit at the vertebral body, and to have a more modest effect at the proximal femur, suggesting that HRT may be a more effective means of reducing the risk of vertebral fractures than hip fractures (Christiansen et al., 1981; Duan et al., 1997; Hillard et al., 1994; Lufkin et al., 1992).

Several randomized controlled trials have clearly demonstrated a dose-response relationship between the dose of estrogen and BMD. (Ettinger et al., 1992; Field et al., 1998; Harris et al., 1991; Speroff et al., 1996) The effects of cyclical treatment with estrone sulfate (0.3, 0.625, 1.25 mg), and calcium carbonate, on spinal trabecular bone density were compared with a placebo in 120 postmenopausal women in the 2-year, multicenter, double-blind study (Harris et al., 1991). The data suggest that 0.625 mg and 1.25 mg of estrone sulfate had different effects than placebo and 0.3 mg of estrone sulfate, given with supplemental calcium, are effective doses for the prevention of spinal bone loss. In a double-blind, dose-ranging, RCT, over an 18-month period, the degree of protection against postmenopausal bone loss afforded by micronized estradiol in dosages of 0.5, 1.0 and 2.0 mg was tested

(Ettinger et al., 1992). Micronized estradiol had a continuous skeletal dose-response effect in the range of 0.5 to 2.0 mg and calcium intake positively modified the skeletal response to 1.0 mg micronized estradiol. Three dosages of transdermally administered estradiol on markers of bone loss in 127 women who had recently undergone a surgical menopause was examined in a 2-year double-blind, RCT study (Field et al., 1998). Biochemical indicators of bone metabolism in urine and serum were periodically assessed, as was bone mineral content of the lumbar spine and radius. After 2 years of therapy, a significant dose–response relationship was detected.

Estrogen plays the dominant role in the prevention of bone loss at the time of menopause. In a study examining the effects of estrogen and medroxyprogesterone in the first year following premenopausal ovariectomy, significant bone loss occurred with ovariectomy (Prior et al., 1997). Estrogen therapy reduced the loss while medroxyprogesterone did not. In a study designed to examine the effect of hormone replacement therapy (HRT) and low-dose vitamin D supplementation on the prevention of bone loss in non-osteoporotic early postmenopausal women, low-dose vitamin D supplementation had only a minor effect in the prevention of osteoporosis and did not give any benefit additional to that of HRT alone (Komulainen et al., 1997). This is true at the spine and hip. In a 1-year study, Blake et al., demonstrated that calcium therapy alone leads to ongoing bone loss while estrogen therapy with either a continuous low dose (conjugated estrogens 0.3 mg/day and medroxyprogesterone 2.5 mg/day) or a moderate dose, cyclical (conjugated estrogens 0.625 mg/day and medroxyprogesterone 5 mg/day) regimen prevented this loss of bone (Blake et al., 1993).

Studies have been performed examining the route of administration on bone density (Hillard et al., 1994; Stevenson et al., 1990). They have demonstrated that transdermal estradiol 0.05 mg/day and oral conjugated equine estrogens 0.625 mg/day prevented bone loss in the spine and hip. However, in one study of 3 years' duration, 12% of women on either transdermal or oral treatment lost a significant amount of bone from the femoral neck by 3 years despite adequate compliance (Hillard et al., 1994). They concluded that women taking therapy primarily for hip fracture prevention may require a follow-up bone density measurement to establish the efficacy of treatment.

HRT and vertebral fractures

Most randomized controlled trials have been performed to demonstrate BMD benefit in both primary and secondary prevention. Only one RCT has reported a fracture benefit in postmenopausal women with established osteoporosis (Lufkin et al., 1992). In a high risk group of postmenopausal women with at least one vertebral fracture, treatment with estradiol and medroxyprogesterone acetate resulted in both an increase in BMD and a reduction in vertebral fractures. There were eight new vertebral fractures occurring in seven women in the HRT-treated group and 20 fractures in 12 placebo-treated women over the 1-year course of the trial. This corresponds with a 61% reduction in fracture risk with HRT (Lufkin et al.,1992). Further support comes from a case control study of estrogen exposure compared to no estrogen therapy (Maxim et al.,1995). Estrogen depletion following bilateral oophorectomy increases the risk for vertebral and wrist fracture (Melton et al., 1996).

HRT and hip fractures

The effects of HRT on reducing hip fractures have been documented in a number of retrospective and prospective cohort and case-control studies (Cauley et al., 1995; Kiel et al., 1987; Naessén et al., 1990; Paganini-Hill et al., 1981; Spector et al., 1992; Weiss et al., 1998). The Study of Osteoporotic Fractures examined a sample of postmenopausal women from four communities who were 65 years of age and older. After a multivariate-adjusted analysis, current users of estrogen had a 40% decreased risk for hip fractures, a 71% risk reduction in wrist fractures, and a 34% risk reduction in all non-spinal fractures when compared with women who had never used estrogen (Cauley et al., 1995). Previous use of estrogen for more than 10 years or use begun soon after menopause had no substantial effect on the risk for fractures (Cauley et al., 1995). Some studies suggest that there is a trend toward greater hip fracture reduction with longer duration of HRT treatment (Paganini-Hill et al., 1981; Weiss et al., 1998). Oophorectomized women appeared to experience the greatest benefit (Paganini-Hill et al., 1981). Estrogen treatment regimens incorporating progesterone have recently been shown to be of benefit as well (Spector et al., 1992). These results suggest that, for protection against fractures, estrogen should be initiated soon after menopause and continued indefinitely.

Effects of hormone replacement therapy on other systems

HRT and cardiovascular disease

Over the past 15 years, there has been evidence that has pointed to a protective effect of hormone therapy with respect to coronary heart disease. This is felt to be, in part, related to the beneficial effects on lipids. Evidence from a literature review of more than 100 articles supported the theory that estrogen reduced the risk of atherosclerosis and myocardial infarction (Wren, 1992). The review suggested that estrogen resulted in a reduction of up to 50% in myocardial infarction, a reduction in the incidence of hypertension, and an improvement in blood flow. For the most part, the literature suggests that HRT may account for up to a 50% reduction in heart disease with relative risk estimates ranging from 0.81 to 0.56 (Falkeborn,

1992; Grady et al., 1992; Grodstein & Stamfer, 1996; Hully et al., 1998; Stamfer et al., 1991). The impact of HRT on cardiovascular disease using up to 16 years of follow-up in 59 337 women from the Nurses' Health Study, who were 30 to 55 years of age at baseline was studied (Grodstein & Stamfer, 1996). This study demonstrated a 40% decrease in the risk of major coronary heart disease among women who took estrogen alone as compared to women who did not use hormones. The multivariate adjusted reduction in relative risk for major coronary heart disease was 61% in women who took estrogen with a progestin as compared to women who did not use hormones. There was no significant association between stroke and use of either combined hormones or estrogen alone. They concluded that the addition of a progestin did not appear to attenuate the cardioprotective effects of postmenopausal estrogen therapy (Grodstein & Stamfer, 1996).

Despite the almost overwhelming evidence of cardiovascular benefit from these prospective observational studies and meta-analyses, a recent randomized controlled trial of the Heart and Estrogen/progestin Replacement Study (HERS) in 2763 postmenopausal women with known coronary artery disease did not reduce the rate of coronary heart disease events (Hully, et al. 1998). Indeed, in these women with significant coronary artery disease, there were more events in the hormone-treated group in the first year of follow-up than in the control group. Over time, however, these findings reversed, such that the longer the duration of hormone use, the less likely it was that a cardiovascular event occurred. It would seem that a key research question that needs to be addressed is the determination of those that are at risk for an early event following institution of hormone therapy and the identification of those who are likely to benefit from long-term treatment. If these groups can be identified, and if they are mutually exclusive, then one might be better able to offer less ambiguous advice. The HERS findings serve to remind us of the limitations of observational studies and to call into question the estimates of cardiovascular benefit obtained from estrogen or hormone replacement therapy in secondary prevention. The results of this study should not be extrapolated to estrogen and HRT in primary prevention. Any conclusions about primary prevention need to be reserved until randomized trials such as the Women's Health Initiative are completed.

HRT and venous thromboembolism

Studies have reported an increase in the relative risk of venous thromboembolism in the first year of estrogen use; however, this observation was not a universal finding (Daly et al., 1996; Gutthann et al., 1997; Hully et al., 1998; Jick et al., 1996). In the HERS study 12 /1383 placebo-treated women and 34/1380 hormone-treated women, followed for on average 4.1 years, developed deep venous thrombosis. This places the hormone-treated group at around three times the risk for developing deep venous thrombosis (Hully et al., 1998).

HRT and breast cancer

One of the most significant deterrents to more widespread use of postmenopausal HRT is the fear of increased risk of breast cancer. Mills et al. evaluated the incidence of breast cancer in HRT users vs. non-users over a 6-year period and reported a RR of 1.39 (95%CI, 1.00 to 1.94) (Mills et al., 1989). A meta-analysis of 39 epidemiological studies found no increased risk for breast cancer in women who ever took estrogen for ≤5 years (Grady et al., 1992). However, in users of estrogen of 8 years or more a RR of 1.25 (95% CI, 1.04 to 1.51) was found (Grady et al., 1992). The Nurses' Health Study found that women currently taking HRT had an increased risk of breast cancer compared with women who had never taken estrogen (Colditz et al., 1995). The greatest risk was in women who had been taking estrogen plus a progestin for 5 or more years, with a 46% increase in breast cancer. The increase was most pronounced among women over the age of 55. Recently, a re-analysis of data from 51 epidemiological studies of 52 705 women with breast cancer and 108 411 women without breast cancer showed a RR of 1.35 (95% CI, 1.21 to 1.49) for developing breast cancer with HRT (Collaborative Group on Hormonal Factors in Breast Cancer, 1997). The concomitant use of a progestin has not been shown to have either a beneficial or an adverse effect on risk of breast cancer (Goddard, 1992; Stamfer et al., 1991; Wren, 1992).

HRT and endometrial cancer

Recent RCTs of combination estrogen and progesterone therapy have demonstrated an increased endometrial proliferation and hyperplasia occurred with increasing unopposed estrogen doses. The combination of a progestational agent and estrogen effectively protects the endometrium against hyperplasia (Speroff et al., 1996; Weinstein et al., 1990). Continuous low dose regimens are also effective and offer the added benefit of reducing the amount of bleeding experienced (Blake et al., 1993; Weinstein et al., 1990).

The effects of smoking on HRT

Smoking has been associated with increased rates of cardiovascular disease in women and hip fractures. The absolute risk of death in a woman's lifetime has been estimated to be 31% from coronary heart disease, 2.8% from breast cancer and 2.8% from hip fracture (Cauley et al., 1995; Cummings et al., 1989). There has been some question of the protective effects of hormone replacement in these women. The Nurses' Health Study has shown that the greatest risk reduction for death from coronary artery disease was in current hormone users who had at least one major cardiovascular risk factor, including current smoking. The observed reduction was 49% in deaths from all causes (relative risk, 0.51; 95% confidence interval, 0.45 to 0.57) The benefit to women with no risk factors was low (RR, 0.89; 95 % CI, 0.62 to 1.28) (Grodstein et al., 1997; Grodstein & Stamfer, 1996).

An association between hip fractures and smoking has been found in a prospective study of 9516 women. Current smokers were found to have twice the risk of hip fracture as non-smokers or past smokers. Women who smoked were generally in poorer health and weighed less than their peers. They were less likely to exercise and had decreased neuromuscular function (Cummings et al., 1989).

A recent meta-analysis found current smokers' relative risk for hip fracture was 1.71 (95% CI, 1.05 to 1.30). By age 80, when hip fractures occur, the risk had increased by 71%. There was no association between the risk of hip fracture and smoking in premenopausal women.

Smoking may increase the risk for fracture by decreasing estradiol levels. There is some thought that hormone replacement may be less effective in smokers. In one study there were lower estrogen levels among postmenopausal women who smoked compared to non-smokers. This was thought to be due to increased hepatic metabolism of estradiol (Jensen et al., 1985). The relative risk of hip fracture in non-smoking women who were taking estrogen was 0.37 as compared to 1.26 in women who smoked (Kiel et al., 1992). In a large prospective study, women who smoked and received hormone replacement had a similar risk reduction for wrist, spine and hip fracture when compared to non-smokers (0.39 for wrist; 0.66 for all non-spinal) (Cauley et al., 1995).

HRT and dementia

In recent years there has been growing interest in the use of hormones in patients with Alzheimer's disease. The prevalence of dementia in Canada has been estimated at 8.0% in those over 65 years and 34.5% among those aged 85 years and over (Canadian Study of Health and Aging Working Group, 1994). Potential mechanisms include possible changes in apolipoprotein E and amyloid levels, stimulation of nerve growth factors and improved cerebral blood flow and cerebral glucose utilization. Estrogen may also increase neurotransmitters particularly acetylcholine which is necessary for memory and learning (Paganini-Hill, 1997). The clinical studies have been limited. They are often retrospective, case series or case control designs. Despite the limitations, in eight recently conducted studies, six found a significantly reduced risk of Alzheimer's disease amongst estrogen users. They estimated a protective effect amongst current users of estrogen to be 50% less than women who have never used HRT. The relative risks have ranged between 0.3 and 0.7 (Paganini-Hill, 1997). The Women's Health Initiative has added an ancillary study to examine the effect of estrogen in a prospective randomized control. A small short-term study demonstrated that estrogen significantly improved cognitive function, dementia symptoms, and regional cerebral blood flow in women with mild-to-moderate dementia (Ohkura et al., 1994).

HRT and mortality

While many experts feel that the overall benefits of HRT on cardiovascular risk and osteoporosis outweigh the risks for the development of breast and endometrial malignancy, there has been very little long-term prospective data to support this contention. Recently, data derived from the Nurses' Health Study were published (Grodstein et al., 1997). Many conclusions have been drawn from this study (Charney et al., 1998). Current use of HRT seems to be associated with lower mortality, particularly from coronary heart disease. Protection appears to be greatest amongst those with the highest risk for coronary heart disease. The overall protective effects seem to be attenuated but are still present after 10 years. Finally, the cessation of HRT returns a women to the risk of a women who never used HRT after only 5 years (Charney et al., 1998).

Decision making and hormone replacement therapy

Given the enormity of the data on HRT, the balance between risks and benefits of therapy and the need for further information, how does the clinician help the individual patient make a decision about HRT? One way to help with this complex decision-making has been to simplify the outcome to life expectancy. Using a mathematical model that takes into account the life expectancy in postmenopausal women with different risk profiles for heart disease, breast cancer, hip fracture and endometrial cancer and the effects of HRT on life expectancy estimated for women with various risks for heart disease, osteoporosis and breast cancer, decisions regarding HRT may be made (Col et al., 1997). In this model, HRT increases the life expectancy for all women. The greatest increase in life expectancy is seen in those with the greatest risk for coronary heart disease and the lowest risk for breast cancer. Women who did not have an increase in their life expectancy were those who were at low risk for coronary heart disease and high risk for breast cancer. Unfortunately, this model does not take into account quality of life and other factors that affect women and their decisions about HRT.

Another approach has been to develop a self-administered decision aid for postmenopausal women considering HRT (O'Connor et al., 1998). Women were guided through an illustrated booklet by an audiotape. The booklet contained detailed information about HRT benefits and risks tailored to a woman's clinical risk, and a values clarification exercise to promote informed decision-making consistent with their own personal values. In a before and after study they were able to show that women had better general knowledge and more realistic personal expectations of HRT benefits and risks. They also felt more certain, informed, clear about values, and supported in their decision-making. Changes in preference occurred in the group of women who were uncertain about HRT, with equal numbers ultimately accepting or declining HRT. These types of decision aids are useful in helping women make decisions about this complex personal issue.

Conclusions

There is little doubt that hormone replacement therapy is beneficial in the prevention of fractures. While there is only one randomized controlled trial demonstrating the prevention of vertebral fractures in those at high risk for fracture, there are a number of well-designed cohort studies that confirm a treatment effect. These studies demonstrate fracture prevention in the hip, wrist and all other fractures, not just vertebral fractures. Other studies demonstrate that bone density actually increases in the first years following institution of therapy. There is a dose–response with higher doses being more effective than lower doses in increasing bone density. Older women with lower bone density respond as well as, if not better than, younger women commencing hormone therapy. Both oral and transdermal routes of administration are effective. The beneficial effects of hormone therapy on bone may be abrogated by smoking, the theory being that smoking reduces estradiol levels.

Other benefits of hormone replacement therapy include the control of menopausal and urogenital symptoms and the potential cardiovascular and neurocognitive benefits. On the other side of the coin is the increase in gall bladder disease, deep venous thrombosis, pulmonary emboli, the increase in endometrial cancer and the potential increase in risk of breast cancer. Healthcare professionals need to educate their patients about these risks and benefits in order to help them in making decisions about hormone replacement therapy. Given the complexity of this decision, it might prove useful to consider the use of decision aids.

REFERENCES

Adami, S., Suppi, R., Bertoldo, F., Rossini, M., Residori, M., Maresca, V., & Lo Casio, V. (1989). Premenopausal ovariectomy-related bone loss: a randomized, double-blind, one-year trial of conjugated estrogen or medroxyprogesterone acetate. *Bone Miner.*, 7, 79–86.

Blake, J. M., Chambers, L. F., Roberts, J. G., & Webber, C. E. (1993). A one-year prospective comparison of calcium supplementation, low dose continuous, and moderate dose cyclical oestrogen and progestagen replacement therapy in the protection of bone mass. *J. Obstet. Gynecol.*, **13**, 185–92.

Canadian Study of Health and Aging Working Group (1994). Canadian Study of health and aging: study methods and prevalence of dementia. *Can. Med. Assoc. J.*, **150**, 899–913.

Cauley, J. A., Seeley, D. G., Ensrud, K., Ettinger, B., Black, D., & Cummings, S. R. (1995). Estrogen replacement therapy in older women. *Ann. Intern. Med.*, **122**, 9–16.

Charney, P., Walsh, J. M. E., & Nattinger, A. B. (1998). Update in women's health. *Ann. Intern. Med.*, **129**, 551–8.

Christiansen, C., Christiansen, M. S., & Transbøl, I. (1981). Bone mass in postmenopausal women after withdrawal of oestrogen/gestagen replacement therapy. *Lancet*, **i**, 459–61.

Col, N. F., Eckman, M. H., Karas, R. H., Pauker, S. G., Goldberg, R. J., Ross, E. M., Orr, R. K., & Wong, J. B. (1997). Patient-specific decisions about hormone replacement therapy in post-menopausal women. *JAMA*, **277**, 1140–7.

Colditz, G. A., Hankinson, S. E., & Hunter, J. (1995). The use of estrogens and progestins and the risk of breast cancer in postmenopausal women. *N. Engl. J. Med.*, **332**, 1589–93.

Collaborative Group on Hormonal Factors in Breast Cancer (1997). Breast cancer and hormone replacement therapy: collaborative reanalysis of data from 51 epidemiological studies of women 52,705 women with breast cancer and 108,411 women without breast cancer. *Lancet*, **350**, 1047–59.

Cummings, S. R., Black, D. M., & Rubin, S. M. (1989). Lifetime risks of hip, Colles', or vertebral fracture and coronary heart disease among white postmenopausal women. *Arch. Intern. Med.*, **149**, 2445–8.

Daly, E., Vessey, M.P., Hawkins, M. M., Carson, J. L., Gough, P., & Marsh, S. (1996). Risk of venous thromboembolism in users of hormone replacement therapy. *Lancet*, **348**, 977–80.

Duan, Y., Tabensky, A., DeLuca, V., & Seeman, E. (1997). The benefit of hormone replacement therapy on bone mass is greater at the vertebral body than posterior processes or proximal femur. *Bone* **21**, 447–51.

Eiken, P., Kolthoff, N., & Nielsen, S.P. (1996). Effect of 10 years' hormone replacement therapy on bone mineral content in postmenopausal women. *Bone*, **19**, 1915–35.

Ettinger, B., Genant, H., Steiger, P., & Madvig, P. (1992). Low-dosage micronized 17β- estradiol prevents bone loss in postmenopausal women. *Am. J. Obstet. Gynecol.*, **166**, 479– 88.

Falkeborn, M. (1992). The risk of acute myocardial infarction with oestrogen and oestrogen–progestin replacement. *Br. J. Obst. Gyn.*, **99**, 821–8.

Field, C. S., Ory, S. J., Wahner, H. W., Herrmann, R. R., Judd, H. L., & Riggs, B. L. (1998). Preventive effects of transdermal 17β- estradiol on osteoporotic changes after surgical meno-pause: A two-year placebo-controlled trial. *Am. J. Obstet. Gynecol.*, **168**, 1110–20.

Goddard, M. K. (1992). Hormone replacement therapy and breast cancer, endometrial cancer and cardiovascular disease: risks and benefits. *Br. J. Gen. Pract.*, **42**, 120–5.

Grady, D., Rubin, S., Petitti, D. B., Fox, C. S., Black, D., Ettinger, B., Ernster, V. L., & Cummings, S. R. (1992). Hormone therapy to prevent disease and prolong life in postmenopausal women. *Ann. Intern. Med.*, **117**, 1016–87.

Grodstein, F. & Stamfer, M. J. (1996). Postmenopausal estrogen and progesterone use and the risk of cardiovascular disease. *N. Engl. J. Med.*, **334**, 453–61.

Grodstein, F., Stamfer, M. J., Colditz, G. A., Willett, W. C., Manson, J. E., Joffe, M., Rosner, B., Fuchs, C., Hankinson, S. E., Hunter, D. J., Hennekens, C. H., & Speizer, F. E. (1997). Postmenopausal hormone therapy and mortality. *N. Engl. J. Med.*, **336**, 1769–75.

Gutthann, S. P., Rodriguez, L. A. G., Castellague, J., & Oliart, A. D. (1997). Hormone replacement therapy and risk of venous thromboembolism: population based case-control study. *Br. Med. J.*, **314**, 800.

Harris, S. T., Genant, H. K., Baylink, D. J., Gallagher, J. C., Katz, S., Karp, S., McConnell, M. A., Green, E. M., & Stoll, R. W. (1991). The effects of estrone (ogen) on spinal bone density of postmenopausal women. *Arch. Intern. Med.*, **151**, 1980–4.

Hillard, T. C., Whitcroft, S. J., Marsh, M. S., Ellerington, M. C., Lees, B., Whitehead, M. I., & Stevenson, J. C. (1994). Long-term effects of transdermal and oral hormone replacement therapy on postmenopausal bone loss. *Osteoporos. Int.*, **4**, 341–8.

Honjo, H., Ogino, Y., & Tanaka, K. (1993). An effect of conjugated estrogen to cognitive impairment in women with senile dementia-Alzheimer's type: a placebo-controlled double blind study. *J. Jpn. Menopause Soc.*, **1**, 167–71.

Hully, S. B., Grady, D., Bush, T., Furberg, C., Herrington, D., Riggs, B., Vittinghoff, E., and the Heart and Estrogen/progestin Replacement Study Research Group (1998). Randomized trial of estrogen plus progestin for secondary prevention of coronary heart disease in postmenopausal women. *JAMA*, **280**, 605–13.

Jensen, J., Christiansen, C., & Røtbro, P. (1985). Cigarette smoking, serum estrogens, and bone loss during hormone-replacement therapy early after menopause. *N. Engl. J. Med.*, **313**, 973–5.

Jick, H., Derby, L. E., Myers, M. W., Vasilakis, C., & Newton, K. M. (1996). Risk of hospital admission for idiopathic venous thromboembolism among users of postmenopausal oestrogens. *Lancet*, **348**, 981–3.

Jilka, R. L. (1998). Cytokines, bone remodelling, and estrogen deficiency: a 1998 update. *Bone*, **23**, 75–81.

Jilka, R. L., Takahashi, K., Williams, D. C., & Manolagas, S. C. (1998). Loss of estrogen upregulates osteoblastogenesis in the murine bone marrow: evidence for autonomy from factors released during bone resorption. *J. Clin. Invest.*, **101**, 1942–50.

Kiel, D. P., Baron, J. A., Anderson, J. J., Hannan, M. T., & Felson, D. T. (1992). Smoking eliminates the protective effect of oral estrogens on the risk for hip fracture among women. *Ann. Intern. Med.*, **116**, 716–21.

Kiel, D. P., Felson, D. T., Anderson, J. J., Wilson, P. W. F., & Moskowitz, M. A. (1987). Hip fractures and the use of estrogens in postmenopausal women. The Framingham Study. *N. Engl. J. Med.*, **317**, 1169–74.

Komulainen, M., Tuppurainen, M. T., Kroger, H., Heikkinen, A. M., Puntila, E., Alhava, E., Honkanen, R., & Saarikoski, S. (1997). Vitamin D and HRT: no benefit additional to that of HRT alone in prevention of bone loss in early postmenopausal women. A 2.5 year randomized placebo-controlled study. *Osteoporos. Int.*, **7**, 116–27.

Lufkin, E. G., Wahner, H. W., O'Fallon, W. M., Hodgson, S. F., Kotowicz, M. A., Lane, A. W., Judd, H. L., Capla, R. H., & Riggs, B. L. (1992). Treatment of postmenopausal osteoporosis with transdermal estrogen. *Ann. Intern. Med.*, **117**, 1–9.

Maxim, P., Ettinger, B., & Soitalny, G. M. (1995). Fracture protection provided by long-term estrogen treatment. *Osteoporos. Int.*, **5**, 23–9.

Melton, L. J., Crowson, C. S., Malkasian, G. D., & O'Fallon, W.M. (1996). Fracture risk following bilateral oophorectomy. *J. Clin. Epidemiol.*, **49**, 1111–15.

Mills, P. K., Beeson, W. L., Phillips, R. L., & Fraser, G. E. (1989). Prospective study of exogenous hormone use and breast cancer in seventh-day adventists. *Cancer*, **64**, 591–7.

Nachtigall, L. E., Nachtigall, R. H., Nachtigall, R. D., & Beckman, E. M. (1979). Estrogen replacement therapy I: a 10-year prospective study in the relationship to osteoporosis. *Obstet. Gynecol.*, **53**, 277–81.

Naessén, T., Persson, I., Adami, H. O., Bergström, R, & Bergkvist, L. (1990). Hormone replacement therapy and the risk for first hip fracture. A prospective, population-based cohort study. *Ann. Intern. Med.*, **113**, 95–103.

O'Connor, A. M., Tugwell, P., Wells, G. A., Elmslie, T., Jolly, E., Hollingworth, G., McPherson, R., Bunn, H., Graham, I., & Drake, E. (1998). A decision aid for women considering hormone therapy after menopause: decision support framework and evaluation. *Pat. Educat. Counseling*, **33**, 267–79.

Ohkura, T., Isse, K., Akazawa, K., Hamamoto, M., Yaoi, Y., & Hagino, N. (1994). Evaluation of estrogen treatment in female patients with dementia of the Alzheimer type. *Endocr. J.*, **41**, 361–71.

Paganini-Hill, A. (1997). Does estrogen replacement therapy protect against Alzheimer's disease? *Osteoporos. Int.* (Suppl. 1), S12–S17.

Paganini-Hill, A., Ross, R. K., Gerkins, V. R., Henderson, B. E., Arthur, M., & Mack, T. M. (1981). Menopausal estrogen therapy and hip fractures. *Ann. Intern. Med.*, **95**, 28–31.

Prior, J. C., Vigna, Y. M., Wark, J. D., Eyre, D. R., Lentle, B. C., Li, D. K. B., Eberling, P. R., & Atley, L. (1997). Premenopausal ovariectomy-related bone loss: a randomized, double-blind, one-year trial of conjugated estrogen or medroxyprogesterone acetate. *J. Bone Miner. Res.*, **12**, 1851–63.

Spector, T. D., Brennan, P., Harris, P. A., Studd, J. W. W., & Silman, A. J. (1992). Do current regimes of hormone replacement therapy protect against subsequent fractures? *Osteoporos. Int.*, **2**, 219–24.

Speroff, L., Rowan, J., Symons, J., Genant, H., & Wilborn, W. (1996). The comparative effect on bone density, endometrium, and lipids of continuous hormones as replacement therapy (CHART study): a randomized controlled trial. *JAMA*, **276**, 1397–403.

Stamfer, M. J., Colditz, G. A., & Willett, W. C. (1991). Postmenopausal estrogen replacement therapy and cardiovascular disease: ten-year follow-up from the nurses' study. *N. Engl. J. Med.*, **325**, 756–62.

Stevenson, J. C., Cust, M. P., Ganger, K. F., Hillard, T. C., Lees, B., & Whitehead, M.I. (1990). Effects of transdermal versus oral hormone replacement therapy on bone density in spine and proximal femur in postmenopausal women. *Lancet*, **335**, 265–9.

The Writing Group for the PEPI Trial (1996). Effects of hormone therapy on bone mineral density. Results from the postmenopausal estrogen/progestin interventions (PEPI) trial. *JAMA*, **276**, 1389–96.

Weinstein, L., Bewtra, C., & Gallagher, C. (1990). Evaluation of a continuous combined low-dose regimen of estrogen-progestin for treatment of the menopausal patient. *Am. J. Obstet. Gynecol.*, **162**, 1534–42.

Weiss, N. S., Ure, B. L., Ballard, J. H., Williams, A. R., & Daling, J. R. (1998). Decreased risk of fractures of the hip and lower forearm with postmenopausal use of estrogen. *N. Engl. J. Med.*, **1980**, 1195–8.

Wren, B. G. (1992). The effect of oestrogen on the female cardiovascular system. *Med J. Aust.*, **157**, 204–8.

21

Selective estrogen receptor modulators

Felicia Cosman and Robert Lindsay

Introduction

Estrogens are frequently prescribed to perimenopausal and postmenopausal women for control of menopausal symptoms such as hot flashes, vaginal dryness, and memory disturbances. More recently, estrogens have been recognized and used for long-term protection against chronic diseases related to estrogen deficiency, most notably osteoporosis and heart disease. Estrogens have diverse multisystemic effects (Ettinger, 1998) including those on the central nervous system and have, therefore, been implicated in maintaining normal cognitive function and possibly reducing the risk of Alzheimer's disease (Henderson, 1997). Estrogens have also been linked to a reduced risk of colorectal cancer. Use of estrogens is limited, however, due to stimulatory effects on both the uterus and the breast, as well as some troublesome side-effects. In the uterus, there may be an increase in the risk of uterine cancer even when progestins are given appropriately (Beresford et al., 1997). Furthermore, the body of epidemiologic data suggests an increase in the risk of breast cancer, at least after long-term (>5–10 years') use (Collaborative Group, 1997). The increased risk of deep venous thrombosis has also been recently described in epidemiologic studies. Side-effects such as breast tenderness and engorgement, vaginal bleeding with many hormone replacement regimens, and a perception that hormone use is associated with weight gain, headaches, and nausea are other symptoms which limit estrogen use. Further questions about the outcomes of continuous combined estrogen and progestin use were raised by the HERS trial (Hulley et al., 1998).

Agents which retain some of the benefits of estrogen, particularly on the skeleton and on the cardiovascular system, while not increasing the risk of uterine and breast cancer, and avoiding some of estrogen's side-effects, therefore, would be beneficial to many postmenopausal women. Drugs in the class called selective estrogen receptor modulators (SERMs) hold this promise (Cosman & Lindsay, 1999).

SERMs: definition

SERMs were previously called antiestrogens, but this term is a misnomer since most of these agents retain some estrogen agonist activity in addition to some estrogen antagonist activity (Wakeling, 1997). A better term, therefore, is mixed estrogen agonist/antagonist or partial agonist antiestrogens. The term SERM implies that these agents have agonist properties on some estrogen receptive tissues and antagonist properties on other estrogen receptive tissues. There are several drugs currently under development which are actually pure estrogen antagonists, as far as we know, and do not appear to exert any estrogen agonist effects throughout the body. These medications might be useful in the future for breast cancer treatment or perhaps benign endometrial diseases such as endometriosis or uterine fibroids. The SERMs which are currently in clinical use include clomifene, tamoxifen, raloxifene and toremifene.

SERMs: mechanism of action

The major actions of the SERMs occur through interaction with the estrogen receptor of which two different subtypes have so far been identified (ER-alpha and ER-beta) (Kulper et al., 1996). These receptor subtypes appear throughout the body with perhaps a predominance of ER-alpha expression in the reproductive tissues and a predominance of ER-beta expression in non-reproductive tissues. SERMs can have agonist activity by binding to one receptor subtype and antagonist activity at the other receptor subtype. Raloxifene, for example, appears to exert antagonist activity on the breast and uterus through the ER-alpha receptor and agonist activity on the skeleton and hepatic lipoprotein production through the ER-beta receptor. The mechanisms of SERM action are more complex, however, since certain agents can have antagonist effects in one tissue type where the ER-alpha subtype is predominant and partial agonist effects in another tissue where ER-alpha is predominant. Tamoxifen is one such example where on the breast, effects are largely antagonistic, but on the uterus, tamoxifen acts as a partial agonist. Furthermore, many organs, such as the central nervous system, contain both alpha and beta receptors, and it is, therefore, difficult to predict how a SERM will act in that tissue (Enmark et al., 1997).

There are also postreceptor differences when various SERMS or estrogens bind to the estrogen receptor. The ultimate conformations achieved by the interaction with SERMS or estrogen and the estrogen receptor are highly variable. These variable conformations bind different auxiliary proteins with different affinities. These auxiliary proteins act as either co-repressors or co-activators which inhibit or potentiate subsequent genomic action (Baker & Jaffe, 1995; Brzozowski et al., 1997).

Some of the purest antiestrogens might be unable to achieve an appropriate functional conformation to result in any transcriptional activity or might reduce estrogen receptor density by increasing turnover of the ligand–receptor complex. Finally, certain SERMs can promote transcription of genetic material through a receptor distinct from the usual estrogen response element (Yang et al., 1996, 1997).

Due to all of these different levels of mechanistic complexity, it is understandable that each SERM can produce its own unique spectrum of activity throughout the body. Therefore, not only do we need to compare the SERMs in terms of which tissue is having predominantly an antagonist effect and in which tissue it is showing a predominantly agonist effect, we also have to compare the various potencies of the estrogen-like effects and the various potencies of the estrogen antagonist effects.

SERMs currently in clinical use: (Fig. 21.1)

Clomifene

Clomifene was one of the first SERMs identified and is a non-steroidal triphenylethylene compound. This agent is actually a mixture of *cis*- and *trans*-isomers with the *cis*-isomer possessing estrogen agonist activity and the *trans*-isomer possessing estrogen antagonist activity (Baker & Jaffe, 1995). This medication was originally studied as a possible morning-after pill, but was found to be an ovulation inducer and is now used almost solely as a fertility-enhancing agent. The ovulation induction activity appears to be the result of estrogen antagonist effects in the central nervous system, particularly at the hypothalamic–pituitary axis where it stimulates gonadotropin secretion. This medication also appears to have activity against breast cancer but, since it has higher toxicity with chronic use and the effect on breast cancer was not as strong as seen with tamoxifen, the clinical development for this indication was discontinued many years ago (Clark & Markaverich, 1982). There have been no human studies investigating clomifene on the skeleton. Several cohort studies indicate a possible increase in the risk of ovarian cancer when clomifene is used repeatedly for fertility purposes (Rossing et al., 1994).

Tamoxifen

Tamoxifen is in the same class of compound as clomifene (triphenylethylene) and was also studied first as a possible postcoital contraceptive agent. Similarly to clomifene, however, it was shown to induce ovulation, but was not subsequently developed for this purpose. Like clomifene, it has estrogen antagonist effects on the hypothalamic–pituitary axis, resulting in increased gonadotropin production and in postmenopausal women can increase menopausal symptoms such as hot flashes due to this effect.

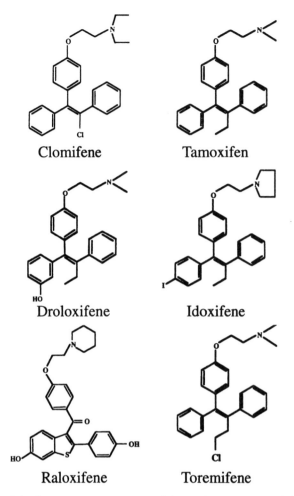

Clomifene   Tamoxifen

Droloxifene   Idoxifene

Raloxifene   Toremifene

Fig. 21.1   Selective estrogen receptor modulators (SERMs) currently in clinical use or clinical development.

Tamoxifen has been developed primarily as an adjuvant chemotherapy for treatment of breast cancer. In an abundance of clinical trials, it has been shown to decrease the risk of development of breast cancer on the contralateral side, reduce rate of recurrence and increase disease-free survival in breast cancer patients at all stages of the disease (Early Breast Cancer Trialists' Collaborative Group, 1998; Osborne, 1998). It also has been shown recently to prevent the development of breast cancer in women with 'high risk' but without previous breast cancer. In that study, The Breast Cancer Prevention Trial, women were considered to be at high risk if they were nulliparous, had menarche before the age of 12, had a first-degree relative with breast cancer, had previous breast disease including atypical hyperplasia or cancer *in situ* or were aged 60 years or older (Fisher et al., 1998). Because the breast cancer incidence was reduced by approximately 45% in those taking tamoxifen, this breast cancer prevention trial was terminated early at 4.5 years. Several European studies investigating tamoxifen as a breast cancer prevention agent remain ongoing currently, but so far have yielded different results.

As the dominant action on the breast was estrogen antagonist, it was thought that tamoxifen would also have estrogen antagonist activity on the skeleton. Early retrospective and ultimately prospective studies in patients with breast cancer treated with tamoxifen, however, did not demonstrate these negative effects and, in fact, showed neutral or even positive effects on the skeleton. For example, Love et al., studied 140 patients with breast cancer randomly assigned to receive tamoxifen or a placebo for 2 years. Bone mass in the lumbar spine increased significantly in the Tamoxifen treated group compared with losses seen in the placebo group (Love et al., 1992). The difference between the placebo group and the tamoxifen-treated group at the end of 2 years was approximately 3% in the spine. In the radius, bone density decreased in both groups to a similar degree, about 1%/year. Studies have also been performed in normal postmenopausal women without a history of breast cancer. Grey et al., studied 57 postmenopausal women and showed that spine BMD increased about 2.1% in tamoxifen treated compared with placebo treated patients over a 2-year period. However, there was only a minimal effect on total body bone mineral (0.5% at 2 years) and no effect on bone mass of the hip in that study (Grey et al., 1995b). Powles et al., studied 125 premenopausal women and 54 postmenopausal women (Fig. 21.2). In the premenopausal women, tamoxifen had a negative effect on bone mass, whereas in postmenopausal women, tamoxifen induced small bone gains in both the spine and hip regions (Powles et al., 1996). This study indicated that, in a normal premenopausal woman with premenopausal estrogen levels, tamoxifen exerts a net antiestrogenic effect, whereas when estrogen levels are very low as seen in postmenopausal women, tamoxifen exerts a net estrogenic effect. In the National Cancer Institute sponsored Breast Cancer Prevention Trial, bone mineral density was not performed, however, peripheral fracture incidence was shown to be reduced by about 20% but results were not quite statistically significant (Fisher et al., 1998). These data do not include vertebral deformity incidence, since routine spine X-rays were not performed, and therefore this fracture effect might under-estimate the ultimate potency of tamoxifen to prevent bone fractures.

Tamoxifen does exert effects that are estrogen-like on serum lipoproteins and perhaps against heart disease. Heart disease outcomes were reported in two studies of breast cancer patients using adjuvant tamoxifen. Fatal MI was about 60% less common in tamoxifen receiving patients than in placebo patients in the Scottish Breast Cancer Study (McDonald & Stewart, 1991). In the Swedish Study, the incidence of cardiac disease requiring hospitalization was 30% less common in those receiving tamoxifen after breast cancer surgery than in those who did not receive

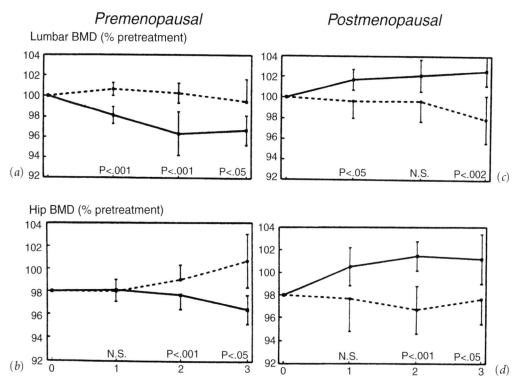

Fig. 21.2   Bone mineral density (BMD) changes in normal premenopausal women (left) and normal menopausal women (right) during treatment with tamoxifen —— 20 mg/d vs. placebo ----- in a breast cancer prevention trial (Powles et al., 1996).

tamoxifen (Rutqvist & Mattsson, 1993). Not all investigations have been consistent with regard to cardiac disease outcomes, however. In the NCI sponsored Breast Cancer Prevention Trial, no reduction in MI risk was seen (Fisher et al., 1998). An insignificant effect on cardiovascular mortality was also seen in a study where tamoxifen was used as adjuvant therapy for breast cancer (Constantino et al., 1997). Primate studies do indicate, however, that tamoxifen can inhibit progression of coronary artery atherosclerosis (Williams et al., 1997).

Tamoxifen has been shown to reduce total cholesterol by about 12%, LDL cholesterol by 20%, and lipoprotein a by about 34% (Grey et al., 1995a; Shewmon et al., 1994). No positive effect on HDL is generally seen and triglyceride levels usually do not change or increase slightly. Also, tamoxifen appears to reduce serum fibrinogen significantly (Powles et al., 1996; McDonald & Stewart, 1991). It is not known whether tamoxifen exerts lipoprotein-independent mechanisms for reducing coronary arteriosclerosis such as reducing LDL oxidation or affecting coronary vasodilation through nitric oxide, prostacyclin or endothelin-1 production.

Tamoxifen could therefore, be potentially useful in postmenopausal women to prevent breast cancer, heart disease, and osteoporosis and has recently received FDA approval for prevention of breast cancer. Its use is limited, however, by several problems. It is a partial estrogen agonist in the uterus and has been shown to increase the risk of both malignant and non-malignant conditions including endometrial and endocervical polyps, fibroids, adenomyosis, and endometrial hyperplasia. The risk of uterine cancer increases two–three-fold on average (Fisher et al., 1998). It also increases the frequency of ovarian cysts, but has not been shown to increase the risk of ovarian cancer (Cohen et al., 1993; Fisher et al., 1994; Jaiyesimi et al., 1995; Thylan, 1995). There is also some concern that tamoxifen might increase the risk of hepatocellular carcinoma on the basis of an increased risk of hepatic tumors and DNA adducts in rodents (Hard et al., 1993). There has not yet been, however, demonstration of an increase in hepatocellular carcinoma in humans. The risk of deep venous thrombosis is also increased in women on tamoxifen (Rutqvist & Mattsson, 1993) and various types of ocular toxicity (Heier et al., 1994) and thrombocytopenia have also been described as potential adverse effects. There are some troubling side-effects in addition, including an increased frequency of hot flushes in postmenopausal, as well as premenopausal women, given tamoxifen.

Raloxifene

Raloxifene is in a distinct drug class from either clomifene or tamoxifen. It is also non-steroidal, but is a benzothiophene compound. This drug was originally developed over two decades ago for treatment of breast cancer, but was dropped for this indication when tamoxifen was shown to be so effective for this purpose. It does have some advantages over tamoxifen, however, in that it might be even more potent as an estrogen antagonist on the breast, although there are as yet no direct head-to-head comparisons. There is a study, recently started by the National Cancer Institute, to evaluate the potency of tamoxifen vs. raloxifene for breast cancer prevention (STAR Study). Furthermore, raloxifene appears to have an advantage over tamoxifen by resulting in less estrogenic uterine stimulation.

In a short-term preliminary trial of raloxifene in 251 healthy postmenopausal women, raloxifene was tested against estrogen and placebo. In general, bone turnover in raloxifene-treated patients was reduced similarly to that seen with estrogen, although doses of raloxifene in this study were all much higher than those used in subsequent studies (Draper et al., 1996). Urinary calcium was reduced in raloxifene groups similarly to that of estrogen. The effects of raloxifene on calcium metabolism and bone histomorphometry also suggest similar changes to those seen with estrogen. Data from rodent studies indicate that the protection of bone mass by raloxifene is associated with an increase in bone strength (Turner et al., 1994).

Human studies for raloxifene are now quite extensive and include both the

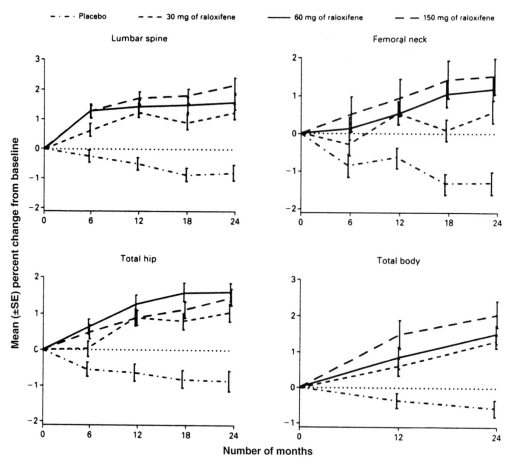

Fig. 21.3   Bone mineral density (BMD) changes in the lumbar spine, femoral neck of the hip, total hip and total body over 2 years during treatment with placebo or raloxifene in normal postmenopausal women (Delmas et al., 1997).

prevention studies in approximately 1200 early postmenopausal women, a study comparing raloxifene with unopposed conjugated equine estrogen which includes over 600 women, and the More Study, Multiple Outcomes of Raloxifene Evaluation in over 7700 women. Data from the Raloxifene for Osteoporosis Prevention Study have now been published on 601 postmenopausal women between the ages of 45 and 60, within 2–8 years from menopause in this multicenter European trial (Delmas et al., 1997; Fig. 21.3). Subjects received one of three raloxifene doses or placebo and bone density, bone turnover, and lipid biochemistry were evaluated over 2 years. Results showed that bone turnover decreased between 20 and 40% over the course of the study. Bone mass increased at all sites with differences of 2–3% between the raloxifene treated subjects and placebo subjects at the end of 2 years. As seen from Powles et al. evaluating normal postmenopausal women given tamoxifen, the effects of raloxifene on the spine and hip were very similar. This similar effect in the spine and hip is distinct from the pattern usually seen with anti-resorptive therapy such as estrogen or alendronate where the spinal bone mass increment is about twice that of the hip bone mass increment. Data from the MORE Osteoporosis Treatment Study suggests that raloxifene reduces vertebral fracture occurrence by about 30 to 50% at 3 years. There has been no signifi-cant effect on peripheral fracture demonstrated yet for raloxifene (Ettinger et al., 1999).

Recent data from the MORE Study indicate that raloxifene may be even more potent as a breast cancer prevention agent than tamoxifen (Cummings et al., 1999). Overall raloxifene reduced the risk of invasive breast cancer by 76%.

Similar to tamoxifen, raloxifene has an estrogen agonist effect on serum lipo-proteins but the pattern and the potency of the effect are somewhat different com-pared to those induced by estrogen. In a study comparing raloxifene to continuous, daily combined hormone replacement therapy (HRT; conjugated equine estrogen 0.625 mg + medroxyprogesterone acetate 2.5 mg), LDL cholesterol was lowered 12 to 14% by both raloxifene and HRT (Walsh et al., 1998). Lipoprotein a was lowered 7 to 8% by raloxifene compared to a 19% reduction by HRT. Raloxifene produced no increment in HDL whereas HRT increased total HDL by 11%. There was an increase in the HDL-2 subclass induced by raloxifene but the effect was only about one-half of the increment seen with HRT on HDL-2 (33% rise). Although these differences in cardiovascular disease intermediates suggest that HRT might be a better protector against atherosclerotic disease than raloxifene, there are two vari-ables which indicate that raloxifene could be superior. Raloxifene lowers serum fibrinogen by 12 to 14%, whereas there was no effect on fibrinogen for HRT. Furthermore, raloxifene does not increase serum triglyceride levels, whereas HRT increased them by 20%. Based on biochemical changes alone, therefore, it is difficult to predict the theoretical potency of atherosclerosis protection by raloxi-fene compared with HRT. Furthermore, serum lipoproteins are only one mecha-nism by which estrogens and SERMs could protect against heart disease. There are no human studies evaluating non-lipoprotein-related effects of raloxifene. However, in primates, treatment with conjugated equine estrogen reduced coro-nary artery plaque size by 70%, whereas raloxifene had no effect on plaque size (Clarkson et al., 1998). In contrast, in the ovariectomized rabbit model, raloxifene did reduce aortic cholesterol accumulation (Bjarnason et al., 1997). Clinical trial data looking at heart disease outcomes in humans is lacking for raloxifene. The effect of continuous combined HRT on heart disease outcomes from the HERS trial showed no significant overall effect (Hulley et al., 1998). A study evaluating both fatal myocardial infarction as well as non-fatal cardiac disease has been started, comparing raloxifene to placebo (raloxifene use for the heart; RUTH). This study will enrol approximately 10 000 postmenopausal women over the age of 55 at risk for heart attack or with known coronary artery disease and will be conducted over 7½ years.

In contrast to both tamoxifen and estrogen, raloxifene does not appear to stimulate uterine tissue. In the Multicenter European Osteoporosis Prevention Study 400 women had serial transvaginal ultrasound over the 2-year treatment period and there was no significant increase in endometrial thickness in raloxifene-treated subjects and no difference was seen compared with placebo treated subjects (Delmas et al., 1997). Like both estrogen and tamoxifen, however, raloxifene does increase the risk of deep venous thrombosis and like tamoxifen, raloxifene increases hot flashes slightly (Evista Product Circular, 1997). Effects on other organ systems such as the brain and urogenital tissues are unknown.

Toremifene

Toremifene, a chlorinated derivative of tamoxifen, has recently been approved for treatment of breast cancer. It appears to have perhaps even more potent effects on breast cancer, which are similar to those of tamoxifen and similar stimulatory effects on uterine tissue. Toremifene does not appear to increase rodent hepatic tumor production (Hard et al., 1993). Little is known about skeletal and cardiovascular effects.

Conclusions

This study of drugs in the SERM class has just begun. Many of the ultimate health outcomes, such as heart attack and fracture, are unknown. Long-term effects on other tissues, such as the perineal tissues and the central nervous system are also completely unknown. The apparent ability of these agents to dramatically reduce the risk of breast cancer is very exciting. These drugs have tremendous potential for reducing a variety of other chronic diseases in women associated with aging and estrogen deficiency and are likely to be of increasing importance as the number of women in the postmenopausal phase of life continues to increase.

REFERENCES

Baker, V. L. & Jaffe, R. B. (1995). Clinical uses of antiestrogens. *Obstet. Gynecol. Survey*, 51, 45–59.

Beresford, S. A., Weiss, N. S., Voigt, L. F., & McKnight, B. (1997). Risk of endometrial cancer in relation to use of oestrogen combined with cyclic progestogen therapy in postmenopausal women. *Lancet*, 349, 458.

Bjarnason, N. H., Haarbo, J., Byrjalsen, I., & Christiansen, C. (1997). Raloxifene inhibits aortic accumulation of cholesterol in ovariectomized, cholesterol-fed rabbits. *Circulation*, **96**, 1964–9.

Brzozowski, A. M,. Pike, A. C. W., Dauter, Z., Hubbard, R. E., & Bonn, T. (1997). Molecular basis of agonism and antagonism in the oestrogen receptor. *Nature*, **389**, 753–8.

Clark, J. H. & Markaverich, B. M. (1982). The agonistic–antagonistic properties of clomiphene: a review. *Pharmacol. Ther.*, **15**, 467–519.

Clarkson, T. B., Anthony, M. S., & Jerome, C. P. (1998). Lack of effect of raloxifene on coronary artery atherosclerosis of postmenopausal monkeys. *J. Clin. Endocrinol.*, **83**, 721–6.

Cohen, I., Rosen, D. J. D., Altaras, M., Beyth, Y., Shapira, J., & Yigael, D. (1993). Tamoxifen treatment in premenopausal breast cancer patients may be associated with ovarian overstimulation, cystic formations and fibroid overgrowth. *Br. J. Obstet. Gynecol.*, **100**, 567–70.

Collaborative Group on Hormonal Factors in Breast Cancer. (1997). Breast cancer and hormone replacement therapy: collaborative reanalysis of data from 51 epidemiological studies of 52 705 women with breast cancer and 108 411 women without breast cancer. *Lancet*, **350**, 1047–59.

Constantino, J. P., Kuller, L. H., Ives, D. G,. Fisher, B., & Dignam, J.(1997).Coronary heart disease mortality and adjuvant tamoxifen therapy. *J. Natl. Cancer Inst.*, **89**, 776–82.

Cosman, F. & Lindsay, R. (1999). Selective estrogen receptor modulators: clinical spectrum. *Endocr. Rev.*, **20**(3), 418–34.

Cummings, S., Eckert, S., Krueger, K., Grady, D., Powles, T. J., Cauley, J. A., Norton, L., Nickelsen, T., Bjarnason, N. H., Morrow, M., Lippman, M. E., Black, D., Glusman, J. E., Costa, A., & Jordan, V. C. (1999). The effect of raloxifene on risk of breast cancer in postmenopausal women. Results from the MORE Randomized Trial. *JAMA*, **281**, 2189–97.

Delmas, P. D., Bjarnason, N. H., Mitlak, B. H., Ravoux, A-C., Shah, A. S., Huster, W. J., Draper, M., & Christiansen, C. (1997). Effects of raloxifene on bone mineral density, serum cholesterol concentrations, and uterine endometrium in postmenopausal women. *N. Engl. J. Med.*, **337**, 1641–7.

Draper, M. W., Flowers, D. E., Huster, W. J., Neild, J. A., Harper, K. D., & Arnaud, C. (1996). A controlled trial of raloxifene (LY139481) HCl: impact on bone turnover and serum lipid profile in healthy postmenopausal women. *J. Bone Miner. Res.*, **11**, 835–42.

Early Breast Cancer Trialists' Collaborative Group. (1998). Tamoxifen for early breast cancer: an overview of the randomized trials. *Lancet*, **351**, 1451–67.

Enmark, E., Pilto-Huikko, M., Grandien, K., Lagercrantz, S., Lagercrantz, J., Fried, G., Nordenskjold, M., & Gustafsson, J-A. (1997). Human estrogen receptor-gene structure, chromosomal localization, and expression pattern. *J. Clin. Endocrinol.*, **82**, 4258–65.

Ettinger, B. (1998). Overview of estrogen replacement therapy: a historical perspective. *PSEBM*, **217**, 2–5.

Ettinger, B., Black, D. M., Mitlak, B. H., Knickerbocker, R. K., Nickelson, T., Genant, H. K., Christiansen, C., Delmas, P. D., Zanchetta, J. R., Stakkestad, J., Gluer, C. C., Krueger, K., Cohen, F. J., Eckert, S., Ensrud, K. E., Avioli, L. V., Lips, P., & Cummings, S. R. (1999). Reduction of vertebral fracture risk in postmenopausal women with osteoporosis treated with raloxifene. Results from a 3-year randomized clinical trial. *J. Am. Med. Ass.*, **282**, 637–45.

Evista (Raloxifene hydrocholoride) Product Circular (1997). Eli Lilly and Company, Indianapolis, IN.

Fisher, B., Costantino, J. P., Redmond, C. K., Fisher, E. R., Wickerham, D. L., & Cronin, W. M. (1994). Endometrial cancer in tamoxifen-treated breast cancer patients: findings from the National Surgical Adjuvant Breast and Bowel Project (NSABP) B-14. *J. Natl Cancer Inst.*, **86**, 527–37.

Fisher, B., Costantino, J. P., Wickerham, D. L., Redmond, C. K., Kavanah, M., Cronin, W. M., Vogel, V., Robidoux, A., Dimitrov, N., Atkins, J., Daly, M., Wieand, S., Tan-Chiu, E., Ford, L., & Wolmark, N. (1998). Tamoxifen for prevention of breast cancer: report of the National Surgical Adjuvant Breast and Bowel Project P-1 Study. *J. Natl. Cancer Inst.*, **90**, 1371–88.

Grey, A. B., Stapleton, J. P., Evans, M. C., & Reid, I. R. (1995a). The effect of the anti-estrogen tamoxifen on cardiovascular risk factors in normal postmenopausal women. *J. Clin. Endocrinol. Metab.*, **80**, 3191–5.

Grey, A. B., Stapleton, J. P., Evans, M. C., Tatnell, M. A., Ames, R. W., & Reid, I. R. (1995b). The effect of the antiestrogen tamoxifen on bone mineral density in normal late postmenopausal women. *Am. J. Med.*, **99**, 636–41.

Hard, G. C., Iatropoulos, M. J., Jordan, K., Radi, L., Kaltenberg, D. P., Imondi, A. R., & Williams, G. M. (1993). Major differences in the hepatocarcinogenicity and DNA adduct forming ability between toremifene and tamoxifen in female Crl: CD(BR) rats. *Cancer Res.*, **53**, 3919–24.

Heier, J. S., Dragoo, R. A., Enzenauer, R. W., & Waterhouse, W. J. (1994). Screening for ocular toxicity in asymptomatic patients treated with tamoxifen. *Am. J. Ophthalmol.*, **117**, 772–5.

Henderson, V. W. (1997). The epidemiology of estrogen replacement therapy and Alzheimer's disease. *Neurology*, **48**, S27–S35.

Hulley, S., Grady, D., Bush, T., Furberg, C., Herrington, D., Riggs, B., & Vittinghoff, E. (1998) Randomized trial of estrogen plus progestin for secondary prevention of coronary heart disease in postmenopausal women. Heart and Estrogen/progestin Replacement Study (HERS) Research Group. *JAMA*, **280**, 605–13.

Jaiyesimi, I. A., Buzdar, A. U., Decker, D. A., & Hortobagyi, G. N. (1995). Use of tamoxifen for breast cancer: twenty-eight years later. *J. Clin. Oncol.*, **113**, 513–29.

Kulper, G. G. J. M., Enmark, E., Pelto-Huikko, M., Nilsson, S., & Gustafsson, J-A. (1996). Cloning of a novel estrogen receptor expressed in rat prostate and ovary. *Proc. Natl Acad. Sci., USA*, **93**, 5925–30.

Love, R. R., Mazess, R. B., Barden, H. S., Epstein, S., Newcomb, P. A., Jordan, V. C., Carbone, P. P., & DeMets, D. L. (1992). Effects of tamoxifen on bone mineral density in postmenopausal women with breast cancer. *N. Engl. J. Med.*, **326**, 852–6.

McDonald, C. C. & Stewart, H. J. (1991). Fatal myocardial infarction in the Scottish adjuvant tamoxifen trial. The Scottish Breast Cancer Committee. *Br. Med. J.*, **303**, 435–7.

Osborne, C. K. (1998). Drug therapy. Tamoxifen in the treatment of breast cancer. *N. Engl. J. Med.*, **339**, 1609–18.

Powles, T. J., Hickish, T., Kanis, J. A., Tidy, A., & Ashley, S. (1996). Effect of tamoxifen on bone mineral density measured by dual energy x-ray absorptiometry in healthy premenopausal and postmenopausal women. *J. Clin. Oncol.*, **14**, 78–84.

Rossing, M. A., Daling, J. R., Weiss, N. S., Moore, D. E., & Self, S. G. (1994). Ovarian tumors in a cohort of infertile women. *N. Engl. J. Med.*, **331**, 771–6.

Rutqvist, L. E. & Mattsson, A., for the Stockholm Breast Cancer Study Group. (1993). Cardiac and thromboembolic morbidity among postmenopausal women with early stage breast cancer in a randomized trial of adjuvant tamoxifen. *J. Natl Cancer Inst.*, **85**, 1398–406.

Shewmon, D. A., Stock, J. L., Rosen, C. J., Heiniluoma, K. M., Hogue, M. M., Morrison, A., Doyle, E. M., Ukena, T., Weale, V., & Baker, S. (1994). Tamoxifen and estrogen lower circulating lipoprotein(a) concentrations in healthy postmenopausal women. *Arterioscler. Thromb.*, **14**, 1586–93.

Thylan, S. (1995). Tamoxifen treatment and its consequences. *Hum. Reprod.*, **10**, 2174–8.

Turner, C. H., Sato, M., & Bryant, H. U. (1994). Raloxifene preserves bone strength and bone mass in ovariectomized rats. *Endocrinology*, **135**, 2001–5.

Wakeling, A. E. (1997). Clinical implications of target organ-specific actions of selective antiestrogens. In *Estrogens and Antiestrogens, Basic and Clinical Aspects*, ed. R. Lindsay, D. W. Dempster, & V. C. Jordan, pp. 165–73. Philadelphia: Lippincott-Raven Publishers.

Walsh, B. W., Kuller, L. H., Wild, R. A., Paul, S., Farmer, M., Lawrence, J. B., Shah, A. S., & Anderson, P. W. (1998). Effects of raloxifene on serum lipids and coagulation factors in healthy postmenopausal women. *JAMA*, **279**, 1445–55.

Williams, J. K., Wagner, J. D., Zhang, L., Golden, D. L., & Adams, M. R. (1997). Tamoxifen inhibits arterial accumulation of LDL degradation products and progression of coronary artery atherosclerosis in monkeys. *Arterioscler. Thromb. Vasc. Biol.*, **17**, 403–8.

Yang, N. N., Venugopalan, M., Hardikar, S., & Glasebrook, A. (1996). Identification of an estrogen response element activated by metabolites of 17-B-estradiol and raloxifene. *Science*, **273**, 1222–5.

Yang, N. N., Venugopalan, M., Hardikar, S., & Glasebrook, A. (1997). Correction: raloxifene response needs more than an element. *Science*, **275**, 1249.

22

Bisphosphonate therapy of osteoporosis

Frederick R. Singer and Payam Minoofar

Preclinical history

About 100 years ago German chemists discovered that inorganic pyrophosphate could prevent deposition of calcium salts from solution. This observation was the basis of the industrial use of polyphosphates for prevention of calcium carbonate deposition in pipes.

The first biological effect of a pyrophosphate analog was demonstrated in 1968 when Fleisch and his associates in Switzerland found that these agents could inhibit vitamin D-induced aortic calcification in rats (Schibler et al., 1968). Subsequent collaboration of the Swiss investigators with Dr M. D. Francis and his colleagues at Procter and Gamble resulted in the development of bisphosphonates which could be applied to the treatment of a variety of human disorders, the most common of which is osteoporosis.

Chemistry

The bisphosphonates, which were initially termed diphosphonates, are compounds which have two C–P bonds. The compounds are referred to as geminal bisphosphonates if the two bonds are found on the same carbon atom (P–C–P), although this class of compounds is usually simply termed bisphosphonates.

The bisphosphonates are analogs of inorganic pyrophosphate whose core structure has a P–O–P structure. The substitution of an alkyl group confers resistance to hydrolysis to the bisphosphonates whereas inorganic pyrophosphate is highly susceptible to hydrolysis by pyrophosphatases such as alkaline phosphatase.

A great variety of bisphosphonates have been synthesized beginning with etidronate (Fig. 22.1). This has been made possible because the core P–C–P structure allows modification of the two lateral chains on the carbon atom and esterification of the phosphates. These compounds can form soluble and insoluble complexes and aggregates with metal ions. Therefore, considerable care has been taken in the intravenous use of these agents in clinical studies so as to avoid toxic effects. There

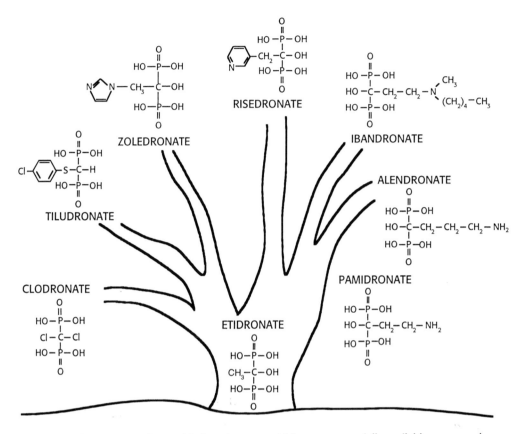

Fig. 22.1 The structure of some bisphosphonates which are commercially available or are under intensive clinical investigation. The least potent, etidronate, clodronate and tiludronate have no amino group on the R² side chain. The presence of an amino group on R² in various configurations confers increased potency on pamidronate, alendronate, risedronate, ibandronate and zoledronate in order of increasing potency.

is evidence of bisphosphonate binding to plasma proteins, but the details of this are incomplete.

Pharmacology

The bisphosphonates are most commonly administered orally although the bio-availability is low. Intestinal absorption ranges from <1% to 10% and may be variable. The low absorption may be a consequence of low lipophilicity and strong negative charge, which reduces transcellular transport and paracellular transport, respectively. Absorption is further reduced if the drug is taken with meals, calcium, iron, or even coffee or orange juice. Consequently, it is strongly recommended that these drugs be taken only with water and that they be taken in the morning 30–120 minutes before breakfast. However, it has been noted that etidronate can be clinically effective if taken at other times of the day if no food or medications are taken 2 hours before or after the drug.

After oral or intravenous administration the half-life of the bisphosphonate ranges from 30 minutes to 2 hours. The bisphosphonates rapidly bind to the skeleton in proportion to the vascularity and rate of bone formation at different sites. This accounts for the standard use of radiolabeled bisphosphonates for bone scans in nuclear medicine departments. Depending on the specific bisphosphonate, 20–80% of the circulating drug binds to bone and the majority of the remaining is excreted unchanged into the urine. The renal clearance of bisphosphonates is quite high, and there is some evidence for active secretion. A small proportion of these drugs may be taken up by the liver and spleen. This uptake may represent phagocytosis of bisphosphonate–metal complexes or aggregates by macrophages in the reticulo-endothelial system. It is possible that aggregates forming in the blood after intravenous infusion of large doses may deposit in the kidney and impair renal function.

The deposition of bisphosphonates in the skeleton is a complex process which as yet is not well defined in man. Clearly, deposition occurs at sites of bone formation but alendronate appears to accumulate preferentially under osteoclasts in rat bone (Sato et al., 1991). Saturation of skeletal uptake in humans does not appear to occur in the doses used to treat human disorders. It is of interest that, despite continuing uptake of a bisphosphonate over time, the maximum biologic effects occur relatively rapidly, are dose dependent and do not increase with time. Discontinuation of treatment generally is followed by a prolonged duration of effect. This presumably represents, at least in part, the effects of stored bisphosphonate in bone. The skeletal half-life of the drugs has been estimated to range from 3 months to a year in rodents. In humans, who have much lower bone turnover, estimates of half-life have been as high as 10 years or more.

The pharmacological actions of bisphosphonates can be divided into physicochemical effects and biological effects. The physicochemical effects mimic those of inorganic pyrophosphate. The drugs bind strongly to calcium phosphate crystals and inhibit crystal formation, aggregation and dissolution. They also inhibit the formation and aggregation of calcium oxalate crystals.

The main biological effect which accounts for the clinical success of these drugs is inhibition of bone resorption (Fleisch et al., 1969). Inhibition of osteoclastic bone resorption has been demonstrated in vitro by studying isolated osteoclasts, in vivo in animals and in vivo in clinical studies. The structural diversity of available bisphosphonates is associated with a great range of potencies. Etidronate is the least potent bisphosphonate with a therapeutic dose of 200–400 mg. Zoledronate produces a substantial decrease in bone resorption at a dose of under 1 mg given intra-venously. The P–C–P motif accounts for binding of bisphosphonates to hydroxya-patite whereas the R^2 side chain structure determines the antiresorptive potency. The addition of a primary amino group confers much greater potency than seen with the earlier bisphosphonates which lacked an amino group. Even greater potency is exhibited by the newer analogs which have methylation of the amino group or inclusion of the group within a heterocyclic ring.

In vivo the effect on bone resorption can be demonstrated within 24–48 hours. Over a longer period of time there is a secondary decrease in rate of bone forma-tion. The much earlier decrease in bone resorption promotes an increase in calcium balance and bone density. At higher doses of bisphosphonates an impairment of bone mineralization followed by osteomalacia may occur (King et al., 1971). This has almost only been observed clinically in patients treated with etidronate. Etidronate is the only bisphosphonate in which this undesirable effect is seen at doses near the therapeutic range.

Mode of action

There appear to be a variety of mechanisms whereby bisphosphonates produce their inhibition of bone resorption (Rogers et al., 1997). Considerable evidence suggests that the mechanisms of inhibition differ amongst the growing number of bisphosphonates.

In Table 22.1 the proposed mechanisms of action to account for inhibition of bone resorption are listed. The effects of bisphosphonates on bone cells are felt to be potentiated by the concentration of the drugs at the internal surfaces of the bone. It is envisioned that the release of drug by osteoclast activity is an important means of inducing intracellular biochemical changes in the cells which reduce osteoclast function. These changes include inhibition of protein synthesis, inhibition of gly-colysis, inhibition of several protein tyrosine phosphatases as well as increasing the level of protein phosphorylation by inhibiting protein phosphatase activity. Inhibition of proton-pumping ATPases may also reduce acidification of the resorp-tion cavity beneath osteoclasts. Russell and colleagues have reported experiments in amoebae of a slime mold which divides bisphosphonates into two classes with respect to mechanisms of inhibition of resorptive activity (Rogers et al., 1997). Clodronate and other bisphosphonates that are quite similar in structure to pyro-phosphate can be metabolized to an analog of ATP which appears to induce apop-tosis of osteoclasts. The amino-containing bisphosphonates are not metabolized but instead appear to inhibit enzymes of the mevalonate pathway and thereby disrupt osteoclast function.

In other in vitro experiments the amino-containing bisphosphonates have been

Table 22.1. Proposed modes of action for inhibition of bone
resorption by bisphosphonates

(i)   Direct inhibition of function of mature osteoclasts
(ii) Induction of osteoclast apoptosis
(iii) Osteoblast-mediated inhibition of osteoclast recruitment
(iv) Inhibition of differention of precursors into osteoclasts

demonstrated to inhibit transformation of osteoclast precursors into mature osteo-clasts (Boonekamp et al., 1986). How important this mechanism is in compari-son with direct inhibition of osteoclast function or induction of cell death is unknown.

Since osteoblasts are known to be local regulators of adjacent osteoclast function, studies have been designed to determine if osteoclast function might be mediated through the osteoblast. Bisphosphonates have now been shown to induce secretion of an osteoclast inhibitor by osteoblasts (Vitté et al., 1996). It has also been con-cluded that the ability of alendronate to inhibit osteoclastic activity is not depen-dent on release of the drug from bone surfaces and that a variety of cell types in bone (osteoblasts, stromal cells) could assist in promoting the effects of bisphos-phonates on bone resorption (Owens et al., 1997).

Although it is quite clear that there is a secondary decrease in bone formation in animals or patients treated with bisphosphonates, some investigators have felt that bone formation might be increased by these drugs in certain circumstances. The first direct experimental evidence consistent with this hypothesis has recently been published (Giuliani et al., 1998). In human bone marrow cultures alendronate stimulated the formation of colony forming units for osteoblasts in the presence of dexamethasone and also colony forming units for fibroblasts, an early source of osteoblast progenitors. In addition, formation of mineralized nodules was observed. These effects were associated with an increase in the concentration of basic fibroblast growth factor in the cultures, a known stimulator of osteoblastic activity. Therefore, it is possible that bisphosphonate therapy may produce a modest degree of bone formation in vivo.

Treatment and prevention of postmenopausal osteoporosis

In postmenopausal osteoporosis an increase in bone resorption is a major manifes-tation of the estrogen-deficient state which generally occurs in women over 50 years of age. This usually is reversed by estrogen replacement therapy but in the great majority of eligible women long-term estrogen is not accepted. The effectiveness of the bisphosphonates in controlling bone resorption in postmenopausal women has been repeatedly documented since 1990 and these drugs are now widely available for use in the postmenopausal woman who refuses or cannot tolerate estrogen.

Etidronate

Two randomized double-blind, placebo-controlled studies published in 1990 demonstrated the effects of etidronate in women with postmenopausal osteoporosis (Storm et al., 1990; Watts et al., 1990). A small study in Denmark involved 66 women who were followed for nearly a 3-year period (Storm et al., 1990). They received placebo or a 400 mg daily oral dose of etidronate for 2 weeks followed by 13 weeks without drug and then a repetition of this regimen ten times. The intermittent program was chosen to minimize the chance of osteomalacia occurring in the study patients. Oral calcium and vitamin D supplementation were provided throughout the study. In the treated patients the lumbar spine density rose by 5.3% whereas there was a 2.7% decrease in the placebo group. Bone biopsies revealed no evidence of osteomalacia.

The second study was a large multicenter trial in the United States with a more complex design carried out over 2 years (Watts et al., 1990). In this study, cyclic etidronate for 2 weeks was again used but another arm of the study was the administration of an oral phosphate supplement 3 days before the etidronate. At the end of 2 years mean spine density rose 4.2% in those who received etidronate alone and 5.2% in the group who also received phosphate. The difference between the two groups was not significant. The rate for new vertebral fractures was reduced by 50% in the etidronate-treated patients as compared to those who received phosphate alone or placebo. The results of an extension of this study were reported in 1993 (Harris et al., 1993). Three years of blinded treatment were followed by a fourth year of unblinded treatment. The increase in lumbar spine density which peaked at year 2 was maintained through the fourth year. An increase in hip density was of a lesser degree but was also sustained over the 4 years. In patients with three or more fractures at study entry there was a reduced vertebral fracture rate. No serious adverse effects were documented.

Estrogen replacement therapy has been shown to produce an additive effect on bone mineral density of the spine and hip when administered with cyclical etidronate therapy (Wimalawansa, 1995, 1998). In postmenopausal women averaging about 52 years of age the combination therapy increased vertebral density by 10.9% and hip density by 7.25% after 4 years (Wimalawansa, 1995). No evidence of osteomalacia was found in iliac crest bone biopsies. However, 3/9 patients treated with intermittent cyclic etidronate did exhibit evidence of osteomalacia (two had focal lesions and one had generalized osteomalacia in the biopsy).

A 4-year trial of estrogen replacement therapy with cyclical etidronate was also done in postmenopausal women with established osteoporosis who averaged 64.9 years (Wimalawansa, 1998). Bone mineral density increased by 10.4% in the lumbar spine and by 7% in the hip, a result quite similar to that found in the women of the previous study. In this study no osteomalacia was detected in the biopsies of women who received combination therapy or cyclical etidronate. Patients treated with the combined therapy lost less than 0.5 cm height after 4 years. The study population of 72 patients was not large enough to prove a significant decrease in fracture incidence among the groups of patients who received combination therapy or one of the therapies in isolation.

At the present time regulatory agencies in many countries (including Canada, France, Germany, Italy, United Kingdom) have approved etidronate for the treatment of osteoporosis. Although it has not been approved in the United States, it is widely prescribed.

Clodronate

Clodronate was the second bisphosphonate to undergo clinical evaluation in patients with bone disorders characterized by increased bone resorption. The drug has been approved throughout the world for use in bone disease associated with malignancy and in a few countries for Paget's disease of bone. As of 1997 the drug was only approved for treatment of osteoporosis in Italy. In an Italian study reported in 1993, 400 mg clodronate given cyclically by mouth for 30 days followed by 60 days with no treatment produced a 3.88% increase in lumbar spine density after 12 months treatment of postmenopausal women (Giannini et al., 1993). The spine density decreased 2.34% in untreated patients. In another study from Italy a 200 mg intravenous infusion of clodronate was administered to 235 women with postmenopausal osteoporosis every 3 weeks for 6 years (Filipponi et al., 1996). The lumbar spine density increased 5.69%. When compared to historical control subjects the incidence of vertebral fractures decreased after 3 years. A more recent study from Finland reported that three intravenous infusions of 300 mg clodronate given one week apart prevented bone loss 24 months later (Heikkinen et al., 1997).

Pamidronate

Pamidronate, the first potent aminobisphosphonate is approved in many countries for intravenous treatment of hypercalcemia of malignancy, bone metastases and Paget's disease of bone. In South America and several Asian countries an oral form is approved for osteoporosis. Development of the oral form has proved difficult because of gastrointestinal irritation from some preparations. When tolerated, oral pamidronate can increase spinal and hip bone density similar to the effects of etidronate and clodronate. In a recent study in England, 300 mg pamidronate daily for

4 weeks every 4 months or 150 mg for 4 weeks every 2 months increased lumbar spine density 2.8% and 3.0%, respectively, after 2 years (Less et al., 1996). The lower dose given more frequently was better tolerated by the postmenopausal women who participated in this study.

Alendronate

Large multicenter trials have been done to investigate the effects of oral alendronate on bone density as well as fracture prevalence in postmenopausal females. In 1995, a dose-finding study of 188 women with low bone density in the United States revealed that 10 mg of alendronate given daily for 2 years produced excellent results (Chestnut et al., 1995). Biochemical markers of bone turnover were suppressed by approximately 50%, lumbar spine density increased by an average of 7.21% and total hip density increased by an average of 5.27%. A second worldwide study evaluated 994 postmenopausal women taking several doses of alendronate for 3 years (Liberman et al., 1995). The 10 mg dose again produced an excellent response as lumbar spine density increased by an average of 8.8% and femoral neck density by an average of 5.9%. Overall, treatment with a variety of doses of alendronate and 500 mg of calcium produced a 48% decrease in the proportion of women with new vertebral fractures as compared to the control group who received 500 mg calcium daily. It was somewhat surprising to note that there was a further slight increase in lumbar spine and femoral neck densities between year 2 and 3. This could represent an unexpected anabolic effect of a bisphosphonate or possibly is consistent with the reversal of negative bone balance at individual remodeling units.

To more definitively examine the effects of alendronate on fracture prevention a randomized trial was conducted on 2027 postmenopausal women with at least one existing vertebral fracture in 11 metropolitan areas of the United States (Black et al., 1996). The first 24 months of the study the patients received 5 mg of alendronate or placebo daily. After it was appreciated that 10 mg was a more effective dose all treated patients received 10 mg daily during the last year of the study. All subjects received a 500 mg calcium supplement if their dietary intake of calcium was less than 1000 mg. Bone density increased to a similar degree as in previous studies. In the women who received alendronate, 8% had one or more new morphometric vertebral fractures compared with 15% in the placebo-calcium group. Clinical fractures, i.e., those requiring medical attention, occurred in 5% of the placebo-calcium patients and 2.3% of those treated with alendronate (Fig. 22.2). The risk of hip or wrist fractures was also reduced by about 50%. Overall, the drug was well tolerated with there being no significant difference in adverse experiences between the placebo and drug groups. When the data were further analyzed, the reduction in fracture risk was present in those of advanced age, ≥75 years as well as in the group with the lowest bone mineral density (Ensrud et al., 1997).

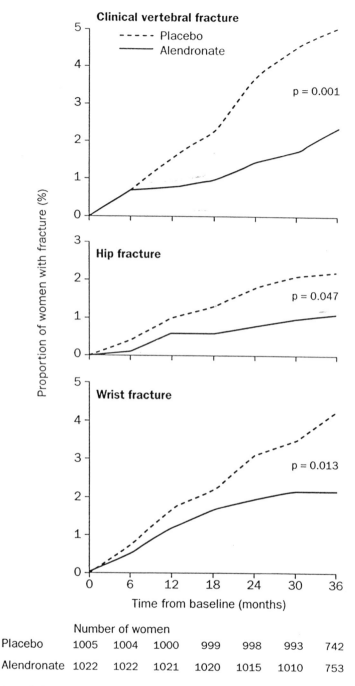

Fig. 22.2   Cumulative proportions of postmenopausal women 55–81-year-old women with clinical vertebral fracture, hip fracture or wrist fracture during a 3-year study treated with a placebo or alendronate (5 mg for 2 years, 10 mg for 1 year). Most women also received a 500 mg calcium supplement to adjust calcium intake to about 1000 mg. From Black et al. (1996), reproduced by permission of *The Lancet*.

The efficacy of alendronate is now well established in postmenopausal women treated continuously for three years. What is not known is how long should treatment continue. One study has been reported which should aid in defining appropriate patterns of alendronate therapy in postmenopausal women who permanently refrain from estrogen use. In the previously discussed study of 188 postmenopausal women with low lumbar spine bone density (Chestnut et al., 1995) follow-up biochemical and bone density evaluations were made for one or two years after discontinuation of the alendronate (Stock et al., 1997). It was encouraging to learn that the difference in bone density between alendronate and placebo groups at the end of treatment was maintained for at least 1 year after 5 or 10 mg of alendronate daily for 2 years, although biochemical markers of bone turnover had partially returned toward pretreatment levels. With time, it should be possible to define optimum intermittent long-term treatment courses for postmenopausal osteoporosis which take advantage of the skeletal storage of alendronate.

One large study of the effects of alendronate therapy in postmenopausal women under 60 years of age has been reported (Hosking et al., 1998). The effects of 2.5 mg or 5 mg of alendronate or placebo on bone mineral density was evaluated in 1174 women. Another group of women received either alendronate or open-label estrogen–progestin therapy. The 5 mg alendronate dose increased lumbar spine density by an average of 3.5% and hip density by an average of 1.9%, whereas estrogen–progestin therapy produced responses 1–2% greater. Bone density fell in the placebo group. This study documented the efficacy of 5 mg alendronate as an alternative to estrogen–progestin in preventing bone loss in early postmenopausal women.

Risedronate

Risedronate, another potent aminobisphosphonate, has proven to be effective in a randomized, double-blind, placebo-controlled trial of 2458 postmenopausal women with at least 1 vertebral fracture (Harris et al., 1999). An oral dose of 5 mg daily increased bone mineral density of the lumbar spine by 5.4% and density of the femoral neck by 1.6% after 3 years. This was associated with a 41% reduction in cumulative incidence of new vertebral fractures and a 39% reduction in nonvertebral fractures.

Prevention of glucocorticoid – induced bone loss

Osteoporosis is a major complication of chronic glucocorticoid therapy. Impaired bone formation appears to be the major abnormality responsible for bone loss but there is also evidence of increased bone resorption. There are now numerous published studies which have documented the benefits of bisphosphonates in prevention of bone loss from glucocorticoid therapy.

There are now two randomized trials using cyclical etidronate which demonstrate the efficacy of this therapy (Adachi et al., 1997; Roux et al., 1998). In a Canadian multicenter trial 141 men and women who were started on high dose glucocorticoid therapy no more than 100 days previously were randomized to placebo or 400 mg etidronate for 14 days every 3 months for 1 year (Adachi et al., 1997). All patients received 500 mg calcium for 76 days after each 14-day period. Lumbar spine bone density decreased an average of 3.23.% and trochanter density an average of 2.74% in the placebo group whereas bone density in the same sites increased slightly in the etidronate group. A second multicenter trial in Europe evaluated 117 men and women who had begun high dose glucocorticoid therapy no more than 90 days prior to entering the study (Roux et al., 1998). The same treatment protocol was used as in the Canadian study. The bone density of the lumbar spine decreased an average of 2.79% in the placebo group and increased an average of 0.30% in the etidronate group. This result was very similar to the Canadian study but there was no significant difference between the two groups with respect to hip density measurements. The explanation for the apparent lack of protective effect of etidronate on hip density loss is not apparent but the decrease of femoral neck and trochanter density after one year was only slightly above 1%. In both these studies etidronate was generally given after the onset of glucocorticoid therapy. It might be expected that somewhat better results would be obtained if the bisphosphonate were given at the onset of glucocorticoid therapy.

In addition to etidronate, other bisphosphonates such as pamidronate (Gallacher et al., 1992), clodronate (Herrala et al., 1998) and alendronate (Gonelli et al., 1997; Saag et al., 1998) have been reported to be effective in treating patients on glucocorticoid therapy. In a randomized trial of alendronate 10 mg daily increased bone mineral density of the lumbar spine by 2.9%. Alendronate is now approved for use in steroid-treated patients in the United States (Saag et al., 1998).

Adverse effects of bisphosphonates

Generally, the bisphosphonates have proven to be well tolerated by most patients but adverse effects may occur with considerable variability from one agent to another (Adami & Zamberlan, 1996).

The most common side-effects are in the gastrointestinal tract. Epigastric pain, vomiting, nausea and diarrhea may occur. These are more likely to occur with aminobisphosphonates, particularly pamidronate. Erosive esophagitis has occurred with alendronate therapy but if the drug is taken with adequate water and the patient does not lie down prior to breakfast this can be avoided.

Pamidronate has been reported to cause uveitis, scleritis and episcleritis, possibly in 1/1000 patients. Skin reactions are rare but have occurred with several bisphosphonates and may represent allergic reactions.

Aminobisphosphonates may cause an acute phase reaction within 24 hours of onset of therapy. This may be mediated by release of interleukin-6 and is associated with increased levels of C-reactive protein and a reduction in serum zinc. The absolute lymphocyte count decreases for several days. Pyrexia, malaise, and myalgias mimic an influenza attack. Recovery is usually within 48 hours and recurrence of the reaction is unusual if treatment is continuous.

Renal failure has rarely occurred with the present commonly used bisphosphonate regimens.

In osteoporosis, hypocalcemia has not been a complication of bisphosphonate therapy and clinical osteomalacia has rarely been evident even with etidronate use. Despite the potential of impaired fracture healing due to suppression of the metabolic activity of bone cells, impaired fracture healing has not been implicated as a complication of bisphosphonate therapy.

REFERENCES

Adachi, J. D., Bensen, W. G., Brown, J., Hanley, D., Hodsman, A., Josse, R., Kendler, D. L., Lentle, B., Olszynki, W., Ste-Marie, L. G., Tenenhouse, A., & Chines, A. A. (1997). Intermittent etidronate therapy to prevent corticosteroid-induced osteoporosis. *N. Engl. J. Med.*, **337**, 382–7.

Adami, S. & Zamberlan, N. (1996). Adverse effects of bisphosphonates. A comparative review. *Drug Safety*, **14**, 158–70.

Black, D. M., Cummings, S. R., Karpf, D. B., Cauley, J. A., Thompson, D. E., Nevitt, M. C., Bauer, D. C., Genant, H. K., Haskell, W. L., Marcus, R., Oh, S. M., Torner, J. C., Quandt, S. A., Reiss, T. F., & Ensrud, K. E. (1996). Randomised trial of effect of alendronate on risk of fracture in women with existing vertebral fractures. *Lancet*, **348**, 1535–41.

Boonekamp, P. M., Pals, L. J. A., van Lennep, M. M. L. et al. (1986). Two modes of action of bisphosphonates on osteoclastic resorption of mineralized matrix. *Bone Miner.*, **1**, 27–39.

Chestnut, C. H., McClung, M. R., Ensrud, K. E., Bell, N. H., Genant, H. K., Harris, S. T., Singer, F. R., Stock, J. L., Yood, R. A., Delmas, P. D. et al. (1995). Alendronate treatment of the postmenopausal osteoporotic woman: Effect of multiple dosages on bone mass and bone remodeling. *Am. J. Med.*, **99**, 144–52.

Ensrud, K. E., Black, D. M., Palermo, L., Bauer, D. C., Barrett-Connor, E., Quandt, S. A., Thompson, D. A., & Karpf, D. B. (1997). Treatment with alendronate prevents fractures in women at highest risk. Results from the Fracture Intervention Trial. *Arch. Internal Med.*, **157**, 2617–24.

Filipponi, P., Cristallini, S., Rizzello, E., Policani, G., Fedeli, L., Gregorio, F., Boldrini, S., Troiani, S., & Massonni, C. (1996). Cyclical intravenous clodronate in postmenopausal osteoporosis: results of a long-term clinical trial. *Bone*, **18**(2), 179–84.

Fleisch, H., Russell, R. G. G., & Francis, M. D. (1969). Diphosphonates inhibit hydroxyapatite dissolution in vitro and bone resorption in tissue culture and in vivo. *Science*, **165**, 1262–4.

Gallacher, S. J., Fenner, J. A. K., Anderson, K., Bryden, F. M., Banham, S. W., Logue, F. C., Cowan,

R. A., Boyle, I. T. et al. (1992). Intravenous pamidronate in the treatment of osteoporosis associated with corticosteroid dependent lung disease: an open pilot study. *Thorax*, 47, 932–6.

Giannini, S., D'Angelo, A., Malvasi, L., Castrignano, R., Pati, T., Tronca, R., Liberto, L., Nobile, M., & Crepaldi, G. (1993). Effects of one-year cyclical treatment with clodronate on postmenopausal bone loss. *Bone*, 14, 137–41.

Giuliani, N., Pedrazzoni, M., Negri, G., Passeri, G., Impicciatore, M., & Girasole, G. (1998). Bisphosphonates stimulate formation of osteoblast precursors and mineralized nodules in murine and human bone marrow cultures in vitro and promote early osteoblastogenesis in young and aged mice in vivo. *Bone*, 22, 455–61.

Gonelli, S., Rottoli, P., Cepollaro, C., Pondrelli, C., Cappiello, V., Vagliasindi, M., & Gennari, C. (1997). Prevention of corticosteroid-induced osteoporosis with alendronate in sarcoid patients. *Calcif. Tissue Int.*, 61, 382–5.

Harris, S. T., Watts, N. B., & Jackson, R. D. (1993). Four-year study of intermittent cyclic etidronate treatment of postmenopausal osteoporosis: three years of blinded therapy followed by one year of open therapy. *Am. J. Med.*, 95, 557–67.

Harris, S. T., Watts, N. B., Genant, H. K. et al. (1999). Effects of risedronate treatment on vertebral and nonvertebral fractures in women with postmenopausal osteoporosis. A randomized controlled trial. *JAMA*, 282, 1344–52.

Heikkinen, J. E., Selander, K. S., Kalevi Laitinen, K., Arnala, I., & Vaananen, H. K. (1997). Short-term intravenous bisphosphonates in prevention of postmenopausal bone loss. *J. Bone Miner. Res.*, 12(1), 103–10.

Herrala, J., Puolijoki, H, Lüppo, K., Raitio, M., Impivaara, D., Tala, E., & Nieminen, M. M. (1998). Clodronate is effective in preventing corticosteroid-induced bone loss among asthmatic patients. *Bone*, 22, 577–82.

Hosking, D., Chilvers, C. E., Christiansen, C., Ravn, P., Wasnich, R., Ross, P., McClung, M., Balske, A., Thompson, D., Daley, M., & Yates, A. J. (1998). Prevention of bone loss with alendronate in postmenopausal women under 60 years of age. Early Postmenopausal Intervention Cohort Study Group. *N. Engl. J. Med.*, 338, 485–92.

King, W. R., Francis, M. D., & Michael, W. R. (1971). Effect of disodium ethane-1-hydroxy-1,1-diphosphonate on bone formation. *Clin. Orthop.*, 78, 251–70.

Less, B., Garland, S. W., Walton, C., Ross, D., Whitehead, M. I., & Stevenson, J. C. (1996). Role of oral pamidronate in preventing bone loss in postmenopausal women. *Osteoporos. Int.*, 6, 480–5.

Liberman, U. A., Weiss, S. R., & Bröll, J. (1995). Effect of oral alendronate on bone mineral density and the incidence of fractures in postmenopausal osteoporosis. *N. Engl. J. Med.*, 333, 1437–43.

Owens, J. M., Fuller, K., & Chambers, T. J. (1997). Osteoclast activation: potent inhibition by the bisphosphonate alendronate through a nonresorptive mechanism. *J. Cell. Physiol.*, 172, 79–86.

Rogers, M. J., Watts, D. J., & Russell, R. G. G. (1997). Overview of bisphosphonates. *Cancer*, 80(Suppl), 1652–60.

Roux, C., Oriente, P., Laan, R., Hughes, R. A., Ittner, J., Goemaere, S., Di Munno, O., Pouilles, J. M., Horlait, S., & Cortet, B. (1998). Randomized trial of effect of cyclical etidronate in the prevention of corticosteroid-induced bone loss. *J. Clin. Endocrinol. Metab.*, 83, 1128–33.

Saag, K. G., Emkey, R., Schnizer, T. et al. (1998). Alendronate for the treatment and prevention of glucocorticoid osteoporosis. *N. Engl. J. Med.*, **399**, 292–9.

Sato, M., Grasser, W., Endo, N., Akins, R., Simmons, H., Thompson, D. D., Golub, E., & Rodan, G. A. (1991). Bisphosphonate action. Alendronate localization in rat bone and effects on osteoclast ultrastructure *J. Clin. Invest.*, **88**, 2095–105.

Schibler, D., Russel, R. G. G., & Fleisch, H. (1968). Inhibition by pyrophosphate and polyphosphate of aortic calcification induced by vitamin D_3 in rats. *Clin. Sci.*, **35**, 363–72.

Stock, J. L., Bell, N. H., Chestnut, C. H., Ensrud, K. E., Genant, H. K., Harris, S. T., McClung, M. R., Singer, F. R., Yood, R. A., Pryor-Tillotson, S., Wei, L., & Santora, A. C. (1997). Increments in bone mineral density of the lumbar spine and hip and suppression of bone turnover are maintained after discontinuation of alendronate in postmenopausal women. *Am. J. Med.*, **103**, 291–7.

Storm, T., Thomsborg, G., Stieniche, T., Genant, H. K., & Sorenson, O. H. (1990). Effect of intermittent cyclical etidronate therapy on bone mass and fracture rate in women with postmenopausal osteoporosis. *N. Engl. J. Med.*, **322**, 1265–71.

Vitté, C., Fleisch, H., & Guenther, H. L. (1996). Bisphosphonates induce osteoblasts to secrete an inhibitor of osteoclast-mediated resorption. *Endocrinology*, **137**, 2324–33

Watts, N. B., Harris, S. T., Genant, H. K., Wahnich, R. D., Miller, P. D., Jackson, R. D., Licata, A. A., Ross, P., Woodson, G. C. III, Yanover, M. J., Mysiev, J. W., Kohse, L., Rao, B. M., Steiger, P., Richmond, B., & Chestnut, C. H. (1990). Intermittent cyclical etidronate treatment of postmenopausal osteoporosis. *N. Engl. J. Med.*, **323**, 73–9.

Wimalawansa, S. J. (1995). Combined therapy with estrogen and etidronate has an additive effect on bone mineral density in the hip and vertebrae: four-year randomized study. *Am. J. Med.*, **99**, 36–42.

Wimalawansa, S. J. (1998). A four-year randomized controlled trial of hormone replacement and bisphosphonate, alone or in combination, in women with postmenopausal osteoporosis. *Am. J. Med.*, **104**, 219–26.

23

The action of fluoride on bone

Marc D. Grynpas, Debbie Chachra and Hardy Limeback

Introduction

The fluoridation of municipal water in cities of Canada and the United States for the purpose of reducing dental decay is perhaps the most important and success-ful public health initiative ever undertaken in these countries. Since its inception more than 50 years ago, water fluoridated at 1 ppm has dramatically reduced the incidence of caries, and this positive effect has reached across all socioeconomic groups. However, since fluoride is a mineral-seeking ion, it is incorporated into bone as well as teeth. The response of bone is known to depend on the dose, and studies in both animal models and in humans have assessed the effect of moderate to high doses of fluoride. As a consequence, it is known that moderate doses of fluoride increase bone mass, making fluoride a potential therapy for osteoporosis (see below). However, chronic exposure to high doses of fluoride (>8 mg/day), while rare in North America, can cause skeletal fluorosis, characterized initially by hypermineralization of bone and later by calcification of ligaments, bone deforma-tion, and other crippling symptoms (Kaminsky et al., 1990). Ingestion of low doses of fluoride through water involves somewhat different mechanisms. Typically, indi-viduals receive less than 5 mg/day of fluoride (less than a tenth of the clinical dose), but it accumulates passively in bone mineral over a timespan of decades. This is intrinsically difficult to model in animals, and therefore remains poorly under-stood. The concern is that the ingestion of a subclinical level of fluoride, over a life-time, may have a potentially serious impact on the skeleton; specifically, it may alter the rate of osteoporotic fracture.

Fluoride ingestion

Fluoride is ingested through fluoridated water, food, and oral care products. Municipally fluoridated water generally has a fluoride concentration of 1 ppm (1 mg/l), and the average adult consumption of water is 1.5 l per day. Many foods contain fluoride, notably fish and other marine products, and tea (Singer et al., 1985). Fluoride ingestion from food in individuals over the age of 12 has remained constant at approximately 0.4 mg/day (Burt, 1992). Increasingly, however, the diet of individuals living in non-fluoridated areas is composed of beverages and foods prepared with fluoridated water (Clovis & Hargreaves, 1988). Individuals, especially children (Simard et al., 1989), also ingest fluoride from oral care products, particularly toothpaste. On average, 1 g of toothpaste is used per brushing, and adults typically ingest about 25% of it (Whitford, 1994). In North America, toothpaste is fluoridated at 1000–1100 ppm, resulting in ingestion of 0.25–0.75 mg/day of fluoride. Finally, fluoride supplements are often provided in non-fluoridated areas (Ismail, 1994). Overall fluoride consumption therefore includes other sources as well as fluoridated water, with an estimated adult total intake of fluoride ranging from 1.2 to 2.2 mg/day (Whitford, 1994).

Fluoride in the body

In general, fluoride is not incorporated into fully mineralized bone and accumulates only in bone formed during the period of exposure (Boivin & Meunier, 1993). A mathematical model of fluoride incorporation in the skeleton (Turner et al., 1993) indicates that the total bone fluoride content is linearly related to the daily ingestion of fluoride in adults up to age 55, after which it appears to plateau. However, other research suggests that fluoride can continue to be incorporated into bone through to the eighth decade of life (Ishiguro et al., 1993; Richards et al., 1994; Weatherell, 1969). The incorporation of fluoride can be affected by other factors, notably osteoporosis or impaired renal function. In osteoporosis, as resorption of bone exceeds formation, fluoride is minimally incorporated into bone. In fact, if daily intake is low, patients may actually lose fluoride from bone (Whitford, 1989). Conversely, increased uptake of fluoride by bone results if renal function is impaired, since ingested fluoride is not cleared rapidly from the system (Ekstrand & Spak, 1990). Therefore, fluoride levels in bone can vary greatly. Our preliminary data (given below) show fluoride concentrations in bone ranging from 200 to 2300 ppm, consistent with data from other studies (Ishiguro et al., 1993; Richards et al., 1994; Weatherell, 1969). The concentration of fluoride in bone is generally higher in sites with a higher turnover rate, such as cancellous rather than cortical bone (Ishiguro et al., 1993; Weatherell, 1969), or vertebrae rather than the iliac crest (Turner et al., 1993). It is not known whether these concentrations of fluoride, accumulated slowly over decades, affect the mechanical and other properties of bone.

Fluoride and bone: mechanisms and effects

Effect on bone mineral

Regardless of concentration or dose, fluoride is incorporated into bone mineral during formation, via a physicochemical mechanism. Fluoride substitutes for the hydroxyl group in hydroxyapatite, forming fluorapatite. This substitution, while no means complete (even in highly fluorotic bone, fluoride replaces only about a third of the hydroxyl ions) (Boivin et al., 1989), nevertheless has profound consequences. The fluoride makes the crystal lattice more compact and stable (Grynpas, 1990), and a mixture of fluorapatite and hydroxyapatite has been shown to be less soluble than either component individually (Moreno et al., 1977). The onset of mineralization is also delayed, resulting in increased osteoid formation (Grynpas et al., 1986). The concentrations of other contaminant ions, such as carbonate and magnesium, appear to be affected, although the exact effect remains controversial (Grynpas, 1990). Finally, fluoride shifts the mineralization profile of bone (a histogram of density fractions) towards denser, more mature fractions and fluoride appears to be concentrated in these denser fractions (Grynpas et al., 1986).

Effect on bone cells

While fluoride is passively incorporated into bone mineral at all concentrations, it appears to only affect bone cells at much higher serum levels than would be experienced through drinking fluoridated water alone (Turner et al., 1993). It is well known that high levels of fluoride increase bone mass in patients subjected to fluoride therapy and in fluorotic individuals (discussed further below). This is a result of both the increased resistance to resorption of fluoridated bone mineral, together with a mitogenic effect of these levels of fluoride on osteoblasts. This is supported by work both in vivo (Boivin et al., 1989) and in culture (Gruber & Baylink, 1991). However, the osteoblasts appear to be flattened and moderately active rather than plump, cuboidal and highly secretory. This suggests that, while fluoride is mitogenic and a promoter of differentiation of osteoblast precursors, it is somewhat toxic to individual cells at these concentrations (Bonjour et al., 1993). Nevertheless, the overall effect is of increased bone formation. While the effect of fluoride on osteoclasts is less well understood, there is some in vitro evidence that sodium fluoride decreases the number of resorption lacunae as well as the amount of bone resorbed per osteoclast (Okuda et al., 1990). The net result of these effects is increased bone formation, which accounts for the interest in fluoride as a therapy for osteoporosis.

Effect on bone architecture

Fluoride therapy for osteoporosis results in a marked increase in bone mass. However, osteoporosis-associated bone loss results in loss of connectivity as well as thinning of the remaining trabeculae and both are thought to be mechanically significant. At present, no biological pathway is known to restore the connectivity, and it is therefore thought that all types of therapy are similarly ineffective at doing so (Parfitt, 1982). Accordingly, fluoride therapy has been shown to increase trabecular thickness, but to leave the connectivity unaltered (Aaron et al., 1992). In addition, trabeculae thus formed appear to be resistant to perforation by resorption

(Aaron et al., 1992). Rats who ingested fluoridated drinking water in a range of concentrations (0, 2, 4, 6 mm/l) displayed similar changes to cancellous bone, and the effects were found to be dose dependent (Cheng & Bader, 1990).

Effect on bone mechanical properties

Among the many roles that bone plays in the body, its mechanical function is certainly the most conspicuous and one of the most important. This is highlighted in patients with osteoporosis, which is characterized not by bone loss *per se* but by the loss of the mechanical integrity of bone, as manifested by fracture upon minimal loading. The mechanical function of bone depends not only on the amount of bone present, but also on its organization at the macroscopic (such as the shape of long bones), on the microstructural (the architecture of trabeculae or of Haversian systems) and on the ultrastructural (the intimate association of collagen and mineral) level. Alterations to any one of them can have profound effects. Fluoride, in particular, has a complex, dose-dependent suite of effects on bone, including altering the amount of bone, the structure, and the mineral–collagen interface. These result in changes to the mechanical properties of bone, and by extension, to the fracture risk. Techniques such as dual-energy X-ray absorptiometry or histomorphometry, while useful, cannot assess these integrated factors. In order to quantify changes to mechanical function, one of two approaches must be used. The first approach is epidemiological: the fracture rate in a given population (such as a clinical trial of patients receiving therapy for osteoporosis) can be measured. The second approach, commonly used in animal studies, is to use in vitro mechanical testing techniques as a proxy for fracture risk. The overall picture of the effect of fluoride on mechanical properties that has arisen, based primarily on animal studies, tentatively suggests a dose-dependent effect on mechanical properties: improvement with increasing fluoride content to an optimum point, followed by severely compromised mechanical properties at high concentrations of fluoride (fluorosis).

In vitro studies in animal models

The evidence that emerges from in vitro mechanical testing of bone from animal studies clearly indicates that high doses of fluoride are detrimental to mechanical properties. Controversy remains over whether there is an optimum fluoride dose or concentration that leads to improved bone strength.

A study by Turner et al. (1992) established a weak, biphasic response to fluoride ingestion in young (21-day-old) rats. The rats were fed a low-fluoride diet, and their drinking water was fluoridated at 0, 1, 2, 4, 8, 16, 32, 64, or 128 ppm. The rats were sacrificed after 4 months. The fluoride content of the vertebrae was assessed, and femora were tested in three-point bending. It was found that the peak bone strength occurred with a fluoride intake of 16 ppm, corresponding to a bone fluoride content of 1216 ppm, and decreasing thereafter. A segmented regression model was postulated to describe this biphasic relationship. This work was in agreement with an earlier study (Rich & Feist, 1970). A later study by the same group (Turner et al., 1995) again began with 21-day-old rats, ingesting water fluoridated at 0, 5, 15, or 50 ppm, but followed them through maturity and senescence: 3, 6, 12 or 18 months. In this study, no positive effect of fluoride treatment was observed, although there was a negative effect at higher doses. No effect of fluoride was observed in a similar study (Einhorn et al., 1992), in which femora from rats exposed to drinking water fluoridated at 0, 25, 50 and 75 ppm were tested in torsion. However, the fluoride content of these bones (2026–11 716 ppm) was greater than the peak fluoride content observed by Turner et al. (1992), which may explain the discrepancy. Beary (1969) found a similar decrease in bone strength in rat femora with high fluoride intake (>45 ppm). Søgaard et al. (1994) examined the mechanical properties of vertebrae (primarily cancellous rather than cortical bone). The rats were 3 months of age at the start and ingested water fluoridated at 0, 100 and 150 ppm for 3 months before sacrifice, resulting in fluoride levels of 343, 3295 and 4617 ppm, respectively. While no changes to the failure load or stress were observed, the mechanical parameters corrected for ash content (a measurement of bone quality) were adversely affected. Similarly, Mosekilde et al. (1987) found reduced trabecular bone strength in pigs with an average bone fluoride concentration of 2836 ppm. Finally, a study examining high doses of fluoride in rabbits showed compromised mechanical properties, despite increased bone mass, mineralization and hardness (Chachra et al., 1999b; Turner et al., 1997).

While animal models are useful in providing information about high doses of fluoride, which would be difficult to obtain in humans, there are two major caveats to be considered prior to extrapolating to the human case. The first is that the rate of fluoride incorporation in other species may not be the same as in humans. For example, in rats, the rate of fluoride incorporation is an order of magnitude less than in humans, suggesting that administration of water fluoridated at 1 ppm to humans would be the equivalent of 10 ppm in rats (Turner et al., 1992). The difference is partially accounted for by differences in intestinal absorption between rats and humans (Angmar-Mansson & Whitford, 1982). The second difference is that animal studies typically examine the effect of high doses of fluoride for short times, rather than the low doses and long exposures of humans. While low doses of fluoride are thought to act by altering bone at the level of crystal structure (Grynpas, 1990) and the mineral–collagen interface (Walsh & Guzelsu, 1993), high doses affect bone cells and therefore remodeling processes.

In vitro studies in humans

To date, data correlating fluoride content and bone quality by in vitro mechanical testing in humans are scarce. Richards et al. (1994) examined vertebral trabecular bone cylinders from individuals aged 20 to 91, who were not exposed to artificially fluoridated water, to elucidate changes in bone mechanics and fluoride content with age. They found that the bone mass decreased, as did the bone strength normalized for the bone mass. While the fluoride concentration increased with age, it did not affect the bone quality in a way that was independent of age and gender effects. Preliminary work from our laboratory (Chachra et al., 1999a) suggests that there is no relation between mechanical properties and fluoride content in femoral heads from individuals living in fluoridated and non-fluoridated communities (Fig. 23.1). At the other limit of fluoride exposure, an assessment of the bone quality of iliac bone biopsies from osteoporotic patients who had received fluoride therapy (Søgaard et al., 1994) indicated that there was a reduction in bone strength and bone strength normalized for ash content, and no decrease in bone mass, after 5 years of fluoride therapy at 40–60 mg/day.

Water fluoridation and osteoporosis

Ingestion of water fluoridated to 1.0 ppm has been generally considered to have no detrimental side-effects. However, long-term exposure to fluoride can result in significant fluoride accumulation in the skeleton and there is concern that this may have adverse effects. In addition, it may result in changes to the structure or degree of mineralization of the bone (as is observed with short-term ingestion of higher doses of fluoride), and this may have mechanical consequences. This would, in turn, affect the incidence of osteoporosis, manifested as fracture rate.

Despite the large number of published studies, considerable controversy remains regarding the issue of fluoridated water and fracture risk, with studies indicating an increased, decreased, or unchanged risk of fracture with fluoridated water consumption. A complete review can be found elsewhere (Allolio & Lehmann, 1999). Two studies correlating the regional variation of hip fracture in the United States (Jacobsen et al., 1992) and in England (Cooper et al., 1991) to local water fluoridation showed a slightly increased risk of fracture. Conversely, two studies comparing fracture rates in fluoridated and unfluoridated communities (Lehmann et al., 1998; Simonen & Laitinen, 1985) found a reduced risk of fracture in the fluoridated communities. One study (Phipps et al., 1997) found a reduced vertebral and hip fracture risk, but an increased risk of wrist fracture. Finally, a number of studies (Cauley et al., 1995; Jacobsen et al., 1993; Suarez-Almazor et al., 1993) showed no change in the risk of fracture as a result of water fluoridation. While studies such as these must be interpreted with caution because of the limitations of retrospective epidemiological studies, two conclusions can be drawn from this mass of data. First, that water fluoridation at 1 ppm most likely has no effect on bone mechanical properties, although it is impossible to exclude a small effect. Secondly, that in order to determine if there is a 10–15% increase in fracture rate

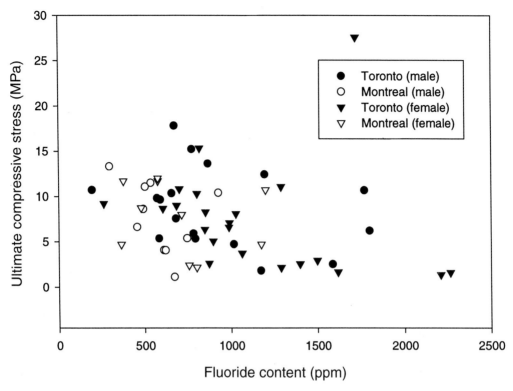

Fig. 23.1   Ultimate compressive stress of bone vs. fluoride content. Femoral heads were obtained from individuals residing in two Canadian cities: Montreal (which has never had fluoridated water) and Toronto (where municipal water has been fluoridated at 1 ppm for more than three decades. Cylindrical specimens of cancellous bone were tested in compression until failure, and the ultimate compressive stress was calculated. Fluoride content of the specimens was then measured by instrumental neutron activation analysis. This graph shows that there is no relationship between fluoride content and bone mechanical properties.

at an appropriate level of certainty would require more than 400000 people enrolled in a cohort study – clearly prohibitive (Allolio & Lehmann, 1999). This suggests that alternative protocols, such as in vitro mechanical testing of human specimens, may be a more appropriate way to determine the effect of water fluoridation on bone quality. Currently, three important questions remain unanswered: the optimum strength of human bone, what bone F levels are associated with this optimum strength and whether the normal accumulation of F in bone has a positive, negative or minimal effect on bone quality.

Endemic skeletal fluorosis, such as in some parts of India where natural water supplies contained fluoride levels of 10–20 ppm, does not occur in North America. There are some areas in North America, however, where a high incidence of bone fractures in people with asymptomatic skeletal fluorosis is possible because the water fluoride level has been found to be as high as 4 ppm, a level which is still considered safe in the US (Gordon & Corbin, 1992) and is set as the upper limit permitted in drinking water. There is evidence that these individuals may have asymptomatic skeletal fluorosis, and are at an increased risk of bone fracture compared to individuals in areas with water fluoridated at 1 ppm (Sowers et al., 1991).

Fluoride as a therapy for osteoporosis

Why use fluoride?

The vast majority of substances used to treat osteoporosis are antiosteoclastic agents. These compounds tend to prevent bone resorption directly: for example, the bisphosphonates (etidronate, pamidronate, alendronate, etc.) bind to bone mineral and block osteoclast resorption at the attachment site. Other compounds, such as estrogens and estrogen receptor modulators (e.g., raloxifene) decrease bone turnover and therefore reduce bone resorption. Calcitonin acts directly on osteoclasts to reduce their resorptive activity. Even calcium can be considered as an antiresorptive agent. While these therapies can sometimes show a slight increase in bone, it is now accepted that this is due to a reduction of the remodeling space and is therefore very limited. Arresting future losses may not always be enough, however, and patients that have already lost a substantial amount of bone require a therapy that restores bone mass. This requires agents that act directly on osteoblasts to form new bone (anabolic agents), either by increasing their number or level of activity or both. There are very few agents that can accomplish this. Androgens and anabolic hormones have very undesirable side-effects. While parathyroid hormone has been shown in rats and humans to increase bone mass, it must be administered by daily injections. Some growth factors such as insulin-like growth factor-I (IGF-I) seem to have some anabolic activity, but in animal studies it has been shown that this activity decreases with age (Danielsen & Flyvbjerg, 1996). The final class of compounds that has been shown to stimulate osteoblastic activity is the salts of trace elements such as fluoride, strontium, and aluminum. Of these, only fluoride salts, which can be taken orally, have been shown today to have a sustained anabolic effect on the skeleton. While fluoride remains the only anabolic treatment for osteoporosis that is presently available, the safety and efficacy of various formulations of fluoride salts have been, and remain, highly controversial.

The evolution of fluoride treatments

Rich and Ensinck (1961) were the first to show that sodium fluoride (NaF) could be used to treat patients with metabolic bone disease. However, to prevent mineralization defects, it was suggested that sodium fluoride be administered in conjunction with calcium and vitamin D. This regimen was shown in 1981

(Harrison et al., 1981) to increase axial bone mass and, since the early 1980s, many countries in Europe have approved the use of sodium fluoride to treat osteoporosis. While a number of clinical trials have demonstrated increases in axial bone density with fluoride, many side-effects were also frequently reported, including gastric distress, joint pain, and stress fractures in the lower limbs. A study by Riggs et al. (1990) showed that, while high doses of sodium fluoride increased spinal bone mass considerably, they did not reduce vertebral fractures and resulted in significant toxicity. This study was criticized for the high dose and for the fluoride preparation used. In a re-analysis of his data, Riggs et al. (1994) showed that the adverse effects may have been caused by the high dose of fluoride. Subsequently, new studies utilizing lower doses, other formulations such as enteric-coated or slow-release sodium fluoride, or monofluorophosphate (MFP) were performed to determine if it was possible to maintain the positive effects of fluoride therapy – increased bone mass and decreased fracture rate – without the negative side-effects. Using a protocol of lower doses of enteric-coated sodium fluoride, together with calcium and vitamin D, Mamelle et al. (1988) demonstrated a decrease in the vertebral fracture rate as well as an increase in bone mass with no gastric side-effects. However, lower limb pain still occurred in the sodium fluoride-treated group. Finally, more recently, Pak et al. (1995) have shown that sustained-release sodium fluoride at even lower doses of fluoride, together with calcium citrate, can reduce vertebral fractures substantially and increase spinal and femoral hip bone mass in patients with established osteoporosis with minimal side-effects. In summary, fluoride therapy over the years has shown an evolution towards lower doses of fluoride, enteric-coated or slow-release formulations, and the addition of calcium and vitamin D.

New understanding of the mode of action of fluoride in osteoporosis

Many problems encountered when using fluoride in the therapy of osteoporosis result from its narrow therapeutic window: the threshold at which fluoride has an effect on bone cells is 95 ng/ml while the toxic threshold is 190 ng/ml in serum (Pak et al., 1997). Similarly, the toxic threshold for skeletal fluoride is between 0.6% and 0.8% of bone mineral. When this threshold is exceeded, bone shows signs of fluorosis, with enlarged lacunae, abnormal bone formation, impaired mineralization and reduced bone strength. Sodium fluoride preparations are rapidly absorbed in the stomach, resulting in high serum concentrations and correspondingly high incorporation of fluoride in regions of active bone formation. Enteric-coated preparations prevent the release of fluoride in the stomach; absorption occurs more slowly in the small intestine, thereby avoiding gastric problems often caused by the release of hydrofluoric acid in the stomach as well as reducing the absorbed dose of fluoride. Slow-release sodium fluoride preparations go even further: the slow absorption through the gastrointestinal tract results in a low, sustained serum concentration which, ideally, is sufficient to stimulate osteoblast activity while minimizing the amount of fluoride which is incorporated into bone mineral. This formulation should both eliminate the gastric side-effects (as shown by Pak and others) and the reduction in the quality of bone induced by the incorporation of large amounts of fluoride at sites of bone formation. The rationale for the co-administration of calcium and vitamin D with fluoride is to prevent osteomalacia and stress fractures. In people who respond well to fluoride therapy, new bone matrix is formed at a high rate (Lau & Baylink, 1998). Also, fluoride has a tendency to increase the lag time for mineral (hydroxyapatite) to be deposited on the osteoid of bone, and, in the elderly, calcium absorption is decreased. Taken together, the rapid increase in bone matrix, delay in mineralization, and poor calcium absorption can create osteomalacia, which can induce stress fractures. For this reason, it is necessary to ensure that there is adequate intake of calcium and vitamin D, so that the areas of rapid bone formation induced by the fluoride stimulation of the osteoblasts can be fully and promptly mineralized.

In summary, fluoride therapy is currently the only widely available anabolic therapy for osteoporosis. Increased understanding of the effects of fluoride on the skeleton has led over the years to a therapeutic protocol consisting of low doses of fluoride with carefully controlled absorption rates to maximize its effect on bone cells and minimize its effect on bone mineral. In addition, calcium and vitamin D supplements are required to prevent the negative consequences of rapid bone formation in the presence of poor calcium absorption in the elderly. However, many questions still remain unanswered. Is there a need for a combined anabolic and antiresorptive therapy and how will they interact? Why does a sizable proportion of patients fail to respond to fluoride therapy? How long should fluoride therapy last? At what point does the accumulation of fluoride in the skeleton start to have a negative effect on bone quality? Fifty years after the introduction of fluoride in the drinking water and nearly 40 years after the first therapeutic use of fluoride, many clinically relevant questions remain unanswered.

REFERENCES

Aaron, J. E., de Vernejoul, M. C., & Kanis, J. A. (1992). Bone hypertrophy and trabecular generation in Paget's disease and in fluoride-treated osteoporosis. *Bone Miner.*, **17**, 399–413.

Allolio, B. & Lehmann, R. (1999). Drinking water fluoridation and bone. *Exp. Clin. Endocrinol. Diabetes*, **107**, 12–20.

Angmar-Mansson, B. & Whitford, G. M. (1982). Plasma fluoride levels and enamel fluorosis in the rat. *Caries Res.*, **16**, 334–9.

Beary, D. F. (1969). The effects of fluoride and low calcium on the physical properties of the rat femur. *Anat Rec.*, **164**, 305–16.

Boivin, G. & Meunier, P. J. (1993). Effects of fluoride on bone mineral. *Res. Clin. Forums*, **15**, 13–19.

Boivin, G., Chavassieux, P., Chapuy, M. C., Baud, C. A., & Meunier, P. J. (1989). Skeletal fluorosis: histomorphometric analysis of bone changes and bone fluoride content in 29 patients. *Bone*, **10**, 89–99.

Bonjour, J. P., Caverzasio, J., & Rizzoli, R. (1993). Effects of fluoride on bone cells. *Res. Clin. Forums*, **15**, 13–19.

Burt, B. A. (1992). The changing patterns of systemic fluoride intake. *J. Dent. Res.*, **71**, 1228–37.

Cauley, J. A., Murphy, P. A., Riley, T. J., & Buhari, A. M. (1995). Effects of fluoridated drinking water on bone mass and fractures: the study of osteoporotic fractures. *J. Bone Miner. Res.*, **10**, 1076–86.

Chachra, D., Limeback, H., Gross, A. E., Hutchison, C. H., Zukor, D., Schwartz, M., & Grynpas, M. D. (1999a). Does fluoridated water alter the mechanical and material properties of human bone? *J. Dent. Res.*, **78**, Abstract 3467.

Chachra, D., Turner, C. H., Dunipace, A. J., & Grynpas, M. D. (1999b). The effect of fluoride treatment on bone mineral in rabbits. *Calcif. Tissue Int.*, **64**, 345–51.

Cheng, P. T. & Bader, S. M. (1990). Effects of fluoride on rat cancellous bone. *Bone Miner.*, **11**, 153–61.

Clovis, J. & Hargreaves, J. A. (1988). Fluoride intake from beverage consumption. *Community Dent. Oral Epidemiol.*, **16**, 11–15.

Cooper, C., Wickham, C. A., Barker, D. J., & Jacobsen, S. J. (1991). Water fluoridation and hip fracture. *J. Am. Med. Assoc.*, **266**, 513–14.

Danielsen, C. C. & Flyvbjerg, A. (1996). Insulin-like growth factor I as a predictor of cortical bone mass in a long-term study of ovariectomized and estrogen-treated rats. *Bone*, **19**, 493–8.

Einhorn, T. A., Wakley, G. K., Linkhart, S., Rush, E. B., Maloney, S., Faierman, E., & Baylink, D. J. (1992). Incorporation of sodium fluoride into cortical bone does not impair the mechanical properties of the appendicular skeleton in rats. *Calcif. Tissue Int.*, **51**, 127–31.

Ekstrand, J. & Spak, C. J. (1990). Fluoride pharmacokinetics: its implications in the fluoride treatment of osteoporosis. *J. Bone Miner. Res.*, **5**, S53–61.

Gordon, S. L. & Corbin, S. B. (1992). Summary of workshop on drinking water fluoride influence on hip fracture on bone health. *Osteoporos. Int.*, **2**, 109–17.

Gruber, H. E. & Baylink, D. J. (1991). The effects of fluoride on bone. *Clin. Orthop.*, **267**, 264–77.

Grynpas, M. D. (1990). Fluoride effects on bone crystals. *J. Bone Miner. Res.*, **5**, S169–75.

Grynpas, M. D., Simmons, E. D., Pritzker, K. P., Hancock, R. V., & Harrison, J. E. (1986). Is fluoridated bone different from non-fluoridated bone? In *Cell Mediated Calcification and Matrix Vesicles*, ed. S. Yousef Ali, pp. 409–14. Elsevier Science Publishers.

Harrison, J. E., McNeill, K. G., Sturtridge, W. C., Bayley, T. A., Murray, T. M., Williams, C., Tam, C., & Fornasier, V. (1981). Three-year changes in bone mineral mass of postmenopausal osteoporotic patients based on neutron activation analysis of the central third of the skeleton. *J. Clin. Endocrinol. Metab.*, **52**, 751–8.

Ishiguro, K., Nakagaki, H., Tsuboi, S., Narita, N., Kato, K., Li, J., Kamei, H., Yoshioka, I.,

Miyauchi, K., & Hosoe, H. (1993). Distribution of fluoride in cortical bone in human rib. *Calcif. Tissue Int.*, **52**, 278–82.

Ismail, A. I. (1994). Fluoride supplements: current effectiveness, side effects, and recommendations. *Community Dent. Oral Epidemiol.*, **22**, 164–72.

Jacobsen, S. J., Goldberg, J., Cooper, C., & Lockwood, S. A. (1992). The association between water fluoridation and hip fracture among white women and men aged 65 years and older. A national ecologic study. *Ann. Epidemiol.*, **2**, 617–26.

Jacobsen, S. J., O'Fallon, W. M., & Melton, L. J. (1993). Hip fracture incidence before and after the fluoridation of the public water supply, Rochester, Minnesota. *Am. J. Public Health*, **83**, 743–5.

Kaminsky, L. S., Mahoney, M. C., Leach, J., Melius, J., & Miller, M. J. (1990). Fluoride: benefits and risks of exposure. *Crit. Rev. Oral Biol. Med.*, **1**, 261–81.

Lau, K. H. & Baylink, D. J. (1998). Pros and cons of fluoride therapy. *Osteologie*, **7**, 157–63.

Lehmann, R., Wapniarz, M., Hofmann, B., Piper, B., Haubitz, I., & Allolio, B. (1998). Drinking water fluoridation: bone mineral density and hip fracture incidence. *Bone*, **22**, 273–8.

Mamelle, N., Meunier, P. J., Dusan, R., Guillaume, M., Martin, J. L., Gaucher, A., Prost, A., Zeigler, G., & Netter, P. (1988). Risk–benefit ratio of sodium fluoride treatment in primary vertebral osteoporosis. *Lancet*, **ii**, 361–5.

Moreno, E. C., Kresak, M., & Zahradnik, R. T. (1977). Physicochemical aspects of fluoride-apatite systems relevant to the study of dental caries. *Caries Res.*, **11**, 142–71.

Mosekilde, L., Kragstrup, J., & Richards, A. (1987). Compressive strength, ash weight, and volume of vertebral trabecular bone in experimental fluorosis in pigs. *Calcif. Tissue Int.*, **40**, 318–22.

Okuda, A., Kanehisa, J., & Heersche, J. N. (1990). The effects of sodium fluoride on the resorptive activity of isolated osteoclasts. *J. Bone Miner. Res.*, **5**, S115–20.

Pak, C. Y., Sakhaee, K., Adams-Huet, B., Piziak, V., Peterson, R. D., & Pointdexter, J. R. (1995). Treatment of postmenopausal osteoporosis with slow-release sodium fluoride. Final report of a randomized controlled trial. *Ann. Intern. Med.*, **123**, 401–8.

Pak, C. Y., Sakhaee, K., Rubin, C. D., Zerwekh, J. E., & Collaborators (1997). Sustained-release sodium fluoride in the management of established postmenopausal osteoporosis. *Am. J. Med. Sci.*, **313**, 23–32.

Parfitt, A. M. (1982). The coupling of bone formation to bone resorption: a critical analysis of the concept and of its relevance to the pathogenesis of osteoporosis. *Metab. Bone Dis. Relat. Res.*, **4**, 1–6.

Phipps, K. R., Orwoll, E. S., Mason, J. D., & Cauley, J. A. (1997). Community water fluoridation, fractures and bone mineral density. *J. Bone Miner. Res.*, **12**, 127.

Rich, C. & Ensinck, J. (1961). Effect of sodium fluoride on calcium metabolism of human beings. *Nature*, **191**, 184–5.

Rich, C. & Feist, E. (1970). The action of fluoride in bone. In *Fluoride in Medicine*, ed. T. L. Vischer, pp. 70–87. Bern: Hans Huber.

Richards, A., Mosekilde, L., & Søgaard, C. H. (1994). Normal age-related changes in fluoride content of vertebral trabecular bone – relation to bone quality. *Bone*, **15**, 21–6.

Riggs, B. L., Hodgson, S. F., O'Fallon, W. M., Chao, E. Y., Wahner, H. W., Muhs, J. M., Cedel, S.

L., & Melton, L. J. (1990). Effect of fluoride treatment on the fracture rate in postmenopausal women with osteoporosis. *N. Engl. J. Med.*, 322, 802–9.

Riggs, B. L., O'Fallon, W. M., Lane, A., Hodgson, S. F., Wahner, H. W., Muhs, J., Chao, E., & Melton, L. J. (1994). Clinical trial of fluoride therapy in postmenopausal osteoporotic women: extended observations and additional analysis. *J. Bone Miner. Res.*, 9, 265–75.

Simard, P. L., Lachapelle, D., Trahan, L., Naccache, H., Demers, M., & Brodeur, J. M. (1989). The ingestion of fluoride dentifrice by young children. *ASDC J. Dent. Child.*, 56, 177–81.

Simonen, O. & Laitinen, O. (1985). Does fluoridation of drinking-water prevent bone fragility and osteoporosis? *Lancet*, ii, 432–4.

Singer, L., Ophaug, R. H., & Harland, B. F. (1985). Dietary fluoride intake of 15–19-year-old male adults residing in the United States. *J. Dent. Res.*, 64, 1302–5.

Søgaard, C. H., Mosekilde, L., Richards, A., & Mosekilde, L. (1994). Marked decrease in trabecular bone quality after five years of sodium fluoride therapy – assessed by biomechanical testing of iliac crest bone biopsies in osteoporotic patients. *Bone*, 15, 393–9.

Sowers, M. R., Clark, M. K., Jannausch, M. L., & Wallace, R. B. (1991). A prospective study of bone mineral content and fracture in communities with differential fluoride exposure. *Am. J. Epidemiol.*, 133, 649–60.

Suarez-Almazor, M. E., Flowerdew, G., Saunders, L. D., Soskolne, C. L., & Russell, A. S. (1993). The fluoridation of drinking water and hip fracture hospitalization rates in two Canadian communities. *Am. J. Public Health*, 83, 689–93.

Turner, C. H., Akhter, M. P., & Heaney, R. P. (1992). The effects of fluoridated water on bone strength. *J. Orthop. Res.*, 10, 581–7.

Turner, C. H., Boivin, G., & Meunier, P. J. (1993). A mathematical model for fluoride uptake by the skeleton. *Calcif. Tissue Int.*, 52, 130–8.

Turner, C. H., Garetto, L. P., Dunipace, A. J., Zhang, W., Wilson, M. E., Grynpas, M. D., Chachra, D., McClintock, R., Peacock, M., & Stookey, G. K. (1997). Fluoride treatment increased serum IGF-I, bone turnover, and bone mass, but not bone strength, in rabbits. *Calcif. Tissue Int.*, 61, 77–83.

Turner, C. H., Hasegawa, K., Zhang, W., Wilson, M., Li, Y., & Dunipace, A. J. (1995). Fluoride reduces bone strength in older rats. *J. Dent. Res.*, 74, 1475–81.

Walsh, W. R. & Guzelsu, N. (1993). The role of ions and mineral–organic interfacial bonding on the compressive properties of cortical bone. *Biomed. Mater. Eng.*, 3, 75–84.

Weatherell, J. A. (1969). *Mineral Metabolism in Pediatrics*, Chapter 4, ed. D. Bartwell & W. L. Burand, Oxford: Blackwell.

Whitford, G. M. (1989). The metabolism and toxicity of fluoride. In *Monographs in Oral Science*, 13. Basel: Karger.

Whitford, G. M. (1994). Intake and metabolism of fluoride. *Adv. Dent. Res.*, 8, 5–14.

24

PTH peptides as anabolic agents in bone

Anthony B. Hodsman

Introduction

The conventional endocrine actions of parathyroid hormone (PTH) include the following properties:

(i) PTH(1–84) and its truncated (1–34) amino terminal fragment, are released from the gland in a pulsatile fashion. Baseline secretion occurs continuously, but the excretion rates rise and fall under the influence of the tightly regulated feedback system described in detail in the section on 'Mechanism of action.' The two most important regulators are the ambient circulating levels of ionized calcium and the vitamin D metabolite, $1, 25 (OH)_2D_3$ (calcitriol).

(ii) interacting with the PTH/PTHrP receptor, PTH exerts its characteristic actions via the adenylate cyclase signaling pathway:

(a) by its action on bone to increase remodeling rates, it increases osteoclastic bone resorption (in this case an indirect effect requiring mediation by osteoblasts), and increases release of calcium to support blood calcium levels.

(b) by its action on renal tubules to modulate renal calcium and phosphate excretion together with regulation of calcitriol formation via the 1-α-cholecalciferol hydroxylase.

While detailed discussion of these actions is presented in other sections of this book, none of these suggests why this 'bone resorbing hormone' may be a potent anabolic agent in both normal and osteopenic states.

In 1931, Pehue et al. described a severe case of osteosclerosis leading to death (due to anemia) in an 8-year-old boy with hypertrophied parathyroid glands (Pehue et al., 1931). Subsequently Selye was able to mimic this serendipitous finding in young male rats given low doses of PTH-extract (Selye, 1932). Over 40 years later Reeve and his co-workers reported the experimental application of synthetic hPTH(1–34) as a potent anabolic agent in treating patients with severe osteoporosis (Reeve et al., 1976, 1980). Even now, there are very few published clinical studies of this agent, with most being short-term uncontrolled cohort studies. There is no published randomized controlled trial evaluating the merits of PTH analogs against placebo, although there are several randomized controlled studies which report the benefits of a PTH analog in patients with osteoporosis but in which both groups received a bone-active drug, either calcitriol (Neer et al., 1991), calcitonin (Hodsman et al., 1997b) estrogen (Lindsay et al., 1997), or nafarelin (Finkelstein et al., 1994). All consistently confirm the potent anabolic properties of PTH peptides.

Mechanism of action

Cellular level

Clearly, the use of exogenous PTH does not simulate the physiological pulsatile secretion of the endogenous hormone. Continuous infusion of PTH in rats leads to a predominantly resorptive action on bone (Tam et al., 1981). Similar conclusions were drawn from continuous infusions in patients with osteoporosis, in whom biochemical markers of bone formation were suppressed during the 24 h infusion, while those of bone resorption increased steadily (Hodsman et al., 1993). Daily subcutaneous injections of PTH are consistently anabolic for bone in animals and human subjects; at the same time endogenous PTH secretion is subject to prolonged suppression (Hodsman et al., 1993). Indeed, there is a case report of a patient developing functional endogenous hypoparathyroidism after cessation of PTH injections used to treat her osteoporosis (Audran et al., 1987). Since exogenous hPTH(1–34) causes infrequent antibody responses to the peptide (Hodsman et al., 1997b; Lindsay et al., 1997), it is possible that daily injections of PTH might also alter endogenous PTH regulation.

It is likely that the anabolic action of PTH requires the adenylate cyclase signaling pathway but not the alternative phospholipase C pathway. Although the natural PTH peptides, hPTH(1–34) and hPTH(1–84) activate both pathways, the truncated N-terminal peptide hPTH(1–31) amide acts through the adenylate cyclase pathway exclusively but is equipotent in its bone anabolic properties (Whitfield et al., 1996).

There is reasonable evidence that PTH stimulates local osteoblast-based production of the insulin-like growth factor system (Dempster et al., 1993), although the molecular mechanisms by which this interaction operates remain obscure. The anabolic effects of PTH also result in multilayered stacking of osteoblasts at sites of bone formation (Dobnig & Turner, 1995; Hodsman et al., 1993; Watson et al., 1995); the origin of these cells is unknown as shown by the diversity of hypotheses in Table 24.1.

Tissue level

With the emerging clinical data, interest in developing a commercially viable PTH product has grown rapidly over the past 10 years. Modern fermentation techniques

Table 24.1. Hypothetical sources of osteoblast activity after anabolic doses of exogenous PTH

  (i) Increased recruitment of osteoprogenitor cells from marrow precursors.

 (ii) PTH-responsive postmitotic cells which have been recruited to the site by chemotaxis.

(iii) Bone lining cells which have been induced to re-enter proliferative cycles and pile up.

(iv) Inhibition of osteoblast apoptosis, thus prolonging the functioning lifespan of the osteoblast as an active synthetic unit.

---

have resulted in the possibility of relatively inexpensive large-scale commercial production. Extensive preclinical evaluation of these peptides has been necessary before proceeding with clinical trials. The ovariectomized (OVX) adult rat has been widely accepted as a model for human postmenopausal osteoporosis. Acute estrogen deficiency closely parallels the early rapid phase of postmenopausal bone loss, including:

(i) increases in both bone resorption and activation frequency.

(ii) a relative deficiency in bone formation leading to a negative remodeling balance (Kalu, 1991; Frost & Jee, 1992; Wronski et al., 1989).

Histologic studies have demonstrated that intermittent daily s.c.injections of hPTH(1–34):

(i) prevent the marked reduction in trabecular bone volume following OVX(Liu & Kalu, 1990).

(ii) restore reduced trabecular bone volume previously induced by OVX, even more effectively than estrogen or bisphosphonates (Shen et al., 1992; Wronski et al., 1993) .

The increase in bone formation rate is primarily due to an increase in both total mineralization surfaces and mineral apposition rates; it occurs within a week of initiation of treatment (Meng et al., 1996).

Measurement of bone mineral density (BMD) in PTH-treated rats has demonstrated corresponding increments in both long bones (primarily cortical sites) (Mosekilde et al., 1994a) and vertebrae (primarily a trabecular site) (Mosekilde et al., 1994a). The quality of bone produced by PTH appears to confer enhanced biomechanical strength. Numerous studies of load-to-failure rates in both vertebral bodies, and femurs have shown that bone from PTH-treated, OVX rats consistently performs better than that from intact, untreated rats (Li et al., 1995; Meng et al., 1996; Shen et al., 1995).

Clinical pharmacology

The published clinical literature of PTH peptides as anabolic treatment for osteoporosis dates back to 1976. Due to the limited supply of the drug, almost all have utilized synthetic hPTH(1–34) and most have reported dosing in 'units.' However the purity and specific activity of this peptide cannot be relied upon in the older literature. Using highly purified synthetic hPTH(1–34) reported doses of 500 units (the most commonly used dose) should be equivalent to approximately 40 micrograms or 10 nmol of pure peptide.

Following subcutaneous injection of hPTH(1–34), plasma concentrations rise rapidly, reaching a peak at 15–20 minutes, (T_{max}), before decaying to baseline by 180–240 minutes with a $T_{1/2}$ of about 70 minutes (Kent et al., 1985; Lindsay et al., 1993). In a detailed review of the current literature, approximately 10% of patients treated with hPTH(1–34) appear to develop antibodies (Hodsman et al., 1997a), half of whom withdrew from therapy because of urticarial reactions or local irritation at the injection site. While such an immune response to a naturally occurring human-sequence peptide may seem high, these reports derive from either impure peptide sources, or peptide formulated in heavily gelatinized vehicle. The most meaningful data on the immunogenicity of PTH peptide must await its assessment in currently ongoing clinical trials using highly purified commercially developed peptides.

Following subcutaneous injections of hPTH(1–34), serum calcium levels demonstrate a delayed rise above baseline by approximately 4 hours, and peak at 6–8 hours (Hodsman et al., 1993; Lindsay et al., 1993). This increment is usually within the physiological reference range. By 24 hours, serum calcium levels have returned to baseline in all but a small minority of patients (less than 10%). However this suggests that clinical doses of PTH above the equivalent of 500 units by daily injection may need to be adjusted for individual safety. Accompanying the rise in serum calcium, mild hypercalciuria is commonly seen (Hodsman et al., 1993; Lindsay et al., 1993).

Clinical protocols

As previously stated, published clinical protocols have been heterogeneous. The majority of studies have empirically used dietary calcium supplements, although the requirement for this is unproven. Indeed, increments in circulating calcitriol have been shown as part of the biological response to injected hPTH(1–34) (Hodsman & Fraher, 1990; Lindsay et al., 1993), together with increased fractional absorption of (unsupplemented) dietary calcium (Hodsman & Fraher, 1990). On the other hand, two of the long-term studies of hPTH(1–34) reported neither a sustained increase in serum calcitriol (Lindsay et al., 1997), nor sustained hypercalciuria (Hodsman et al., 1997b; Lindsay et al., 1997).

Table 24.2 indicates the extent to which investigators have explored concomitant therapy during clinical studies. Only the larger studies are cited.

Table 24.2. Use of concomitant therapy in clinical studies of hPTH(1–34)

Concomitant therapy	Number of subjects	Duration (months)
Calcitriol (Neer et al., 1987;	31	18–27
Reeve et al., 1987)	13	12
Calcitonin (Hesch et al., 1989;	13	14
Hodsman et al., 1997b)	39	24
Estrogen (Reeve et al., 1990;	12	12
Lindsay et al., 1997)	34	36

Clinical outcomes

Bone mineral density

Fig. 24.1 shows the changes in lumbar spine BMD measurements (made by DXA) from several studies in which responses to hPTH(1–34) were followed for up to 3 years (Hodsman et al., 1997b; Lindsay et al., 1997; Neer et al., 1991; Rittmaster et al., 1998). Fig. 24.1 is not a legitimate 'plot' – the studies employed very different protocols (see Table 24.2), and one of them used 28-day cycles of PTH repeating every 3 months (Hodsman et al., 1997b). Nonetheless the changes in bone mass are quite consistent, averaging 8–9% during the first year and a further 3% during the second. These increments are much more rapid than those seen with bisphosphonates (Black et al., 1997). Studies using quantitative computerized tomography of lumbar vertebrae demonstrate increments of 25–100% over baseline (Hesch et al., 1989; Reeve et al., 1990; Slovik et al., 1986)

Fig. 24.2 shows the changes in BMD reported in the 3-year study of Lindsay et al., in which a group of women with osteoporosis had been receiving chronic estrogen treatment for at least 1 year, and were then randomized to receive daily injections of hPTH(1–34), 400 units, plus estrogen – or to continue estrogen alone (Lindsay et al., 1997). Significant increments in BMD were found at three important skeletal sites–lumbar spine (13%), femoral neck (2.7%) and total body calcium (7.8%). Lindsay et al. found no significant changes in radial BMD in keeping with reports from other studies (Hesch et al., 1989; Reeve et al., 1987; Slovik et al., 1986). Only one report from Neer et al. demonstrated an abrupt, but non-progressive, fall in radial BMD during the first year of PTH therapy (Neer et al., 1991). Although this is one of the few studies to use calcitriol as concomitant medication with hPTH(1–34), there is no obvious explanation for this apparently isolated finding of reduced radial bone mass. One possible explanation may relate to the increased remodeling space in cortical bone due to the increased bone turnover induced by PTH therapy.

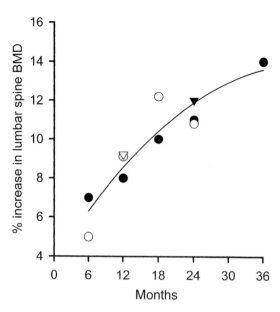

Fig. 24.1   Composite changes in lumbar spine BMD measured by dual-energy X-ray absorptiometry during up to 3 years of therapy with PTH. The plot shows the average reported changes in BMD across time. Individual points represent the mean data for separate publications. ○ Hodsman et al. (1997b), ● Lindsay et al. (1997), △ Rittmaster et al. (1998), ▲ Neer et al. (1991).

Taken together, these findings demonstrate rapid increments in lumbar spine BMD during PTH therapy, with smaller increments in the appendicular skeleton. This contrasts with findings in response to the other important anabolic agent, sodium fluoride, in which significant bone loss may occur in the appendicular skeleton (Hodsman & Drost, 1989; Riggs et al., 1990).

Bone histology

Bone histomorphometry was the primary outcome parameter in the initial clinical reports of the efficacy of hPTH(1–34). In the two cohorts of patients studied by Reeve and co-workers, paired iliac crest biopsies were obtained before and after 6 to 12 months of hPTH(1–34) therapy (Bradbeer et al., 1992; Reeve et al., 1980). Significant increases in trabecular bone volume, trabecular width and mean trabecular osteon wall thickness were consistently found. Static measurements of formation surfaces increased by an average of 10%, and resorption surfaces by an average of 2 to 3%. These early studies contained very little kinetic data based on tetracycline labels. However, the kinetic data of Hodsman et al. indicate that increments in formation and resorption surfaces lead to increased bone formation rates

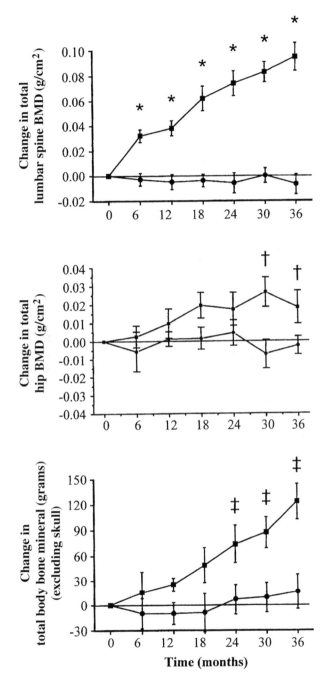

Fig. 24.2   Changes in bone mineral density following hPTH(1–34), 400 IU/day. Data are modified from Lindsay et al. (1997), and show two groups of patients, one treated with estrogen alone (●) and the other treated with estrogen plus PTH (■). *, P<0.001 vs. estrogen; †, P<0.05 vs. estrogen; ‡, P<0.02 vs. estrogen.

(three-fold) and remodeling activation frequency (two-fold) and occurs within 2 to 4 weeks of initiating hPTH(1–34) therapy(Hodsman et al., 1993). Therefore, the available histological evidence indicates that the anabolic effects of PTH are associated with sharp increases in bone turnover as well as increased bone formation. Thus the remodeling balance between resorption and formation is altered from negative to strongly positive.

Biochemical markers of bone turnover

Biochemical markers of bone turnover have provided important surrogate measures of the underlying changes in bone tissue. On the other hand, the findings have left open still more unanswered questions of the anabolic mechanisms of action for PTH. The histological studies in both animal models and osteoporotic subjects all suggest a marked increase in bone turnover. Not surprisingly, sharp increases in the urinary excretion of several markers of bone resorption have been reported in response to PTH therapy. Increases in urinary hydroxyproline (OH–Pro), or N-telopeptides (NTX) vary from 25–100% over baseline (Finkelstein et al., 1994; Hodsman et al., 1993, 1997b; Lindsay et al., 1997; Reeve et al., 1980). In longer-term studies of 2 to 3 years' duration the initial rise in urinary NTX excretion appears to peak at 6 months and gradually returns towards baseline over the next 18 months (Hodsman et al., 1997b; Lindsay et al., 1997). This pattern is very similar, whether PTH is given by continuous daily injections (Lindsay et al., 1997), or by cyclical 28-day courses (Hodsman et al., 1997b).

Biochemical indices of bone formation have included total serum alkaline phosphatase (tAP), bone specific serum akaline phosphatase (BSAP), osteocalcin (OC),and procollagen I carboxypeptides (PICP). The magnitude of the increments in bone formation markers over baseline are very similar to those seen for urinary OH–Pro (Finkelstein et al., 1994; Hodsman et al., 1993, 1997b; Lindsay et al., 1997; Reeve et al., 1980). Similar patterns of response over time have also been demonstrated, with peak increments at 6 months, followed by a gradual decline towards baseline thereafter (Hodsman et al., 1997b; Lindsay et al., 1997).

These changes in bone turnover markers are very different to those seen with other treatments for osteoporosis. Thus, antiresorptive agents such as estrogen or bisphosphonates produce predominantly a reduction in bone resorption markers (Garnero et al., 1994; Riis et al., 1995), reflecting the primary underlying histologic response of reduced bone turnover. On the other hand, another anabolic agent, sodium fluoride, causes only inconsistent increases in serum tAP and/or OC (Hodsman & Drost, 1989; Riggs et al., 1990).

In summary, the consistent increases in both bone resorption and formation markers in response to PTH supports the histological evidence for a marked increase in bone turnover. Since BMD increases over the same time period, the remodeling balance must remain positive. Although the subsequent decline in turnover markers over 18–36 months may suggest the development of skeletal resistance to PTH, longitudinal BMD measurement has neither confirmed nor refuted this hypothesis. Moreover, the reported changes in bone resorption markers have not been helpful in addressing the hypothesis that concurrent use of antiresorptive agents may enhance the effectiveness of PTH treatment by selectively suppressing bone resorption.

PTH peptides used with antiresorptive drugs

As noted previously, the clinical protocols involving PTH have been very heterogeneous. Only one randomized placebo-controlled trial has been performed, with hPTH(1–84). The primary outcome of this trial, BMD, has been published only in outline (Rittmaster et al., 1998). Other investigators have employed antiresorptive agents as co-therapy. In the randomized trial of Hodsman et al. sequential calcitonin (75 units s.c.) was given daily for 6 weeks after each 4-week cycle of hPTH(1–34) to one of the two groups (Hodsman et al., 1997b). The study was designed to evaluate specifically the hypothesis that an antiresorptive drug would enhance the effect of cyclical PTH alone; the results clearly showed no benefit. The earlier study by Hesch et al. was also a variant of cyclical hPTH(1–38) and calcitonin, but there were no true controls in this study (Hesch et al., 1989).

In the study of Reeve et al., daily hPTH(1–34) injections were combined with concurrent estrogen therapy (Reeve et al., 1991). Compared with historical controls given hPTH(1–34) alone (Reeve et al., 1980), calcium balance studies were significantly more positive and the hypercalciuria seen with the 'unopposed' PTH therapy was largely abolished. These findings suggest that estrogen may modify the bone resorptive action of PTH without antagonizing its anabolic function. In the randomized trial of Lindsay et al., women previously treated with estrogen for at least 1 year were randomized to continue estrogen alone, or to continue estrogen with the addition of daily hPTH(1–34) injections. However, there is no way to tell if the PTH-treated arm would have had a different outcome had they not received estrogen concurrently (Lindsay et al., 1997).

The bisphosphonates are a more potent, and bone-specific group of drugs. No clinical studies have been published to date in which a bisphosphonate was included as concurrent medication. However, this hypothesis has been tested in the osteopenic rat model. Combination therapy with risedronate provided no additional benefits to PTH alone in the mature OVX rat when vertebral BMD and strength was assessed (Mosekilde et al., 1994b). Other animal studies actually suggest that bisphosphonates may blunt the anabolic effects on bone. This has been found for pamidronate (Cheng et al., 1995), tiludronate(Delmas et al., 1995) and cimadronate (Mashiba et al., 1997). There is therefore no experimental evidence to support the role for concomitant therapy with bisphosphonates and PTH.

As a clinical side-bar to this argument, Cosman et al. have recently performed a short-term study in which postmenopausal women with osteoporosis, previously treated with alendronate, were randomized to continue alendronate alone or to receive hPTH(1–34) in a dose of 400 units s.c./day in addition to alendronate (Cosman et al., 1998). After the 6 weeks of PTH therapy, biochemical markers of bone formation (serum OC and PICP) increased significantly, with no change in the patients continuing on alendronate alone. In contrast to the bone formation markers, biochemical markers of bone resorption did not change significantly among the two groups. These clinical data suggest that concurrent therapy with a bisphosphonate does not block the anabolic effect of PTH whilst minimizing its antiresorptive actions. While these early clinical data do not provide evidence for an enhanced effect on bone mass and ultimately fracture reduction, they are encouraging with respect to the potential clinical flexibility of using PTH with other bone-active agents .

The current therapeutic question of clinical importance relates to the need for maintenance therapy. The strategic value of PTH remains its ability to effect rapid increments in bone mass, and hopefully an equally rapid reduction in future fracture risk. As an injectable drug, it is not an ideal candidate for prolonged (5 to 10 years') use. Moreover, if skeletal 'tachyphylaxis' does develop over 2 to 3 years, this compound would not be an ideal drug to maintain gains in bone mass achieved following initiation of treatment. In the rat, cessation of PTH treatment leads to rapid losses of bone (Gunness-Hey & Hock, 1989), an effect that is also seen clinically after cessation of anabolic treatment with sodium fluoride (Talbot et al., 1996).

Given that PTH therapy increases bone turnover, the total skeletal remodeling space will increase proportionately. Assuming that bone loss might occur independently after cessation of PTH treatment, the combination of an enlarged remodeling space and rapid bone loss might expose the skeleton to rapid losses of bone mass. Here, the use of bisphosphonates as maintenance therapy confers many advantages.

(i)   As oral agents, long-term acceptance by patients will aid in compliance.
(ii) There is established data on long-term safety with this class of drugs (5 to 7 years).
(iii) Their role in rapidly reducing bone turnover is well established (Liberman et al., 1995). This should allow for refilling of the remodeling space followed by a further and ongoing increase in BMD.

There are two clinical studies of bisphosphonates used as maintenance therapy following cessation of PTH therapy, both reported only in abstract form. Hodsman et al., used 28-day cycles of clodronate (400 mg/day) repeating every 3 months. This failed to prevent small declines in bone mass during the first year, but lumbar BMD stabilized in the second year and remained higher than baseline BMD (prior to initiation of PTH therapy) (Hodsman et al., 1995). Rittmaster et al. presented preliminary data on 77 patients previously participating in a 1-year randomized trial of hPTH(1–84) or placebo (Rittmaster et al., 1998). After 12 months of maintenance treatment with alendronate (10 mg p.o./day), BMD increased further in patients previously treated with PTH in both the lumbar spine (approximately 6%), and femoral neck (approximately 3%). However, these increments were no larger than those seen in previously placebo-PTH-treated patients.

The available data suggest that maintenance of bone mass following cessation of PTH therapy will require therapeutic intervention over and above dietary calcium supplements. The logical approach suggests the use of antiresorptive agents and the current generation of potent bisphosphonates seem to be effective.

Side effects

Close to 200 patients with osteoporosis have been treated with PTH and reported in the clinical literature(Hodsman et al., 1997a). Of these, no deaths have occurred. As discussed on p. 334, about 10% of patients have apparently developed antibodies to the injected hPTH(1–34), of whom half discontinued therapy. Several patients described mild nausea and arthralgia in one study (Finkelstein et al., 1994). Mild hypercalcemia and hypercalciuria have been observed, but neither has resulted in documented clinical consequences, and no increased incidence of renal calculus formation has been reported to date. Hodsman et al. have raised an issue about the long-term safety of PTH on renal function (Hodsman et al., 1997b). In this report, 39 patients were treated with cyclical high dose hPTH(1–34) (800 units per day for 28-day cycles/four times per year over 2 years). This patient population experienced a significant 10% increase in serum creatinine (albeit within the normal range of age-related serum creatinine). Thus, PTH-induced hypercalciuria might conceivably affect renal function.

Conclusions

After 25 years of sporadic clinical, and latterly intensive experimental research, PTH holds the promise of an important new anabolic agent for the reversal of osteoporosis. It has an apparently low side-effect profile and the great majority of patients respond rapidly to the drug. Randomized placebo-controlled clinical trials designed to address fracture-reduction are in progress and should definitively address the efficacy of this drug.

The spectrum of clinical utility over and above postmenopausal osteoporosis has not been widely explored. PTH is effective at preventing bone loss in young women undergoing premature menopause induced by the gonadotrophin antagonist, nafarelin (Finkelstein et al., 1994). Other conditions causing osteoporosis, such as glucocorticoid-induced osteoporosis have not been explored.

The utility of co-therapy or maintenance management with antiresorptive drugs (e.g., estrogens and bisphosphonates) holds promise. The analog, hPTH (1–31) amide apparently has comparable anabolic effects on bone, but little effect on serum and urinary calcium. The potential clinical application of such analogs may further enhance the safety profile of PTH (Hodsman et al., 1999; Whitfield et al., 1996). Alternative delivery systems such as aerosolized inhalation and absorption through the pulmonary capillaries(Patton et al., 1994), may enhance the convenience of PTH therapy.

It is to be hoped that the PTH family of peptides have a promising future. However, the same comment was made 25 years ago of the other potent bone anabolic drug, sodium fluoride. Therefore, the place of PTH in the management of osteoporosis must await appropriately conducted placebo-controlled randomized clinical trials. It is unlikely that the results of these studies will be available within the next 2–3 years.

REFERENCES

Audran, M., Basle, M. F., Defontaine, A., Jallet, P., Bidet, M. T., Ermias, A., Tanguy, G., Pouplard, A., Reeve, J., Zanelli, J., & Renier, J. C. (1987). Transient hypoparathyroidism induced by synthetic human parathyroid hormone-(1–34)-treatment. *J. Clin. Endocrinol. Metab.*, **64**, 937–43.

Black, D. M., Cummings, S. R., Karpf, D. B., Cauley, J. A., Thompson, D. E., Nevitt, M. C., Bauer, D. C., Genant, H. K., Haskell, W. L., Marcus, R., Ott, S. M., Torner, J. C., Quandt, S. A., Reiss, T. F., & Ensrud, K. E. (1997). Randomised trial of effect of alendronate on risk of fracture in women with existing vertebral fractures. *Lancet*, **348**, 1535–41.

Bradbeer, J. N., Arlot, M. E., Meunier, P. J., & Reeve, J. (1992). Treatment of osteoporosis with parathyroid peptide (hPTH 1–34) and oestrogen: increase in volumetric density of iliac cancellous bone may depend on reduced trabecular spacing as well as increased thickness of packets of newly formed bone. *Clin. Endocrinol.*, **37**, 282–9.

Cheng, P. T., Chan, C., & Muller, K. (1995). Cyclical treatment of osteopenic ovariectomized adult rats with PTH(1–34) and pamidronate. *J. Bone Miner. Res.*, **10**, 119–26.

Cosman, F., Nieves, J., Woelfert, L., Shen, V., & Lindsay, R. (1998). Alendronate does not block the anabolic effect of PTH in postmenopausal osteoporotic women. *J. Bone Miner. Res.*, **13**, 1051–5.

Delmas, P. D., Vergnaud, P., Arlot, M. E., Pastoureau, P., Meunier, P. J., & Nilssen, M. H. L. (1995).

The anabolic effect of human PTH (1–34) on bone formation is blunted when bone resorption is inhibited by bisphosphonate tiludronate – Is activated resorption a prerequisite for the in vivo effect of PTH on formation in a remodelling system? *Bone*, **16**, 603–10.

Dempster, D. W., Cosman, F., Parisien, M., Shen, V., & Lindsay, R. (1993). Anabolic actions of parathyroid hormone on bone. *Endocr. Rev.*, **14**, 690–709.

Dobnig, H. & Turner, R. T. (1995). Evidence that intermittent treatment with parathyroid hormone increases bone formation in adult rats. *Endocrinology*, **136**, 3624–38.

Finkelstein, J. S., Klibanski, A., Schaefer, E. H., Hornstein, M. D., Schiff, I., & Neer, R. M. (1994). Parathyroid hormone for the prevention of bone loss induced by estrogen deficiency. *N. Engl. J. Med.*, **331**, 1618–23.

Frost, H. M. & Jee, W. S. S. (1992). On the rat model of human osteopenias and osteoporoses. *Bone Miner.*, **18**, 227–36.

Garnero, P., Shih, W. J., Gineyts, E., Karpf, D. B., & Delmas, P. D. (1994). Comparison of new biochemical markers of bone turnover in late postmenopausal osteoporotic women in response to alendronate treatment. *J. Clin. Endocrinol. Metab.*, **79**(6), 1693–700.

Gunness-Hey, M., & Hock, J. M. (1989). Loss of the anabolic effect of parathyroid hormone on bone after discontinuation of hormone in rats. *Bone*, **10**, 447–52.

Hesch, R. D., Busch, U., Prokop, M., Delling, G., & Rittinghaus, E. F. (1989). Increase of vertebral density by combination therapy with pulsatile 1–38 hPTH and sequential addition of calcitonin nasal spray in osteoporotic patients. *Calcif. Tissues Int.*, **44**, 176–80.

Hodsman, A. B. & Drost, D. J. (1989). The response of vertebral bone mineral density during the treatment of osteoporosis with sodium fluoride. *J. Clin. Endocrinol. Metab.*, **69**, 932–8.

Hodsman, A. B. & Fraher, L. J. (1990). Biochemical reponses to sequential human parathyoid hormone (1–38) and calcitonin in osteoporotic patients. *Bone Miner.*, **9**, 137–52.

Hodsman, A. B., Fraher, L., & Adachi, J. (1995). A clinical trial of cyclical clodronate as maintenance therapy following withdrawal of parathyroid hormone, in the treatment of postmenopausal osteoporosis (Abstract). *J. Bone Miner. Res.*, **10**, S200.

Hodsman, A. B., Fraher, L. J., Ostbye, T., Adachi, J. D., & Steer, B. M. (1993). An evaluation of several biochemical markers for bone formation and resorption in a protocol utilizing cyclical parathyroid hormone and calcitonin therapy for osteoporosis. *J. Clin. Invest.*, **91**, 1138–48.

Hodsman, A. B., Fraher, L. J., & Watson, P. H. (1997a). Parathyroid hormone: The clinical experience and prospects. In *Anabolic Treatments for Osteoporosis.* ed. J. E. Whitfield & P. Morley. Boca Raton, FL: CRC Press.

Hodsman, A. B., Fraher, L. J., Watson, P. H., Ostbye, T., Stitt, L. W., Adachi, J. D., Taves, D. H., & Drost, D. (1997b). A randomized controlled trial to compare the efficacy of cyclical parathyroid hormone versus cyclical parathyroid hormone and sequential calcitonin to improve bone mass in postmenopausal women with osteoporosis. *J. Clin. Endocrinol. Metab.*, **82**, 620–8.

Hodsman, A. B., Watson, P. H., Drost, D., Fraher, L. J., Holdsworth, D., Thornton, M., Hock, J., & Bryant, H. (1999). Assessment of maintenance therapy with reduced doses of PTH(1–34) in combination with a raloxifene analogue (LY117018) following anabolic therapy in the ovariectomized rat. *Bone*, **24**, 451–5.

Kalu, D. N. (1991). The ovariectomized rat model of postmenopausal bone loss. *Bone Miner.*, **15**, 175–92.

Kent, G. N., Loveridge, N., Reeve, J., & Zanelli, J. M. (1985). Pharmacokinetics of synthetic human parathyroid hormone 1–34 in man measured by cytochemical bioassay and radioimmunoassay. *Clin. Sci.*, **68**, 171–7.

Li, M., Mosekilde, L., Sogaard, C. H., Thomsen, J. S., & Wronski, T. J. (1995). Parathyroid hormone monotherapy and cotherapy with antiresoprtive agents restore vertebral bone mass and strength in aged ovariectomized rats. *Bone*, **16**, 629–35.

Liberman, U. A., Weiss, S. R., Broll, J., Minne, H. W., Quan, H., Bell, N. H., Rodriguez-Portales, J., Downs, R. W., Dequeker, J., Favus, M., Seeman, E., Recker, R. R., Capizzi, T., Santora, A. C., Lombardi, A., Shah, R. V., Hirsch, L. J., & Karpf, D. B. (1995). Effect of oral alendronate on bone mineral density and the incidence of fractures in postmenopausal osteoporosis. *N. Engl. J. Med.*, **333**, 1437–43.

Lindsay, R., Nieves, J., Formica, C., Henneman, E., Woelfert, L., Shen, V., & Dempster, D. (1997). Randomised controlled study of effect of parathyroid hormone on vertebral-bone mass and fracture incidence among postmenopausal women on oestrogen with osteoporosis. *Lancet*, **350**, 550–5.

Lindsay, R., Nieves, J., Henneman, E., Shen, V., & Cosman, F. (1993). Subcutaneous administration of the amino-terminal fragment of human parathyroid hormone-(1–34): kinetics and biochemical response to estrogenized osteoporotic patients. *J. Clin. Endocrinol. Metab.*, **77**, 1535–9.

Liu, C. C. & Kalu, D. N. (1990). Human parathyroid hormone-(1–34) prevents bone loss and augments bone formation in sexually mature ovariectomized rats. *J. Bone Miner. Res.*, **5**, 973–82.

Mashiba, T., Tanizawa, T., Takano, Y., Takahashi, H. E., Mori, S., & Norimatsu, H. (1997). A histomorphometric study on effects of single and concurrent intermittent administration of human PTH(1–34) and bisphosphonate cimadronate on tibial metaphysis in ovariectomized rats. *Bone*, **17**, 273S-8S.

Meng, X. W., Liang, X. G., Birchman, R., Wu, D. D., Dempster, D. W., Lindsay, R., & Shen, V. (1996). Temporal expression of the anabolic action of PTH in cancellous bone of ovariectomized rats. *J. Bone Miner. Res.*, **11**, 421–9.

Mosekilde, L., Danielsen, C. C., & Gasser, J. (1994a). The effect on vertebral bone mass and strength of long term treatment with antiresorptive agents (estrogen and calcitonin), human parathyroid hormone-(1–38), and combination therapy, assessed in aged ovariectomized rats. *Endocrinology*, **134**, 2126–34.

Mosekilde, L., Søgaard, C. H., McOsker, J. E., & Wronski, T. J. (1994b). PTH has a more pronounced effect on vertebral bone mass and biomechanical competence than antiresorptive agents (estrogen and bisphosphonate) – assessed in sexually mature, ovariectomized rats. *Bone*, **15**, 401–8.

Neer, R. M., Slovik, D., Daly, M., Lo, C., Potts, J., & Nussbaum, S. (1991). Treatment of postmenopausal osteoporosis with daily parathyroid hormone plus calcitriol. *Osteoporosis 1993, Int. Suppl.*, S204–5.

Neer, R. M., Slovik, D., Doppelt, S., Daly, M., Rosenthal, D., Lo, C., & Potts, J. (1987). The use of parathyroid hormone plus 1,25-dihydroxyvitamin D to increase trabecular bone in osteoporotic men and postmenopausal women. In *Osteoporosis 1987*, ed. C. Christiansen, J. S. Johansen, & B. J. Riis, pp. 829–35. Kobenhavn, Denmark: Osteopress Aps.

Patton, J. S., Trinchero, P., & Platz, R. M. (1994). Bioavailability of pulmonary delivered peptides and proteins: -interferon, calcitonins and parathyroid hormones. *J. Controlled Release*, **28**, 79–85.

Pehue, M., Policard, A., & Dufort, A. (1931). L'Osteoporose ou maladie des os marmoreens. *La Press Medicale*, **53**, 999.

Reeve, J., Arlot, M., Price, T. R., Edouard, C., Hesp, R., Hulme, P., Ashley, J. P., Zanelli, J. M., Green, J. R., Tellez, M., Katz, D., Spinks, T. J., & Meunier, P. J. (1987). Periodic courses of human 1–34 parathyroid peptide alternating with calcitriol paradoxically reduce bone remodelling in spinal osteoporosis. *Eur. J. Clin. Invest.*, **17**, 421–8.

Reeve, J., Bradbeer, J. N., Arlot, M., Davies, U. M., Green, J. R., Hampton, L., Edouard, C., Hesp, R., Hulme, P., Ashby, J. P., Zanelli, J. M., & Meunier, P. J. (1991). hPTH 1–34 treatment of osteoporosis with added hormone replacement therapy: biochemical, kinetic and histological responses. *Osteoporos. Int.*, **1**, 162–70.

Reeve, J., Davies, U. M., Hesp, R., McNally, E., & Katz, D. (1990). Treatment of osteoporosis with human parathyroid peptide and observations on the effect of sodium fluoride. *Br. Med. J.*, **301**, 314–8.

Reeve, J., Hesp, R., Williams, D., Klenerman, L., Zanelli, J. M., Darby, A. J., Tregear, G. W., Parsons, J. A., & Hume, R. (1976). Anabolic effect of low doses of a fragment of human parathyroid hormone on the skeleton in postmenopausal osteoporosis. *Lancet*, **i**, 1035–8.

Reeve, J., Meunier, P. J., Parsons, J. A., Bernat, M., Bijvoet, O. L. M., Courpron, P., Edouard, C., Klenerman, L., Neer, R. M., Renier, J. C., Slovik, D., Vismans, F. J. F. E., & Potts, J. T. J. (1980). Anabolic effect of human parathyroid hormone fragment on trabecular bone in involutional osteoporosis: a multicentre trial. *Br. Med. J.*, 1340–4.

Riggs, B. L., Hodgson, S. F., O'Fallon, W. M., Chao, E. Y. S., Wahner, H. W., Muhs, J. M., Cedel, S. L., & Melton, L. (1990). Effect of fluoride treatment on the fracture rate in postmenopausal women with osteoporosis. *N. Engl. J. Med.*, **322**, 802–9.

Riis, B. J., Overgaard, K., & Christiansen, C. (1995). Biochemical markers of bone turnover to monitor the bone response to postmenopausal hormone replacement therapy. *Osteoporos. Int.*, **5**, 276–80.

Rittmaster, R. J., Bolognese, M., Ettinger, B., Hanley, D., Hodsman, A. B., Kendler, D. L., & Rosen, C. J. (1998). Treatment of osteoporosis with parathyroid hormone followed by alendronate (Abstract). *Proc. Ann. Meeting Am. Soc. Bone Miner. Res., San Francisco, CA, Dec 1998*.

Selye, H. (1932). A condition simulating human scleroderma in rats injected with parathyroid hormone. *J. Am. Med. Assoc.*, **99**, 108.

Shen, V., Birchman, R., Xu, R., Otter, M., Wu, D., Lindsay, R., & Dempster, D. W. (1995). Effects of reciprocal treatment with estrogen and estrogen plus parathyroid hormone on bone structure and strength in ovariectomized rats. *J. Clin. Invest.*, **96**, 2331–8.

Shen, V., Dempster, D. W., Mellish, R. W. E., Birchman, R., Horbert, W., & Lindsay, R. (1992).

Effects of combined and separate intermittent administration of low-dose human parathyroid hormone fragment (1–34) and 17β-estradiol on bone histomorphometry in ovariectomized rats with established osteopenia. *Calcif. Tissues Int.*, **50**, 214–20.

Slovik, D. M., Rosenthal, D. I., Doppelt, S., Potts, J. T. J., Daly, M. A., Campbell, J. A., & Neer, R. M. (1986). Restoration of spinal bone in osteoporotic men by treatment with human parathyroid hormone (1–34) and 1,25-dihydroxyvitamin D. *J. Bone Miner. Res.*, **1**, 377–81.

Talbot, J. R., Fischer, M. M., Farley, S. M., Libanati, C., Farley, J., Tabuenca, A., & Baylink, D. B. (1996). The increase in spinal bone density that occurs in response to fluoride therapy for osteoporosis is not maintained after the therapy is discontinued. *Osteoporos. Int.*, **6**, 442–7.

Tam, C. S., Heersche, J. N. M., Murray, T. M., & Parsons, J. A. (1981). Parathyroid hormone stimulates the bone apposition rate independently of its resorptive action: differential effects of intermittent and continuous administration. *Endocrinology*, **110**, 506–12.

Watson, P. H., Lazowski, D. A., Han, V. K. M., Fraher, L. J., Steer, B. M., & Hodsman, A. B. (1995). Parathyroid hormone restores bone mass and enhances osteoblast insulin-like growth factor-1 gene expression in ovariectomized rats. *Bone*, **16**, 1–9.

Whitfield, J. F., Morley, P., Willick, G. E., Ross, V., Barbier, J-R., Isaacs, R. J., & Ohannessian-Barry, L. (1996). Stimulation of growth of femoral trabecular bone in ovariectomized rats by the novel parathyroid hormone fragment, hPTH(1–31) (Ostabolin). *Calcif. Tissue Int.*, **58**, 81–7.

Wronski, T. J., Dann, L. M., Scott, K. S., & Cintrón, M. (1989). Long-term effects of ovariectomy and aging on the rat skeleton. *Calcif. Tissue Int.*, **45**, 360–6.

Wronski, T. J., Yen, C-F., & Dann, L. M. (1993). Parathyroid hormone is more effective than estrogen or bisphosphonates for restoration of lost bone mass in ovariectomized rats. *Endocrinology*, **132**, 823–31.

25

Vitamin D and vitamin D analogs as therapeutic agents

Richard Kremer

The concept of supplementary food substances made its appearance earlier in this century. It was then clearly established that both fat- and water-soluble substances can prevent deficiency disease (DeLuca, 1981; DeLuca & Schnoes, 1983). A fat-soluble substance with antirachitic activity termed 'vitamin D' was identified in cod liver oil. Furthermore, it was demonstrated that ultraviolet light could heal rickets (DeLuca, 1981; DeLuca & Schnoes, 1983) by inducing antirachitic activity in the sterol fraction of food (DeLuca, 1981; DeLuca & Schnoes, 1983). This pioneering work provided the means for the prevention and elimination of rickets as a major medical problem.

It is now recognized that the role of vitamin D is much broader than regulation of calcium metabolism as reflected by its effects on the proliferation and differentiation of a variety of cells, including normal, malignant and immune cells (Holick, 1995).

Classical actions of vitamin D

A deficiency of vitamin D results in one of two diseases: either rickets in children or osteomalacia in the adult. The major target tissues of vitamin D in the regulation of calcium metabolism are the intestine, bone and kidney. Parathyroid hormone (PTH) is required for calcium mobilization from bone and for renal conservation of calcium, but vitamin D itself, stimulates intestinal calcium absorption. In bone, vitamin D exerts its effects in concert with PTH. Although it had been believed that vitamin D may play a role in the synthesis of the organic matrix and the mineralization process itself, it was demonstrated that vitamin D does not function directly in either bone growth or mineralization when plasma calcium and phosphorus levels are maintained in the normal range (DeLuca, 1985). By maintaining calcium and phosphorus within the normal range, vitamin D promotes the deposition of calcium hydroxyapatite into the bone matrix.

Metabolism of vitamin D

Vitamin D consists of two forms, vitamin D_2 (ergocalciferol) of plant origin and vitamin D_3 (cholecalciferol) the animal form of the compound.

It is now well known that 7-dehydrocholesterol is metabolized in the skin to vitamin D_3 by irradiation with ultraviolet light, while vitamin D_2 is derived from food or food supplements. Both are then converted in the liver into 25-dihydroxyvitamin D [25(OH)D] and subsequently activated further to form the final active metabolite $1\alpha,25$-dihydroxyvitamin D [$1\alpha,25(OH)_2D$] by hydroxylation at the carbon-1 position. The other important pathway is 24R-hydroxylation, which is now established as the first step for the inactivation of vitamin D. This reaction is catalyzed by 24R-hydroxylase, and its activity intimately regulated by $1\alpha,25(OH)_2$ D, PTH and/or phosphorus levels. After conversion of $1\alpha,25(OH)_2D$ into $1\alpha,24,25(OH)_3D$, it is metabolized to 24-oxo-$1\alpha,25(OH)_2D$, then to 24-oxo-$1\alpha,23,25(OH)_3D$ and finally to calcitroic acid. Recently, the enzyme regulating $1\alpha,25(OH)_2D$ production, 1α hydroxylase, was cloned (Takeyama et al., 1997) and this important discovery should help to elucidate the molecular mechanism of regulation by $1\alpha,25(OH)_2D$, PTH and phosphorus, and the pathways of $1\alpha,25(OH)_2D$ degradation and its possible regulation. For a more detailed description of vitamin D metabolism, see Chapter 7, this volume.

Mechanism of action

$1\alpha,25(OH)_2D$ easily penetrates plasma membranes to bind its nuclear receptor, the vitamin D receptor (VDR) (Reichel et al., 1989). Vitamin D responsive elements (VDREs) have been identified in the 5′ upstream region of the osteocalcin, osteopontin, $\beta3$ integrin, 24R-hydroxylase, parathyroid hormone and parathyroid hormone related peptide genes (Haussler et al., 1997). The DNA sequence of VDRE is that of a direct repeat structure with a 3 nucleotide base spacer as exemplified by the sequences shown in Table 25.1 but VDR must form a heterodimer with another nuclear receptor, the retinoid X receptor to be fully active (Zhang et al., 1992).

New actions of vitamin D

The pioneering work of Suda and co-workers (Abe et al., 1981) that demonstrated the differentiation-inducing effect of $1\alpha,25(OH)_2D$ on leukemia cells opened the way for investigating new actions of vitamin D. Since then, various effects of $1\alpha,25(OH)_2D$ have been proposed.

$1\alpha,25(OH)_2D_3$, the physiologically active form of vitamin D_3, is capable of inhibiting proliferation and inducing differentiation in a variety of cells expressing the

Table 25.1. Nucleotide sequence of the reported VDREs

Ligand	Sequence		
Human osteocalcin	GGGTGA	ACG	GGGGCA
Rat osteocalcin	GGGTGA	ATG	AGGACA
Mouse SPP-1 (osteopontin)	GGTTCA	CGA	GGTTCA
Human PTH	TCAACT	ATA	GGTTCA
Chicken PTH	GGGTCA	GGA	GGGTGT
Mouse calbindin-D28K	GGGGGA	TGT	GAGGAG
Rat 24-hydroxylase I	GGTTCA	GCG	GGTGCG
Rat 24-hydroxylase II	AGGTGA	GTG	AGGGCG
Rat PTHrP	GGGTGG	AGA	GGGGTG

vitamin D receptor, notably skin keratinocytes (Hosomi et al., 1983), many cancer cells (De Luca & Ostrem, 1986) and cells of the immune system (Rigby et al., 1984). Initial study of the immunobiology of $1\alpha,25(OH)_2D_3$ led to the finding that $1\alpha,25(OH)_2D_3$ was a potent inhibitor of both T-lymphocyte proliferation and lymphokine production (Manolagas et al., 1998), with its antiproliferative activity mediated primarily through inhibition of interleukin-2 (IL-2) production (Reichel et al., 1987). Cell cycle analysis demonstrated that each of these effects of $1\alpha,25(OH)_2D_3$ inhibited the transition of activated T-cells from the early, G_1 (G_{1A}), to the late, G_1 (G_{1B}) (Rigby, 1998) providing evidence of the specificity of $1\alpha,25(OH)_2D_3$ in regulating T-lymphocyte proliferation. In addition, selective examinations of B-cells have shown that $1\alpha,25(OH)_2 D_3$ inhibits B-cell proliferation and immunoglobulin production in vitro. These studies suggest the potential utility of $1\alpha,25(OH)_2D_3$ as a therapeutic agent in the treatment of graft rejection and autoimmune disease.

While these findings stimulated an interest in the use of $1\alpha,25(OH)_2D_3$ for the treatment of hyperproliferative diseases involving aberrant or incomplete terminal cell differentiation (i.e., psoriasis and cancer) and disorders of the immune system, the use of pharmacologically active doses of $1\alpha,25(OH)_2D_3$ is restricted by its potent hypercalcemic effects. Recently side chain analogs of $1\alpha,25(OH)_2D_3$ have been developed and have highly potent antiproliferative and/or immunoregulatory activity with more favorable therapeutic ratios to $1\alpha,25(OH)_2D_3$.

Analogs of $1\alpha,25(OH)_2D_3$

Since the discovery of new actions of $1\alpha,25(OH)_2D_3$, many scientists have tried to synthesize non-calcemic vitamin D analogs which separate the newly identified

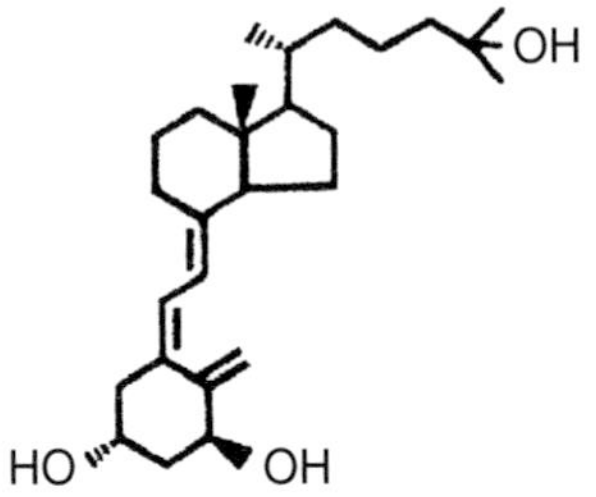

$1\alpha,25(OH)_2D_3$

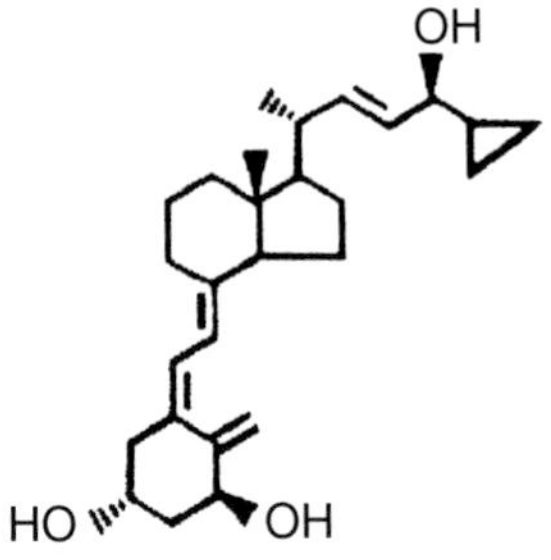

Calcipotriol
(MC 903)

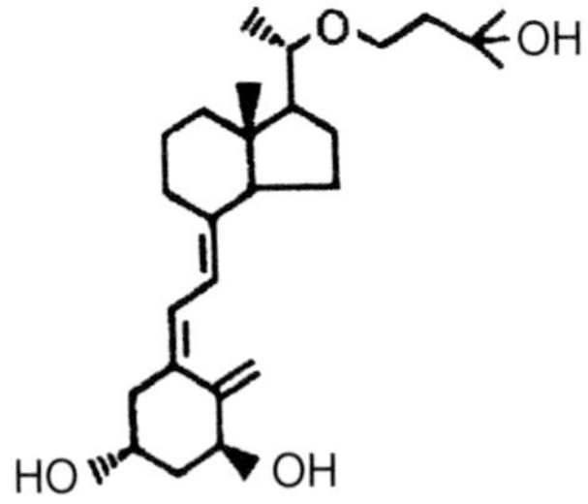

22-oxa-$1\alpha,25(OH)_2D_3$

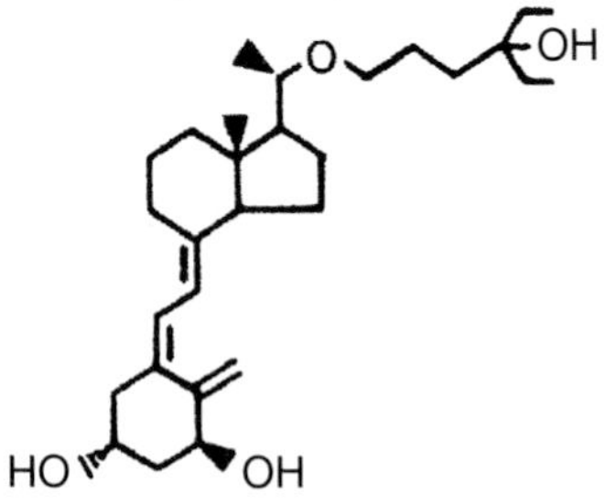

KH 1060

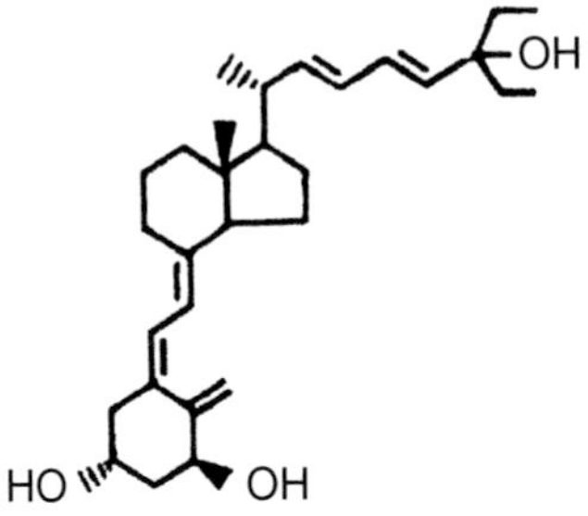

EB 1089

Fig. 25.1 Structure of the most common vitamin D analogs.

effect from the hypercalcemia effect. The mechanisms of selectivity of the new vitamin D analogs are unknown but may be related, at least in part, to the different pharmacokinetics of the analogs, such as the difference in metabolic clearance rate mainly determined by the binding efficacy to serum transport protein, and the different metabolism in both classical (such as the kidney, bone and intestine) and therapeutic (such as tumors, skin and parathyroid) target tissues. In addition, vitamin D analogs may bind with different affinities to the VDR or modulate the interaction of the VDR with RXR or their co-activators. The structure of the most commonly used vitamin D analogs is shown in Fig. 25.1.

Calcipotriol (MC 903), which in vitro is as potent as $1\alpha,25(OH)_2D_3$ in inducing cell differentiation and inhibiting cell proliferation, but which is at least 100 times less active than $1\alpha,25(OH)_2D_3$ in inducing hypercalcemia and hypercalciuria (Binderup & Bramm, 1988). Due to a rapid rate of metabolic degradation, calcipotriol is not suitable for systemic use (Kissmeyer & Binderup, 1991), but it has been shown to be very effective in the topical treatment of psoriasis (Kragballe et al., 1991). Taking advantage of its antiproliferative action, calcipotriol has been tried and proved effective on cutaneous metastatic breast cancer in patients with tumors possessing receptors for $1\alpha,25(OH)_2D_3$ (Bower et al., 1991), but further studies are warranted to determine its full potential in this condition.

Analogs with altered stereochemistry at carbon 20 in the side chain (20-epivitamin D analogs) have been developed and showed potent effects on T-cell activation in vitro. Such analogs as KH 1060, suppress allogeneic MLR reactions at concentrations of $5 \times 10^{-15}M$ and inhibit IL-2 production and IL-1 induced IL-8 release in human T-lymphocytes (Binderup & Bramm, 1988). From this in vivo work (Veyron et al., 1993), it has been clarified that KH 1060 at dosages as low as 0.02 μg/kg/day inhibits skin graft rejection in mice and has a cyclosporine-sparing effect when combined treatment is used. These results suggest that KH 1060 is a very potent analog and may be of potential benefit in the treatment of autoimmune disease as well as in the prevention of graft rejection.

Bone and mineral disorders

Bone remodeling

$1\alpha,25(OH)_2D_3$ influences bone remodeling during growth and in adult life. In vitro studies have shown that $1\alpha,25(OH)_2D_3$ directly affects the differentiation of osteoclasts in the bone marrow (Roodman et al., 1985). Osteoblasts also possess functional VDRs as demonstrated by their abilities to express alkaline phosphatase and osteocalcin in response to $1\alpha,25(OH)_2D_3$. However, it is believed that $1\alpha,25(OH)_2D_3$ does not participate directly in bone mineralization but rather promotes osteoid mineralization by maintaining circulating phosphate and calcium concentrations within the normal range (De Luca, 1985).

Nutritional rickets and osteomalacia

Rickets is a disorder of mineralization of the bone matrix or osteoid in growing bones whereas osteomalacia occurs after the cessation of growth and involves only the bone and not the growth plate. Vitamin D deficiency usually results from lack of adequate sunlight and/or consumption of diet low in fortified foods (Sandstead, 1980; Stamp, 1975). Breast-fed infants who do not receive vitamin D supplementation are also at risk for vitamin D deficiency since breast milk is low in vitamin D content (Sandstead, 1980). Rickets has also been reported in infants receiving total parenteral nutrition (TPN) in which the solution was low in calcium and vitamin D (Klein & Chesney, 1986). The recommended regimens for vitamin D deficiency in these conditions is variable and range from 1500–5000 IU/day orally (Sandstead 1980), 10000–50000 IU/month intramusculary (Sandstead 1980) or 600 IU in 6 divided doses over 1–2 hours (Shah & Finberg, 1994). Alternatively, ultraviolet lamp treatment may also be of great value (Stamp, 1975). In cases of malabsorption it is preferable to use oral preparations of $25(OH)D_3$ (20–30 µg/day), $1\alpha,25(OH)_2D_3$ (0.5–1.5 µg/day) or intra-muscular injection of vitamin D_2 (ergo-calciferol). For prevention of vitamin D deficiency in breast-fed infants, a daily supplementation of 400 IU of vitamin D_2 is recommended and in TPN-fed infants 20–25 IU/kg/day (Koo et al., 1986).

Inherited type of rickets

Hereditary pseudovitamin D deficiency rickets also known as vitamin D-dependent rickets type I is an autosomal recessive disorder. Affected patients have low serum concentrations of $1\alpha,25$-$(OH)_2D$ and normal or high concentrations of $25(OH)D$ (Scriver et al., 1978; Delvin et al., 1981). In these patients physiologic doses of $1\alpha,25(OH)_2D_3$ (0.25 µg to 1 µg/day) but massive doses of vitamin D or $25(OH)D_3$ are required to cure rickets (Fraser et al., 1973). Recently, the $25(OH)D_3$ 1 hydroxylase gene was cloned (Takeyama et al., 1997) and inactivating mutations in the $25(OH)D_3$-1α hydroxylase gene were found to be the cause of pseudovitamin D deficiency rickets (Kitanaka et al., 1998).

Vitamin D-dependent rickets type II (VDDR-II) also called hereditary resistance to $1,25(OH)_2D$ has a pattern of inheritance suggesting autosomal recessive disease. The majority of patients do not respond to any form of vitamin D therapy because of inactivating mutations in the vitamin D receptor (VDR) (Hughes et al., 1988; Liberman et al., 1983; Malloy et al., 1989; Marx et al., 1986). However, mildest forms of the disease have also been reported (Liberman et al., 1983; Takeda et al., 1986). Therapeutic regimen should be adopted for each individual patient. To overcome the vitamin D resistance massive doses of $1\alpha(OH)D_3$ or $1\alpha,25(OH)_2D_3$ up to 6 µg/day should be initiated soon after birth together with up to 3 g of supplemental calcium/day. In cases where this regimen has failed, high doses of intravenous calcium have been used and resulted in clinical, biochemical and histological healing of the condition (Griffin & Zerwekh, 1983; Liberman et al., 1986; Malloy et al., 1990).

X-linked hypophosphatemia vitamin D-resistant rickets

In this condition patients have a reduced phosphate reabsorption in the proximal tubule leading to hypophosphatemia (Eicher et al., 1976) (see Chapter 8, this volume for further details). A mutation in the phosphate-regulating gene with homology to endopeptidases on the X chromosome (PEX gene) has been identified

(The HYP consortium 1995). Patients exhibit inappropriately normal levels of $1\alpha,25(OH)_2D$ in the face of severe hypophosphatemia. Therapeutic intervention combines partial phosphate supplementation and $1\alpha,25(OH)_2D_3$, which in many cases, restores plasma phosphorus levels and corrects the bone disease (Glorieux et al., 1980; Verge et al., 1991).

Osteoporosis

Rationale for supplementing the diets of elderly with calcium and vitamin D is based on studies showing a decreased absorption of calcium (Bullamore et al., 1970) and vitamin D (Barragry et al., 1978) with age as well as a decreased synthesis of vitamin D by the skin (McLaughlin & Holick, 1985) as indicated by a decline of serum 25(OH)D with age. Recent studies indicate that combined calcium and vitamin D supplementation reduces rates of non-vertebral fractures in elderly when living at home (Dawson-Hughes et al., 1997) or in nursing homes (Chapuy et al., 1992). It requires a minimum of 600 IU/day to maintain 25(OH)D levels in healthy young males and it is therefore reasonable to recommend a minimum daily intake of 800 IU in elderly individuals with or without established osteoporosis. However, this amount may be adjusted higher or lower depending on the daily consumption of milk products and sunlight exposure.

Corticosteroid induced bone loss

Corticosteroids are known to decrease intestinal calcium absorption (Kimberg et al., 1971) and therefore contribute to bone loss, a condition frequently encountered in corticosteroid-treated patients (Lubert & Raisz, 1990). It has been suggested that vitamin D_3 (400 to 800 IU/day) and calcium should be given to all patients receiving long-term corticosteroid therapy (Meunier, 1993) and recent studies seem to confirm this suggestion in patients treated with low dose corticosteroids (<10 mg of prednisone/day) (Buckley et al., 1996). Treatment with $1\alpha,25(OH)_2D_3$ (0.25 to 0.5 μg/day) and calcium may be recommended in patients on high dose corticosteroids (>10 mg of prednisone/day) (Sambrook et al., 1993) with close monitoring of blood and urinary calcium concentrations. Other regimens with pharmacologic dosages of vitamin D_3 (50000 IU three times a week) had been recommended in the past (Hahn & Hahn, 1976) but no randomized clinical trials have been devised to study the efficacy of these regimens. The guidelines to treat these patients remains empirical, and new controlled studies are clearly needed in this area.

Hyperparathyroidism

Parathyroid hormone (PTH) plays a major role in maintaining serum calcium levels within a very narrow range (see Chapter 6). Once the serum calcium levels are perturbed, the secretion as well as the synthesis of PTH are adequately regulated. Extracellular calcium as well as $1\alpha,25(OH)_2D_3$ are crucially involved in this process.

Although researchers in the field had long believed that the major modulator of PTH secretion was calcium and that the suppressive effect of $1\alpha,25(OH)_2D_3$ was mediated by its effect on raising serum calcium, $1\alpha,25(OH)_2D_3$ itself suppresses PTH gene expression at the transcriptional level. In vivo in rat model, not only $1\alpha,25(OH)_2D_3$ but also its non-calcemic analogs, OCT and MC 903, are able to suppress the transcription of the PTH gene (Naveh-Many & Silver, 1993). Interestingly, VDR mRNA gradually increases following $1\alpha,25(OH)_2D_3$ administration reaching a peak level at 24 h. Such upregulation of VDR mRNA may well potentiate its inhibitory action on PTH mRNA.

In certain clinical situations, the level of serum PTH is so elevated that deleterious bony lesions occur and worsen the patients' condition. Secondary hyperparathyroidism in chronic renal failure is one such example. The level of PTH mRNA is clearly elevated in secondary hyperparathyroidism and it is not due to enlarged cell number but each parathyroid cell produces a greater amount of PTH mRNA. These studies suggest a rationale for the therapeutic effectiveness of $1\alpha,25(OH)_2D_3$ and its analogs in chronic renal failure.

An insensitivity to the suppressive effect of calcium on PTH secretion is usually observed in uremic patients (probably due to a disorder of the recently discovered calcium sensor). This phenomenon is well known as a shift of set-point from 1.0 mmol/l of calcium in the normal setting to 1.26 mmol/l in the uremic state. Although the precise explanation of this mechanism is as yet unclear, the low level or decreased number of $1\alpha,25(OH)_2D_3$ receptors may play a role in altering the set-point. Chronic administration of $1\alpha,25(OH)_2D_3$ can shift the curve back toward the left. These abnormalities in parathyroid function may contribute to the development and maintenance of hyperparathyroidism in chronic renal failure and provide the basis for the therapeutic effects of $1\alpha,25(OH)_2D_3$ in the treatment of secondary hyperparathyroidism. A newly synthesized vitamin D derivative, $19\text{-NOR-}1\alpha,25(OH)_2D_2$, may exert a more beneficial therapeutic effect on suppressing secondary hyperparathyroidism in chronic renal failure than seen to date, because of certain unique biological characteristics such as the ability to inhibit cell growth of parathyroid cells without inducing a hypercalcemic effect through enhancing gut absorption of calcium (Takahashi et al., 1997).

Vitamin D treatment for malignant osteolysis

In the last several years the principle of differentiation therapy in the prevention and treatment of cancer has received an increasing amount of interest.

Differentiation therapy is based on the observation that many cancer cells are arrested at an early, immature stage of development, and that a number of chemical entities are able to stimulate these cells to differentiate into their mature forms. Encouraging clinical results have recently been observed in patients with acute promyelocytic leukemia, treated with the differentiation-inducing vitamin A metabolite all-*trans*-retinoic acid (Warrell et al., 1991).

The physiologically active form of vitamin D_3, $1\alpha,25(OH)_2D_3$ is a potent inducer of cell differentiation in a number of freshly isolated cancer cells and established cell lines. In tumor-bearing animals, $1\alpha,25(OH)_2D_3$ and its synthetic analog 1-hydroxyvitamin D_3 [$1(OH)D_3$], which undergoes biotransformation in the liver to $1\alpha,25(OH)_2D_3$, have been shown to suppress tumor growth, inhibit metastasis and prolong survival (Eisman et al., 1987; Honma et al., 1983; Sato et al., 1984). Preliminary clinical studies have indicated that oral administration of $1\alpha,25(OH)_2D_3$ or $1\alpha(OH)D_3$ may be of benefit in myelofibrosis, myelodysplastic syndromes and non-Hodgkin's lymphomas (Arlett et al., 1984; Cunningham et al., 1985; Motomura et al., 1991). However, as stated previously, the clinical use of these compounds is limited by their strong effects on calcium metabolism. Administration of more than a few μg per day leads to hypercalcemia (Stern & Bell, 1989). A further limitation is the discovery that certain *ras*-transformed cancer cells are partially resistant to $1\alpha,25(OH)_2D$ growth inhibition requiring 10- to 100-fold higher concentrations of this compound to achieve the same effects (Sebag et al., 1992; Solomon et al., 1998, 1999).

To date, only a few vitamin D analogs useful for systemic administration have been described: $1\alpha,25$-dihydroxy-16-ene-23-yne-vitamin D_3, which has been shown to prolong survival of mice injected with leukemia cells (Zhou et al., 1990); $1\alpha,25$-dihydroxy-16-ene-23-yne-26,27- hexafluorovitamin D_3, which has tumor preventing effects in rats with carcinogen-induced mammary tumors (Anzano et al., 1994); 22-oxa-$1\alpha,25(OH)_2D_3$ (OCT), which is able to delay growth of implanted breast tumors in athymic mice (Abe et al., 1991) and EB 1089. EB 1089 has strong activity as compared to $1\alpha,25(OH)_2D_3$, on the regulation of growth and differentiation of cancer cells in vitro (Yu et al., 1995), coupled with a decreased risk of inducing calcemic effects in vivo (Haq et al., 1993). It also has the ability to inhibit the growth of mammary tumors (Colston et al., 1992) and its skeletal complications (El Abdaimi et al., 1998) in vivo, without causing hypercalcemia.

A proliferative disease involving the bone marrow can also be recognized during development of myeloid leukemias. This myeloproliferative disease, also known as refractory anemia or myelodysplastic syndrome (MDS), appears to be a promising target of $1\alpha,25(OH)_2D_3$ therapy, and in a recent trial a sustained response was obtained in MDS patients (Bloch et al., 1990; Kelsey et al., 1992) with orally administered $1\alpha,25(OH)_2D_3$ in combination with calcium-lowering agents.

Approximately 10% of cancer patients develop malignant hypercalcemia, a potentially life-threatening condition. While some presently available agents offer a degree of relief of the problem, apart from cytotoxic agents, none of the currently available drugs to combat this condition works via affecting the specific mechanism causing the hypercalcemia.

Development of alternative treatment options to manage the condition would be an advancement in the care of cancer patients. It is now felt that, regardless of the presence of cancer cells in bone tissue, cancer-related osteolysis is mediated by factors released from malignant cells. Parathyroid hormone-related peptide (PTHrP) is thought to be the most important mediator of cancer-related hypercalcemia, and is detected by present immunoassays in about 50–80% of hypercalcemic cancer patients (Budayr et al., 1989; Fraser et al., 1993; Henderson et al., 1990). It is most frequently elevated in patients with solid tumors especially in those with squamous (epidermoid) carcinoma. About 50% of hypercalcemia breast cancer patients have elevated levels of PTHrP (Bundred et al., 1991; Grill et al., 1991), and it is also associated with hematologic malignancies, including myelomas and lymphoma (Henderson et al., 1990; Ikeda et al., 1994; Kremer et al., 1996).

PTHrP is expressed by a wide variety of cancer and non-cancer cells (e.g., epithelial and hematopoietic cell lines). In vitro studies in human keratinocytes demonstrated the ability of $1\alpha,25(OH)_2D_3$ to control PTHrP production (Henderson et al., 1991). $1\alpha,25(OH)_2D_3$ could inhibit PTHrP production in a dose-dependent manner in normal human epidermal keratinocytes (NHEK) (Kremer et al., 1991; Yu et al., 1995) and other normal epithelial cells, including human mammary epithelial cells (Sebag et al., 1994). Studies performed in cancer cell lines confirmed these data, but also pointed to a relative resistance of cancer cells to $1\alpha,25(OH)_2D_3$-induced PTHrP inhibition. In malignant cells, 10–100 times higher concentrations of $1\alpha,25(OH)_2D_3$ were required to achieve the same effects as in normal cells (Henderson et al., 1991; Yu et al., 1995). Furthermore, because $1\alpha,25(OH)_2D_3$ causes hypercalcemia at relatively low doses, it has limited applications in clinical practice regarding PTHrP suppression in cancer patients.

Consequently, it seems logical to study new vitamin D analogs with similar, more potent non-classical biological effects as $1\alpha,25(OH)_2D_3$ but with less calcemic activity in vivo. EB 1089 was initially tested in vitro and found to be 10–100 times more potent than $1\alpha,25(OH)_2D_3$ in inhibiting PTHrP expression and production (Yu et al., 1995). This analog was subsequently used in vivo in the rat Leydig cell tumor model, an animal model that mimics human malignancy associated hypercalcemia. In that model, EB 1089 was administered subcutaneously by constant infusion, and was able to prevent the development of hypercalcemia and significantly reduce both tumor mass and circulating levels of PTHrP (Haq et al., 1993). Furthermore, treated non-hypercalcemic animals survived longer than the non-treated hypercalcemic animals. Studies in nude mice implanted with human squamous tumors producing PTHrP that were treated with EB1089 confirmed these results (El Abdaimi et al., 1999).

Recent studies have shown that the PTHrP gene's promoter contains a vitamin D response element (VDRE) (Kremer et al., 1996a and Table 25.1). Consequently, similar to the scenario with $1\alpha,25(OH)_2D_3$, binding of the EB 1089 – vitamin D receptor complex to the VDRE region of the PTHrP gene is thought to be the mechanism inhibiting transcription of the PTHrP gene.

Conclusions

Since its discovery in the early part of this century, vitamin D has evolved from a simple food nutrient to a potent hormone with multiple effects in addition to its classical effect on calcium homeostasis. These new non-classic actions of $1\alpha,25(OH)_2D_3$ have catalyzed considerable research activity to understand the mechanism(s) of these new functions. Emerging from these studies is the discovery of vitamin D analogs with properties indicating their potential usefulness in a variety of clinical disorders. Active basic research aimed at determining structure–function relationships of these analogs will likely expand in the next decade and should help select potential candidates for future clinical applications.

REFERENCES

Abe, E., Miyaura, C., Sakagmi, H., Takeda, M., Konno, K., Yamazaki, T., Yoshiki, S., & Suda, T. (1981). Differentiation of mouse myeloid leukemic cells induced by $1\alpha,25$-hydroxyvitamin D_3. *Proc. Natl Acad. Sci, USA*, **78**, 4990.

Abe, J., Nakano, T., Nishii, Y., Matsumoto, T., Ogata, E., & Ikeda, K. (1991). A novel vitamin D_3 analog, 22-oxa-1,25-dihydroxyvitamin D_3, inhibits the growth of human breast cancer in vitro and in vivo without causing hypercalcemia. *Endocrinology*, **129**, 832–7.

Anzano, M. A., Smith, J. M., Uskokovic, M. R., Peer, C. W., Mullen, L. T., Letterio, J. J., Welsh, M. C., Shrader, M. W., Logsdon, D. L., Driver, C. L., Brown, C. C., Roberts, A. B., & Sporn, M. B. (1994). $1\alpha,25$-dihydroxy-16-ene-23-yne-26,27-hexafluorocholecalciferol (Ro24–5531), a new deltanoid (vitamin D analogue) for prevention of cancer in rat. *Cancer Res.*, **54**, 1653–6.

Arlett, P., Nicodeme, R., Adoue, D., Larregain-Fournier, D., Delsol, G., & Tallec. Y. (1984). Clinical evidence for 1,25-dihydroxycholecalciferol action in myelofibrosis. *Lancet*, i, 1013–14.

Barragry, J. M., Franch, M. W., & Corless, D. (1978). Intestinal chole-calciferol absorption in the elderly and in younger adults. *Clin. Sci. Mol. Med.*, **55**, 213–20.

Binderup, L. & Bramm, E. (1988). Effects of a novel vitamin D analogue MC 903 on cell proliferation and differentiation in vitro and on calcium metabolism in vivo. *Biochem. Pharmacol.*, **37**, 889–95.

Bloch, A., Koeffler, H. P., Pierce, G. B., & Hozumi. M. (1990). Ninth annual Sapporo cancer seminar: cell differentiation and cancer control. *Cancer Res.*, **50**, 1346.

Bower, M., Colston, R. C., Stein, R. C., Hedley, A., Gazet, J. C., Ford, H. T., & Coombes, R. C. (1991). Topical calcitriol treatment in advanced breast cancer. *Lancet*, **337**, 701–2.

Buckley, L., Leib, E. S., Cartularo, K. S., Vacek, P. M., & Cooper, S. M. (1996). Calcium and vitamin D₃ supplementation prevents bone loss in the spine secondary to lower dose corticosteroids in patients with rheumatoid arthritis. *Ann. Int. Med.*, **125**, 961–8.

Budayr, A. A., Nissensan, R. A., Klein, R. F., Pun, K. K., Clark, O. H., Diep, D., Arnaud, C. D., & Strewler, G. J. (1989). Increased serum levels of a parathyroid hormone-like protein in malignancy-associated hypercalcemia. *Ann. Int. Med.*, **111**, 807–12.

Bullamore, J. R., Wilkinson, R., Gallagher, J. C., Nordin, B. E. C., & Marshall, D. H. (1970). Effect of age on calcium absorption. *Lancet*, **ii**, 535–7.

Bundred, N. J., Ratcliffe, W. A., Walker, R. A., Coley, S., Morrison, J. M., & Ratcliffe, J. G. (1991). Parathyroid hormone-related protein and hypercalcemia in breast cancer. *Br. Med. J.*, **1303**, 1506–9.

Chapuy, M. C., Arlot, M. E., Duboeuf, F., Brun, J., Crouzet, B., Arnaud, S., Delmas, P. D., & Meunier, P. J. (1992). Vitamin D₃ and calcium to prevent hip fractures in elderly women. *N. Engl. J. Med.*, **327**, 1637–42.

Colston, K. W., MacKay, A. G., James, S. Y., Binderup, L., Chander, S., & Coombes, R. C. (1992). EB1089: a new vitamin D analog that inhibits the growth of breast cancer cells in vivo and in vitro. *Biochem. Pharmacol.*, **44**, 2273–80.

Cunningham, D., Gilchrist, N. L., Cowan, R. A., Forrest, G. J., McArdle, C. S., & Soukop, M. (1985). Alfacalcidol as a modulator of growth of low grade non-Hodgkin's lymphomas. *Br. Med. J.*, **291**, 1153–5.

Dawson-Hughes, B., Harris, S., Krall, E., & Dallal, G. E. (1997). Effect of calcium and vitamin D supplementation on bone density in men and women 65 years of age or older. *N. Engl. J. Med.*, **337**, 670–6.

DeLuca, H. F. (1981). The transformation of a vitamin into a hormone: the vitamin D story. *Harvey Lect.*, **75**, 333–79.

DeLuca, H. F. (1985). The vitamin D-calcium axis. In *Calcium in Biological Systems*, ed. R. P. Rubin, G. B. Weiss, & J. W. Putney Jr, pp. 491–511. New York: Plenum.

DeLuca, H. F. & Schnoes, H. K. (1983). Vitamin D: recent advances. *Ann. Rev. Biochem.*, **52**, 411–39.

DeLuca, H. F. & Ostrem, V. (1986). The relationship between the vitamin D system and cancer. *Adv. Exp. Med. Biol.*, **206**, 413–19.

Delvin, E. E., Glorieux, F. H., Marie, P. J., & Pettifor, J. M. (1981). Vitamin D dependency: replacement therapy with calcitriol. *J. Pediatr.*, **99**, 26–34.

Eicher, E. M., Southard, J. L., & Scriver, C. R. (1976). Hypophosphatemia: Mouse model for human familial hypophosphatemic (vitamin D-resistant) rickets. *Proc. Natl Acad. Sci., USA*, **73**, 4667.

Eisman, J. A., Barkla, D. H., & Tutton, J. M. (1987). Suppression of in vivo growth of human cancer solid tumor xenografts by 1,25-dihydroxyvitamin D₃. *Cancer Res.*, **47**, 21–5.

El Abdaimi, K., Dion, N., Papavasiliou, V., Cardinal, P. E., Binderup, L., Goltzman, D., Sainte Marie, L. G., & Kremer, R. (1998). The vitamin D analog EB1089 prevents skeletal metastasis and prolongs survival time in nude mice transplanted with human breast cancer cells. ASBMR-IBMS Second Joint Meeting, vol. 23(5), p. 1158. San Francisco, CA. December 1–6.

El Abdaimi, K., Papavasiliou, V., Rabbani, S. A., Rhim, J. S., Goltzman, D., & Kremer, R. (1999). Reversal of hypercalcemia with the vitamin D analogue EB1089 in a human model of squamous cancer. *Cancer Res.*, **59**, 3325-8.

Fraser, D., Kooh, S. W., Kind, H. P., Holick, M. F., Tanaka, Y., & DeLuca, H. F. (1973). Pathogenesis of hereditary vitamin D-dependent rickets: an inborn error of vitamin D metabolism involving defective conversion of 25-hydroxyvitamin D to 1α,25 dihydroxyvitamin D. *N. Engl. J. Med.*, **289**, 817–22.

Fraser, W., Robinson, J., Lawton, R., Durham, B., Gallacher, S., Boyle, I., Beastall, G., & Logue, F. (1993). Clinical and laboratory studies of a new immunoradiometric assay of parathyroid hormone-related protein. *Clin. Chem.*, **39**, 414–19.

Glorieux, F. M., Marie, P. J., Pettifor, J. M., & Delvin, E. E. (1980). Bone response to phosphate salts, ergocalciferol and calcitriol in hypophosphatemic vitamin D-resistant rickets. *N. Engl. J. Med.*, **303**, 1023.

Griffin, J. E. & Zerwekh, J. E. (1983). Impaired stimulation of 25-hydroxyvitamin D-24-hydroxylase in fibroblasts from a patient with vitamin D-dependent rickets, type II. *J. Clin. Invest.*, **72**, 1190–9.

Grill, V., Ho, P., Body, J. J., Johanson, N., Lee, S. C., Kukreja, S. C., Moseley, J. M., & Martin, T. J. (1991). Parathyroid hormone-related protein: elevated levels in both humoral hypercalcemia of malignancy and hypercalcemia complicating metastatic breast cancer. *J. Clin. Endocrinol. Metab.*, **73**, 1309–15.

Hahn, T. J. & Hahn, B. H. (1976). Osteopenia in subjects with rheumatic diseases. Principles of diagnosis and therapy. *Semin. Arthritis Rheum.*, **6**, 165–8.

Haq, M., Kremer, R., Goltzman, D., & Rabbani, S. (1993). A vitamin D analogue (EB 1089) inhibits parathyroid hormone-related peptide production and prevents the development of malignancy-associated hypercalcemia in vivo. *J. Clin. Invest.*, **91**, 2416–22.

Haussler, M. R., Haussler, C. A., Jurutka, P. W., Thompson, P. D., Hsieh, J. C., Remus, L. S., Selznick, S. H., & Whitfield, G. K. (1997). The vitamin D hormone and its nuclear receptor: molecular actions and disease states. *J. Endocrinol.*, **154**, 557–73.

Henderson, J. E., Sebag, M., Rhim, J., Goltzman, D., & Kremer, R. (1991). Dysregulation of parathyroid hormone-like peptide expression and secretion in a keratinocyte model of tumor expression. *Cancer Res.*, **51**, 6521–8.

Henderson, J. E., Shustik, C., Kremer, R., Rabbani, S. A., Hendy, G. N., & Goltzman, D. (1990). Circulating concentrations of parathyroid hormone-like peptide in malignancy and in hyperparathyroidism. *J. Bone Miner. Res.*, **5**, 105–13.

Holick, M. F. (1995). Non calcemic actions of 1,25 dihydroxyvitamin D_3 and clinical applications. *Bone*, **17**, 1075–115.

Honma, Y., Hozumi, M., Abe, E., Konno, K., Fukushima, M., Hata, S., Nishii, Y., DeLuca, H. F., & Suda, T. (1983). 1α,25–Dihydroyvitamin D_3 and 1α-hydroxyvitamin D_3 prolong survival time of mice inoculated with myeloid leukemia cells. *Proc. Natl Acad. Sci., USA*, **80**, 201–4.

Hosomi, J., Hosoi, J., Abe, E., Suda, T., & Kuroke, T. (1983). *Endocrinology*, **113**, 1950–7.

Hughes, M. R., Malloy, P. J., Kieback, D. G., Kesterson, R. A., Pike, J. W., Feldman, D., & O'Malley, B. W. (1988). Point mutations in the human vitamin D receptor gene associated with hypocalcemia rickets. *Science*, **242**, 1702–5.

Ikeda, K., Ohno, H., Hane, M., Yokoi, H., Okada, M., Honma, T., Yamada, A., Tatsumi, Y., Tanaka, T., Saitoh, T., Hirose, S., Mori, S., Takevch, Y., Fukumotos, S., Terukina, S., Iguchi, H., Kiriyama, T., Ogata, E., & Matsumoto, T. (1994). Development of a sensitive two-site immunoradiometric asssay for parathyroid hormone-related peptide: evidence for elevated levels in plasma from patients with adult T-cell leukemia/lymphoma and B-cell lymphoma. *J. Clin. Endocrinol. Metab.*, **79**, 1322–7.

Kelsey, S. M., Newland, A. C., Cunningham, J., Makin, H. K. J., Coldwell, R. D., Mills, M. J., & Grant, I. R. (1992). Sustained haematological response to high-dose oral alfacalcidol in patients with myelodysplastic syndromes. *Lancet*, **340**, 316.

Kimberg, D. V., Baerg, R. D., Gershon, E., & Gravdusius, R. T. (1971) Effect of cortisone treatment on active transport of calcium by the small intestine. *J. Clin. Invest.*, **50**, 1309–21.

Kissmeyer, A-M. & Binderup, L. (1991). Calcipotriol (MC 903): pharmacokinetics in rats and biological activities of metabolites. A comparative study with 1,25(OH)$_2$D$_3$. *Biochem. Pharmacol.*, **41**, 1601–6.

Kitanaka, S., Takeyama, K-I., Murayama, A., Sato, T., Okumura, K., Nogami, M., Hasegawa, Y., Niimi, H., Yanagisawa, J., Tanaka, T., & Kato, S. (1998). Inactivating mutations in the 25-hydroxyvitamin D$_3$ 1α-hydroxylase gene in patients with pseudovitamin D-deficiency rickets. *N. Engl. J. Med.*, **338**, 653–61.

Klein, G. L. & Chesney, R. W. (1986). Metabolic bone disease associated with total parenteral nutrition. In *Total Parenteral Nutrition: Indication, Utilization, Complications and Pathophysiological Considerations*, 1st edn., ed. E. Lebenthal, pp. 431–3. New York: Raven Press.

Koo, W. W. K., Kaplan, L. A., Bendon, R., Succop, P., Tsang, R. C., Horn, J., & Steicher, D. (1986). Response to aluminium in parenteral nutrition during infancy. *J. Pediatr.*, **109**, 877–83.

Kragballe, K., Gjertsen, B. T., DeHoop, D., Karlsmark, T., Van De Karkhof, P. C. M., Larko, O., Tikjob, G., Wieboer, C., Strand, A., & Roel-Petorsen, J. (1991). Double-blind right/left comparison of calcipotriol and betamethasone valerate in treatment of psoriasis vulgaris. *Lancet*, **337**, 193–6.

Kremer, R., Karaplis, A. C., Henderson, J., Gulliver, W., Barnville, D., Hendy, G. N., & Goltzman, D. (1991). Regulation of parathyroid hormone like peptide in cultured normal human keratinocytes: effect of growth factors and 1,25 dihydroxyvitamin D on gene expression and secretion. *J. Clin. Invest.*, **87**, 884–93.

Kremer, R., Sebag, M., Champigny, C., Meerovitch, K., Geoffrey, N. H., White, J., & Goltzman, D. (1996a). Identification and characterization of 1,25-dihydroxyvitamin D$_3$ responsive repressor sequences in the rat parathyroid hormone-related peptide gene. *J. Biol. Chem.*, **27**, 16310–16.

Kremer, R., Shustik, C., Tabak, T., Papavasiliou, V., & Goltzman, D. (1996b). Parathyroid-hormone-related peptide in haematologic malignancies. *Am. J. Med.*, **100**, 406–11.

Liberman, U. A., Eil, C., Holst, P., Rosen, J. F., & Marx, J. S. (1983). Hereditary resistance to 1,25-dihydroxyvitamin D: defective function of receptors for 1,25-dihydroxyvitamin D in cells cultured from bone. *J. Clin. Endocrinol. Metab.*, **57**, 958–62.

Liberman, U. A., Eil, C., & Marx, S. J. (1986). Receptor positive hereditary resistance to 1,25-dihydroxyvitamin D: chromatography of hormone–receptor complexes on DNA-cellulose shows two classes of mutation. *J. Clin. Endocrinol. Metab.*, **62**, 122–6.

Lubert, B. P. & Raisz, L. G. (1990). Glucocorticoid-induced osterporosis: pathogenesis and management. *Ann. Int. Med.*, **112**, 352–64.

McLaughlin, J. & Holick, M. F. (1985). Aging decreases the capacity of human skin to produce vitamin D$_3$. *J. Clin. Invest.*, **76**, 1536–8.

Malloy, P. J., Hochberg, Z., Pike, J. W., & Feldman, D. (1989). Abnormal binding of vitamin D receptors to deoxyribonucleic acid in a kindred with vitamin D dependent rickets, type II. *J. Clin. Endocrinol. Metab.*, **68**, 263–9.

Malloy, P. J., Hochberg, Z., Tiosano, D., Pike, J. W., Hughes, M. R., & Feldman, D. (1990). The molecular basis of hereditary rickets type II: truncated vitamin D receptor in three kindreds. *Mol. Cell Endocrinol.*, **86**, 2017–79.

Manolagas, S. C., Provredini, D. M., & Joubas, C. D. (1998). Interaction of 1,25 dihydroxyvitamin D$_3$ and immune system. *Molec. Cell Endocrinol.*, **43**, 113.

Marx, S. J., Bliziotes, M. M., & Nanes, M. (1986). Analysis of the relation between alopecia and resistance to 1,25-dihydroxyvitamin D. *Clin. Endocrinol.*, **25**, 373–81.

Meunier, P. J. (1993). Is steroid-induced osteoporosis preventable? (Editorial) *N. Engl. J. Med.*, **328**, 1781–2.

Motomura, S., Kanamoria, H., Maruta, A., Kodama, F., & Ohkubo, T. (1991). The effect of 1-hydroxyvitamin D$_3$ for prolongation of leukemic transformation-free survival in myelodysplastic syndromes. *Am. J. Hematol.*, **38**, 67–8.

Naveh-Many, T. & Silver, J. (1993) Effect of calcitriol, 22-oxacalcitriol and calcipotriol on serum calcium and parathyroid hormone gene expresion. *Endocrinology*, **133**, 2724–8.

Reichel, H., Koeffler, H. P., & Norman, A. W. (1989). The role of the vitamin D endocrine system in health and disease. *N. Engl. J. Med.*, **320**, 981–91.

Reichel, H., Koeffler, H. P., Tobler, A., & Norman, A. W. (1987). 1,25 dihydroxyvitamin D$_3$ inhibits interleukin synthesis by normal human peripheral blood lymphocytes. *Proc. Natl Acad. Sci., USA*, **84**, 3385.

Rigby, W. F. C. (1998). The immunobiology of vitamin D. *Immunol. Today*, **9**, 54–8.

Rigby, W. F. C., Stacy, T., & Fanger, M. W. (1984). *J. Clin. Invest.*, **74**, 1451–8.

Roodman, G. D., Ibbotson, K. J., MacDonald, B. R., Kuehl, T. J., & Mundy, G. R. (1985). 1,25(OH)$_2$D$_3$ causes formation of multinucleated cells with osteoclasts characteristics in culture of primate marrow. *Proc. Natl Acad. Sci., USA*, **82**, 8313–17.

Sambrook, P., Birmingham, J., Kelly, P., Kempler, C., Nguyen, T., Pocok, N., & Eisman, J. (1993). Prevention of corticosteroid osteoporosis. A comparison of calcium, calcitriol and calcitonin. *N. Engl. J. Med.*, **328**, 1747–52.

Sandstead, H. H. (1980). Clinical manifestations of certain classical deficiency diseases. In *Modern Nutrition in Health and Disease*, 6th edn., ed. R. S. Goodhart & M. E. Shils, pp. 693–6, Philadelphia: Lea and Febiger.

Sato, T., Takusagawa, K., Asoo, N., & Konno, K. (1984). Effect of 1α-hydroxyvitamin D$_3$ on metastasis of rat ascites hepatoma K-231. *Br. J. Cancer*, **50**, 123–5.

Scriver, C. R., Reade, T. M., DeLuca, H. F., & Hamstra, A. J. (1978). Serum 1,25 dihydroxyvitamin D levels in normal subjects and in patients with hereditary rickets or bone disease. *N. Engl. J. Med.*, **299**, 976–9.

Sebag, M., Henderson, J. E., Goltzman, D., & Kremer, R. (1994). Regulation of parathyroid hormone-related peptide production in normal human mammary epithelial cells in vitro. *Am. J. Physiol.*, **267**(3), C723–30.

Sebag, M., Henderson, J. E., Rhim, J. S., & Kremer, R. (1992). Relative resistance to 1,25-dihydroxyvitamin D$_3$ in a keratinocyte model of tumor progression. *J. Biol. Chem.*, **267**, 12162–7.

Shah, B. R. & Finberg, L. (1994). Single day therapy for vitamin D deficiency rickets: a preferred method. *J. Pediatr.*, **1125**, 487–90.

Solomon, C., Sebag, M., White, J., Rhim, J., & Kremer, R. (1998). Disruption of vitamin D receptor/retinoid X receptor heterodimer formation following ras transformation of human keratinocytes. *J. Biol. Chem.*, **273**, 17573–8.

Solomon, C., White, J. H., & Kremer, R. (1999). MAP kinase inhibits 1,25-dihydroxyvitamin D$_3$-dependent signal transduction by phosphorylation of human RXR on serine 260. *J. Clin. Invest.*, **103**, 1729–35.

Stamp, J. C. B. (1975). Factors in human vitamin D nutrition and in the production and cure of classical rickets. *Proc. Nutr. Soc.*, **34**, 119–30.

Stern, P. H. & Bell, N. H. (1989). Disorders of vitamin D metabolism – toxicity and hypersensitivity. In *Metabolic Bone Disease*, pp. 203–13. CRC Press.

Takahashi, F., Finch, J. L., Denda, M., Dusso, A. S., Brown, A. J., & Slatopolsky, E. (1997). A new vitamin D analog of 1,25(OH)$_2$D$_3$ 19–NOR-1,25(OH)$_2$D$_2$ suppresses serum PTH and parathyroid gland growth in uremic rats without elevation of intestinal vitamin D receptor content. *Am. J. Kidney Dis.*, **30**, 105–12.

Takeda, E., Kuzoda, Y., Saijo, T., Toshima, K., Naito, E., Kobashi, H., Iwakuni, Y., & Miyao, M. (1986). Rapid diagnosis of vitamin D-dependent rickets type II by use of phytohemagglutinin-stimulated lymphocytes. *Clin. Chim. Acta*, **155**, 245–50.

Takeyama, K., Kitanaka, S., Sato, T., Kobori, M., Yanagisawa, J., & Kato, S. (1997). 25-hydroxyvitamin D$_3$, 1α hydroxylase and vitamin D synthesis. *Science*, **277**, 1827–30.

The HYP consortium (1995). A gene (PEX) with homologies to endopeptidases is mutated in patients with X-linked hypophosphatemic rickets. *Nat. Genet.*, **11**, 130–6.

Verge, C. F., Lam, A., Simpson, J. M., Lowell, C. J., Howard, N. J., & Silink, M. (1991). Effect of therapy in X-linked hypophosphatemic rickets. *N. Engl. J. Med.*, **325**, 1843.

Veyron, P., Pamphile, R., Binderup, L., & Touraine, J. L. (1993). Two novel vitamin D analogs, KH1060 and CB966 prolong skin allograft survival in mice. *Transpl. Immunol.*, **1**, 72–6.

Warrell, R. P., Frankel, S. R., Miller, W. H., Scheinberg, D. A., Itri, L. M., Hittelman, W. N., Vyas, R., Andreef, M., Tafuri, A., Jakubowski, A., Gabrilove, J., Gordon, M. S., & Dmitrovsky, E. (1991). Differentiation therapy of acute promyelocytic leukemia with tretinoin (all-*trans*-retinoic acid). *N. Engl. J. Med.*, **324**, 1385–93.

Yu, J., Papavasiliou, V., Rhim, J., Goltzman, D., & Kremer, R. (1995). Vitamin D analogues: new therapeutic agents for the treatment of squamous cancer and its associated hypercalcemia. *Anti-Cancer Drugs*, 5, 101–8.

Zhang, X., Hoffman, B., Tran, P. B. V., Graupner, G., & Fahly, P. (1992). Retinoid X receptor is an auxiliary protein for thyroid hormone and retinoic acid receptors. *Nature*, 355, 441–6.

Zhou, J-Y., Norman, A. W., Chen, D-L., Sun, G-W., Uskokovic, M., & Koeffler, H. P. (1990). 1,25-dihydroxy-16-ene-23-yne-vitamin D$_3$ prolongs survival time of leukemic mice. *Proc. Natl Acad. Sci., USA*, **87**, 3929–32.

Index

DATE DUE

APR 0 3 '02			
JUN 1 7 '03			
SEP 2 0 '04			
MAR 2 3 '05			
APR 1 1 '05			
MAY 0 3 '05			
MAY 0 2 '06			
GAYLORD			PRINTED IN U.S.A.

JUL   '01